Vision, Perception, and Cognition

A Manual for the Evaluation and Treatment of the Adult with Acquired Brain Injury

Fourth Edition

Vision, Perception, and Cognition

A Manual for the Evaluation and Treatment of the Adult with Acquired Brain Injury

Fourth Edition

Barbara Zoltan, MA, OTR/L

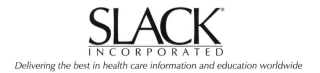

SLACK
INCORPORATED

Delivering the best in health care information and education worldwide

www.slackbooks.com

ISBN: 978-1-55642-738-1

Vision, Perception, and Cognition: A Manual for the Evaluation and Treatment of the Adult with Acquired Brain Injury, Fourth Edition Instructor's Manual is also available from SLACK Incorporated. Don't miss this important companion to this book. To obtain the Instructor's Manual, please visit www.efacultylounge.com.

This book was originally published under the first edition title *Perceptual Dysfunction in the Adult Stroke Patient: A Manual for Evaluation and Treatment* by Ellen Siev and Brenda Freishtat and under the second edition title *The Adult Stroke Patient: A Manual for Evaluation and Treatment of Perceptual and Cognitive Dysfunction, Revised Second Edition* by Barbara Zoltan, Ellen Siev, and Brenda Freishtat.

The procedures and practices described in this book should be implemented in a manner consistent with the professional standards set for the circumstances that apply in each specific situation. Every effort has been made to confirm the accuracy of the information presented and to correctly relate generally accepted practices. The authors, editor, and publisher cannot accept responsibility for errors or exclusions or for the outcome of the material presented herein. There is no expressed or implied warranty of this book or information imparted by it. Care has been taken to ensure that drug selection and dosages are in accordance with currently accepted/recommended practice. Due to continuing research, changes in government policy and regulations, and various effects of drug reactions and interactions, it is recommended that the reader carefully review all materials and literature provided for each drug, especially those that are new or not frequently used. Any review or mention of specific companies or products is not intended as an endorsement by the author or publisher.

SLACK Incorporated uses a review process to evaluate submitted material. Prior to publication, educators or clinicians provide important feedback on the content that we publish. We welcome feedback on this work.

Published by: SLACK Incorporated
                     6900 Grove Road
                     Thorofare, NJ 08086 USA
                     Telephone: 856-848-1000
                     Fax: 856-853-5991
                     www.slackbooks.com

Contact SLACK Incorporated for more information about other books in this field or about the availability of our books from distributors outside the United States.

Library of Congress Cataloging-in-Publication Data

Zoltan, Barbara.
  Vision, perception, and cognition : a manual for the evaluation and treatment of the adult with acquired brain injury / Barbara Zoltan. -- 4th ed.
     p. ; cm.
  Prev. ed. had subtitle: a manual for the evaluation and treatment of the neurologically impaired adult.
  "Previously published under the title Perceptual dysfunction in the adult stroke patient: a manual for evaluation and treatment, by Ellen Siev and Brenda Freishtat; and under the title The Adult stroke patient: a manual for evaluation and treatment of perceptual and cognitive dysfunction, revised second edition, by Barbara Zoltan, Ellen Siev, and Brenda Freishtat."
  Includes bibliographical references and index.
  ISBN-13: 978-1-55642-738-1 (alk. paper)
  ISBN-10: 1-55642-738-7 (alk. paper)
  1. Brain damage--Diagnosis. 2. Brain damage--Patients--Rehabilitation.. I. Title. II. Title: Manual for the evaluation and treatment of the adult with acquired brain injury.
  [DNLM: 1. Brain Injuries--rehabilitation. 2. Cerebrovascular Disorders--rehabilitation. 3. Cognition Disorders--diagnosis. 4. Cognition Disorders--therapy. 5. Vision Disorders--diagnosis. 6. Vision Disorders--therapy. WL 354 Z86v 2006]
  RC387.5.Z65 2006
  616.8'103--dc22

                              2006039599

For permission to reprint material in another publication, contact SLACK Incorporated. Authorization to photocopy items for internal, personal, or academic use is granted by SLACK Incorporated provided that the appropriate fee is paid directly to Copyright Clearance Center. Prior to photocopying items, please contact the Copyright Clearance Center at 222 Rosewood Drive, Danvers, MA 01923 USA; phone: 978-750-8400; website: www.copyright.com; email: info@copyright.com

Printed in the United States of America.

Last digit is print number: 10   9   8   7   6   5

Dedication

This book is dedicated to Les, Adam, and Scott
for their love, patience, and understanding.

Contents

Vision, Perception, and Cognition: A Manual for the Evaluation and Treatment of the Adult with Acquired Brain Injury, Fourth Edition Instructor's Manual is also available from SLACK Incorporated. Don't miss this important companion to this book. To obtain the Instructor's Manual, please visit www.efacultylounge.com.

Acknowledgments

For time and ideas

Susan L. Daniel, OD
Camila E. Dukes, OD, FCOVD
Gordon Muir Giles PhD, OTR, FAOTA
Rick Parente, PhD
Farrell Sheffield, OTR/L, CDRS
Joan Pascale Toglia, PhD, OTR
Mary Warren, MS, OTR/L, SCLV, FAOTA
Robert Williams

For research assistance

Gavin Gruber

About the Author

Barbara Zoltan, MA, OTR/L is a consultant in Southern California. She obtained her bachelor's degree in Occupational Therapy from Tufts University and her master's degree from the University of Southern California. She holds certifications in both sensory integration and neurodevelopmental treatment and has served on the editorial boards of the *Journal of Head Trauma Rehabilitation* and *Occupational Therapy in Health Care*. Her more than 20 years of experience specializing in neurological rehabilitation has included a broad range of research, teaching, administrative and clinical practice. She has published over 20 articles, chapters, and books related to the adult with acquired brain injury.

Foreword

No one is impervious to an acquired brain injury, and the long-term effects can include language, motor, visual, perceptual, and cognitive problems. Occupational therapists, in particular, have developed theoretical frameworks as well as evaluation and intervention strategies that tackle these problems as they affect the client's activities of daily living.

This fourth edition of *Vision, Perception, and Cognition: A Manual for the Evaluation and Treatment of the Adult with Acquired Brain Injury* is an important, evidence-based resource book for both the student and experienced clinician. The book has translated many complex, abstract concepts into practical techniques that are easily applied when working with the adult with acquired brain injury.

At this time, there is no one resource that better takes the reader through the entire process from theory, to evaluation, to intervention as it relates to vision, perception, and cognition. The fourth edition builds on its predecessors with many new, relevant, and timely topics including areas such as neuralplasticity and functional reorganization, visual vestibular processing, and dynamic assessment. The material contained in this book is applicable to any setting from home health care to inpatient rehabilitation.

I know readers will treasure this classic resource and keep it within arm's reach.

Karen Jacobs, EdD, OTR/L, CPE, FAOTA
Clinical Professor
Boston University
Sargent College of Health and Rehabilitation Sciences
Boston, MA

Preface

There are 4.6 million stroke survivors in the United States.[1] More than 700,000 people sustain a cerebral vascular accident (CVA) annually in the United States.[2-5] Of those surviving the initial insult, 50% will live another 5 years, and 75% will be rehabilitated to some degree of independence. Of these new clients, 60% to 70% can expect to become ambulatory, although significant functional return of the affected upper extremity is expected in only 30% to 40%. In addition, there are over 422,000 new cases of traumatic brain injury (TBI) each year.[3,4,6] As many as 5.3 million Americans have a disability as the result of a TBI.

Although the residual behavioral and functional problems that occur as the result of a CVA are generally less severe, they are similar to those of a TBI. In recent years, the term ABI, or acquired brain injury, has been developed. ABI includes both the TBI client, who has sustained an external insult, and the CVA, brain surgery, or arterio-venous malformation (AVM) client, who has sustained an internal insult.[7] Both categories of clients have a sudden onset of damage to the central nervous system (CNS) with resulting neurological dysfunction common to both.[7] The techniques of evaluation and treatment I have included in this book are appropriate for both the TBI and CVA client, and I have, therefore, adopted the new categorical term of ABI for this edition.

Until recently, rehabilitation focused on restoration of motion and compensation for lost functional skills. Visual, perceptual, and cognitive deficits, noted for many years to exist as a result of ABI, have only recently been acknowledged as a cause of continued confusion and lack of rehabilitation progress in many clients even though motor skills have returned. As many as two-thirds of all TBI clients experience some type of cognitive loss.[8] Recent research has clearly shown a significant relationship between visual, perceptual, and/or cognitive loss and functional abilities.[9-11]

Despite the prevalence of ABI clients, the formulation of definitive evaluation and treatment techniques remains incomplete at best. This book was completed after extensive research and clinical experience as well as communication with experts in the field and is intended to reflect the current state of the art in the evaluation and treatment of visual, perceptual, and cognitive processing deficits for the adult ABI client. It is intended to be a resource book, and as such, the material has been documented as closely as possible for future referencing. Occupation-based theoretical information is included as well as specific theoretical information pertaining to each subcomponent skill. The application of this information to practice through specific frames of reference is also provided. Evidence-based practice information discovered through extensive research and communication with experts in the field is presented throughout the book. Specific evaluation and treatment techniques based on this theoretical and evidence-based information are outlined.

Information pertaining to both dynamic and static assessment as well as top-down and bottom-up approaches to evaluation and treatment are described. Finally, information related to the contextual impact on performance is included throughout the book as well as information pertaining to client and family or caregiver education.

It is my goal that this book be useful for both the student and the experienced clinician. It is also my hope that it will foster good clinical reasoning skills and stimulate future research.

Barbara Zoltan, MA, OTR/L

REFERENCES

1. Gillen G. Coping during inpatient stroke rehabilitation: an exploratory study. *Am J Occup Ther.* 2006;60(2): 136-145.
2. Allen CK. Treatment plans in cognitive rehabilitation. *Occup Ther Pract.* 1989;1(1):1-8.
3. American Heart Association. Heart and stroke supplement. 2002. Available at: http://www.americanheart. org. Accessed

4. Joe BE. Accelerating stroke rehab. *OT Week*. 1995;9(42):14-15.
5. McCollough NC III, Sarniento A. Functional prognosis of the hemiplegic. *J Florida Med Assoc*. 1970;56:31-34.
6. Kong KH, Chua KS, Tow AP. Clinical characteristics and functional outcome of stroke patients 75 years old and older. *Arch Phys Med Rehabil*. 1998;79(12):1535-1538.
7. Rundek T, Sacco RL. Outcome following stroke. In: Mohr JP, Choi DW, Grotta JC, Weir B, Wolf PA, eds. *Stroke: Pathophysiology, Diagnosis, and Management*. 4th ed. Philadelphia, Pa: Churchill Livingstone; 2004.
8. Titus MLD, Gall NG, Yerxa EJ, Roberson TA, Mack W. Correlation of perceptual performance and activities of daily living in stroke patients. *Am J Occup Ther*. 1991;45(5):410-417.
9. Edmans JA, Lincoln NB. The frequency of perceptual and body image dysfunction to activities of daily living of persons after stroke. *Am J Occup Ther*. 1995;49(6):551-559.
10. National Center for Injury Prevention and Control. *Traumatic Brain Injury in the United States: A Report to Congress*. Atlanta, Ga: Centers for Disease Control and Prevention; 1999.
11. Suchoff I, Ciuffreda KJ, Kapoor N. An overview of acquired brain injury and optometric implications. In: Suchoff I, Ciuffreda KJ, Kapoor N, eds. *Visual and Vestibular Consequences of Acquired Brain Injury*. Santa Ana, Calif: Optometric Extension Program, Inc; 2001.

RESOURCES

Cicerone KD, Dahlberg C, Kalmar K, et al. Evidence-based cognitive rehabilitation: recommendations for clinical practice. *Arch Phys Med Rehabil*. 2000;81(12):1596-1615.

Dobkin BH. Rehabilitation and recovery of the patient with stroke. In: Mohr JP, Choi DW, Grotta JC, Weir B, Wolf PA, eds. *Stroke: Pathophysiology, Diagnosis, and Management*. 4th ed. Philadelphia, Pa: Churchill Livingstone; 2004.

Farah MJ, Feinberg TE. Consciousness of perception after brain damage. *Semin Neurol*. 1997;17(2):145-152.

Kaplan CP, Corrigan JD. The relationship between cognition and functional independence in adults with traumatic brain injury. *Arch Phys Med Rehabil*. 1994;75:643-647.

Rubio, KB, van Deusen J. Relationship of perceptual and body image dysfunction to activities of daily living of persons after stroke. *Am J Occup Ther*. 1995;49(6):551-559.

Vogenthaler DR. Rehabilitation after closed head injury: a primer. *J Rehab*. 1987;Fall:15-21.

Wolf PA, Clagett P, Easton JD, et al. Preventing ischemic stroke in patients with prior stroke and TIA: a statement for healthcare professionals from the Stroke Council of the American Heart Association. *Stroke*. 1994;30:1991-1994.

CHAPTER 1

THEORETICAL AND ADDITIONAL FACTORS GUIDING EVALUATION AND TREATMENT

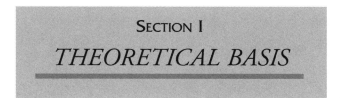

SECTION I
THEORETICAL BASIS

Theory as a Basis for Evaluation and Treatment

Occupational therapy, as with any health profession, requires a conceptual foundation with underlying assumptions to guide practice decisions. These theoretical concepts are generally structured into models. Portions of these models, which are methodological in emphasis, form a frame of reference.[1] The frame of reference is the mechanism that links theory to practice.[2] Occupational therapy contains many frames of reference, depending on the client population or specific area of focus. Although these frames of reference have been effective to some degree, only recently has the profession begun to relate them to an overall theoretical basis for occupational therapy practice.

Every occupational therapist would agree that the profession is based on the concept of human occupation. Referrals are made because of the client's inability to perform daily life tasks, which prevents independence and return to previous life roles. Not all occupational therapists, however, would agree on how to evaluate and treat these inabilities. Many therapists utilize a restorative approach and profess a need to evaluate component skills such as attention, memory, or strength as a means to help clarify the cause of occupational performance deficits and assist in treatment planning. Interventions that aim at restoring cognitive deficits are a standard component of most rehabilitation programs.[3,4] Assumptions of this approach are made based on established clinical and neuroimaging research about the correlation of specific component deficits to the client's problems with occupational performance.[5] In addition, when utilizing a restorative approach, it is now understood that providing structured functional activities which allow transfer of the gains made in performance components, is crucial to success.[6,7] Whenever possible, many occupational therapists are utilizing occupation-based restorative activities.

Issues such as health care costs and time constraints are causing many occupational therapists to shift away from a restorative approach to visual, perceptual, and cognitive deficits, to a more adaptive or compensatory approach.[8] In addition, the restorative approach to evaluating and testing component skills has recently come into question. Some therapists believe this approach to be reductionistic and recommend a more holistic focus of evaluation and treatment.[3,9,10]

Some believe that "…while a certain causal relationship does exist whereby improvement in the microlevel of cognitive components of performance may result in improved occupational performance in real life, a large variance in actual performance abilities cannot be explained by looking at or treating the micro-level alone."[9] These therapists believe that occupational performance should be the primary focus of occupational therapy assessment and treatment. Others believe that while a more top-down approach may place the client in the community earlier, it remains unclear how not addressing performance components will affect long-term neurological and functional recovery.

In recent years, in addition to a restorative and adaptive approach to client care, a "contextual" approach has been added to the mix. Therapists utilizing this approach focus not on the client's deficits but on how the client's environment facilitates or constrains performance. The major assumption of this approach is that the client's deficit only becomes a disability when he or she cannot perform in a given environment. The concept of a "contextual" approach is emerging and is likely to undergo continued refinement.

As with any controversy, critical thinking or questioning often results in an improved perspective. This perspective leads to the incorporation of ideas from many sides and the formation of a solution that is useful and beneficial to all practitioners. Catherine Trombly, for example, answers to the labeling of component skills evaluation as "reductionistic" as follows[11]:

> *If a hierarchical theory of occupational functioning that includes abilities and capacities is accepted, then the assessment process should include these levels… the assessment should not be considered a reductionistic one, but rather an augmentative one that relates and extends each level toward occupational functioning.*

Abreu et al support the need for multiple levels of evaluation and treatment in their description of the quadraphonic approach.[3] They encourage therapists to evaluate the client at both the micro and macro levels of occupational functioning so that abilities and skills can be reliably monitored at both levels. Ben-Yishay and Diller describe cognitive difficulties as "layered and coexistent"[12,13] They also recommend a systematic, multi-model approach to cognitive rehabilitation. Farrell et al, believe the effective remediation of visuo-motor deficits requires a systematic approach within a hierarchical framework.[13] Weinstock-Zlotnik and Hinojosa believe that foundational factors in the bottom-up approach keep the therapist grounded in the very intricacies of physical, psychological, and cognitive function.[14]

As previously mentioned, the overall aim of occupational therapy intervention is the facilitation of the client's ability to participate in activities that are meaningful and productive and, therefore, support participation in daily life.[15] For the adult with acquired brain injury (ABI), the therapist needs to understand how the consequences of brain injury can be minimized so that meaningful participation in daily life can occur.[16,17] This overall goal is compatible with a top-down or bottom-up approach as well as an approach that focuses on the contextual or environmental influence on client performance. All approaches are needed to address the issues our clients present.[6,7,17-20] Treatment should encompass both poles of the component-function continuum.[17] Moyers states as follows[17]:

> *Effective occupational therapy intervention requires manipulation of multiple interventions simultaneously targeting both components of functioning and disability (body*

structure/body function and activity participation) to facilitate occupational perfor-
mance in relevant environments.

For some identified problems, the focus of the intervention plan will be restorative for some compensatory, for others contextual, and yet others will focus on helping the client self-manage performance. A comprehensive intervention program enables clients to be more functional through the use of compensatory strategies, while at the same time working to restore functional capacities.[7]

One factor that must be considered in making a choice between a restorative or adaptive approach is the client's ability to learn.[21] In order to utilize the restorative approach, the client must have some learning capacity.[22] The therapist must identify what modes of input the client can process most easily, what approaches to tasks are still available to the client, and what tasks are still meaningful to the client.[22]

A variety of frames of reference for treatment have been operationalized and fall within either a restorative or adaptive conceptual base. In addition, as just described, concepts related to a "contextual approach" are now emerging. Although the concepts related to a strict contextual approach are not yet fully operationalized, this author believes those that are have value, and they are therefore included in this chapter. In addition, the occupation-based frames of reference described in the "Adaptive Approach" section take into consideration contextual influence on the client's performance. The information presented on Dynamic Assessment and the Dynamic Interactional Approach (DIA) also includes concepts related to contextual influences on performance. The restorative neurodevelopmental treatment (NDT) frame of reference now also incorporates context influences on client performance in its theoretical assumptions. Finally, the subsequent evaluation and treatment sections throughout the book all pose questions or consider environmental or contextual issues related to client performance.

In summary, the goal of occupational therapy is to minimize the consequences of the ABI for those whose deficits cause a disability related to occupational performance. The theoretical basis for evaluation and treatment need not include one level of focus to the exclusion of another. Evaluation and treatment that focus on deficits of components of function thought to be prerequisites of occupational performance have been termed bottom-up assessment. Examining role competence, the tasks that define these roles and what the client can and cannot do, is termed top-down assessment. Some clinicians are utilizing the term contextual approach when focusing on contextual influences on client performance. The combination of top-down and bottom-up approaches to occupational functioning as well as those that consider contextual influences on client performance will give the clearest picture of the client's overall functioning at all levels. The therapist should choose a combination of assessments and treatment to provide the most complete picture of the client in the least amount of time.[1] In order to make these decisions, the therapist must understand the underlying concepts and have a framework for organizing and interpreting information.

In addition, the therapist should utilize his or her clinical reasoning skills to identify relevant evaluation and treatment approaches.[15] The intervention process should be dynamically interrelated with ongoing assessment.[15] Finally, no matter which combination of approaches are utilized, assessment and intervention strategies should be both client-centered and evidence-based, when possible, and have as the ultimate goal effective adaptation, which leads to improved occupational performance.

Information on the restorative and adaptive approaches and associated frames of reference, as well as contextual influence on client performance, are described in Section I of this chapter. Section II provides information on additional factors that guide evaluation and treatment. These topics include client-centered practice, client and family education, the client's learning capacity, evidence-based practice, and clinical reasoning.

RESTORATIVE APPROACH

The restorative (previously called remedial) approach used in rehabilitation focuses on the impairment underlying the client's disability.[15,17,22-25] This approach examines foundational factors that are contributing to the client's limitations, real disabilities, and strengths.[17] It is based on neuroanatomical and neurophysiological models of learning.[26] It aims at changing the individual's psychological, cognitive, physiological, and neurobehavioral capabilities.[15,20] The goal of the restorative approach is to increase and improve the client's ability to process and use incoming information so as to allow increased function in daily life.[12,15,27]

The restorative approach aims at promoting or enhancing brain recovery or reorganization.[27,28] A basic premise or assumption of the restorative approach is that the brain can repair itself by reestablishing synaptic connections or growing new ones.[29] As described in the subsequent sections on plasticity and neuroimaging contained in this chapter, there is now a plethora of neuroscience research that validates this assumption. The injured or damaged brain does indeed display restitution and neuro-organizational capabilities.

Recovery functions of the brain just described have been shown to be experience dependent. When utilizing an approach, activities are chosen that meet the client's current skills and gradually graded for increased complexity in order to facilitate improved performance and abilities. Restorative treatment is often most effective or efficient when there are a few impairments affecting many areas of occupational performance.[7,15,30] Restorative treatment is a bottom-up approach that historically has assumed the client will be able to generalize to activities of daily living (ADLs). It has been assumed that "…if one trains to remediate an impaired core area of cognitive function, the individual will be able to resume competent functioning in those daily life situations that involve these core functions."[12]

Traditionally, the restorative treatment approach involved repeated drills and exercises carried out in the occupational therapy clinic. The assumption was the restoration of specific performance components, which are believed to be subcomponents of occupational performance, would generalize to actual improvement of the occupational performance activity itself. Some past research, however, indicates that a restorative approach to some subcomponent skills has a limited direct effect on the enhancement of functional activities.[12,31] Many rehabilitation professionals have come to believe that this apparent lack of research support is in part due to the amount of transfer of function required from clinic exercises and drills to everyday function. Most contemporary clinicians advocate the use of occupation-based activities in the most naturalistic environments even when the treatment aim is restorative. Even when the occupational therapist is utilizing a restorative approach, the intervention modality is almost always daily occupation.[18] For example, if treating an ABI client with constructional apraxia who repairs telephones for a living, instead of the traditional clinical activities utilizing parquetry blocks and copying block designs, the therapist would now likely address the deficit by having the client work on repairing phones. The goal is still to facilitate improved constructional abilities, which are assumed to take place through experience dependent brain recovery; however, the experience is occupation-based and, therefore, does not require a great deal of transfer of learning. The treatment is a functional or occupation-based restorative treatment.

ADAPTIVE APPROACH

The adaptive approach is a top-down approach that promotes adaptation of and to the environment to capitalize on the client's abilities. Adaptive approaches provide training in actual occupational behavior and are traditionally used when restoration is unlikely.[29] This approach assumes that certain functions cannot be recovered or restored completely.[26] As a top-down approach, the therapeutic process usually starts with a rapport building interview during which strengths and problems of occupational performance are identified.[6]

Adaptive approaches facilitate improved function through compensation. Compensation becomes necessary when the client's skills or abilities cannot meet environmental demands.[32,34] Compensation, which in general terms means a response to loss or deficiency, can involve changing an activity and/or the environment to meet the client's capabilities.[7,15,20,34-36] Additionally, the client can alter his or her behavior in order to perform activities in a different way.[37] Some mechanisms of compensation that the client can utilize can include 1) increasing the time or effort spent on a given task, 2) substituting a different skill that results in successful task completion, 3) developing a new skill to use, 4) modifying client expectations about performing the task, and 5) selecting alternative tasks or goals.[37]

Compensation can be external, which is assistance provided by outside sources, or situational, which is a technique utilized by the client so he or she does not depend on others.[38] In order to utilize situational compensation techniques, the client must have at least some awareness of existing deficits. This awareness may cause the client to be frustrated with his or her performance; however, it can help motivate him or her to learn new strategies. The client's perception of how much control he or she has over the environment will mediate the experience of loss and the effectiveness of compensatory strategies.[39] Compensatory behaviors are most successful when they are overlearned to the point of being automatic.[31] In addition, compensation strategies should be practiced in a variety of different environments.[25] The choice and design of activity or environmental compensations is based on the therapist's understanding of disability and activity analysis[34] as well as his or her understanding of the client's learning style and capabilities. Specific compensatory strategies cannot be forced on the client, and the therapist should explore successful strategies that the client utilized before the brain injury. For example, making lists or organizing work materials.

Frames of Reference Utilizing a Restorative Conceptual Base: Bottom-Up Approaches

NEURODEVELOPMENTAL APPROACH

Neurodevelopmental treatment (NDT) is a comprehensive management approach to motor recovery as it relates to ADLs.[40] Treatment is aimed at giving the client control over his or her movements, with treatment performed in a functional situation whenever possible.[41] Beginning with the original work of Bobath, the NDT approach is a problem solving approach that focuses on the individual as a whole person.[42]

The NDT approach works specifically to inhibit abnormal reflex mechanisms and facilitate normal movement.[41] Tactile and kinesthetic stimulation through handling and movement are provided to encourage contact between the individual and the environment.[43] The client is taught to move normally in all functional tasks. The ultimate goal is to teach the client how to control his or her own movements automatically without the aid of the therapist.[44] Movements of the upper and lower trunk are considered key to postural control and limb function and are therefore facilitated.[6] The therapist works toward the development of a variety of postural sets that make movements easy and automatic.[41] This in turn makes possible the redevelopment of a normal body scheme, leading to improvement in higher level visual perceptual skills.

Proponents of the NDT approach have recently reanalyzed the basic theoretical concept of the approach in conjunction with what is now known as related to motor learning. In a survey of 431 therapists, 89.9% believed that the theoretical concepts of NDT should be revised to include current knowledge related to advances in neuroscience, motor learning, motivation, praxis, etc.[40] The same survey revealed that although many therapists are using handling techniques such as proximal points of control, weight bearing, and weight shifts, others are now providing a more family-centered approach, and are encouraging active client involvement with minimal handling techniques. This shift in emphasis allows the client to initiate and direct his or her own movements.

The Neuro-Developmental Treatment Association (NDTA) has operationalized some of the new concepts, which are now additional basic assumptions of current NDT practice. Although current NDT incorporates many of the original ideas and techniques, new ones have been added based on current information from the motor sciences.[42] Concepts such as the importance of the client's active problem solving, motivation in the coordination of movement for a purpose, and movement repetition are a few examples of concepts now central to the NDT approach.[14,42] The importance of the vestibular and somatosensory systems to movement is now also embedded in NDT. Environment and cognitive processes are also considered part of the process that can affect motor performance. In other words, "...NDT has discarded the idea that the CNS is the most important aspect of motor control and singularly responsible for the appearance of abnormal posture and movement in clients with CNS damage."[42]

As described previously, proponents of NDT now believe that environmental factors will influence motor learning. Which environmental factors are important will depend on the goal of the action or task. Environmental factors can include areas such as timing or spatial components. As Howle states "...the specific requirements of the task in context will influence the selection of combinations from various neural maps that contribute to the final posture and movement ensemble."[42] The interaction among various neural and body systems, the purpose of the task, the individual, and the context will all affect posture and movement.[42] This focus has allowed for additional avenues of intervention.[42]

Cognitive processing will also affect motor learning. Client performance "...in a difficult learning context forces the client to use multiple and variable processes to overcome the difficulty of practice."[45] Performance will be more difficult at the beginning stage, when the client is first acquiring a skill; however, this is beneficial to both retention and learning. Jarus summarizes the key areas to successful motor relearning as follows[45]:

> *Contextual variety, open environment, and low knowledge of results ... facilitate cognitive motor functioning during motor skill acquisition, thereby enhancing retention and transfer.*

The final areas of consideration in motor relearning are movement analysis and handling techniques. It is now believed by many therapists utilizing NDT that movement analysis should include all systems that affect movement. These systems include musculoskeletal, synergistic organization, muscle tone, sensation, automatic reflexes, equilibrium, and perception/cognition. Spasticity, for example, is now considered a neural system impairment that is only one contributing factor to abnormally increased tone.[6,42] The components of the movement analysis include the base of support, alignment, sequencing, and stability/mobility.[6] The ultimate goal for the client is efficient functional movement with a large variety of movement options.[6]

Hands-on facilitation remains a major intervention strategy of NDT; however, neither reflex-inhibiting postures nor reflex-inhibiting patterns are current NDT treatment strategies.[42] Therapists "...now use localized limited inhibition of ineffective posture and movement synergies to redirect movement during facilitation of function."[42] These handling and inhibition techniques are applied precisely during early practice and are combined with trial and error and independent movement.[42]

In summary, NDT practice still includes many of the original concepts and techniques outlined by Bobath. The theory base, however, has recently changed to include concepts drawn from motor learning such as organization of movement, environmental influence on movement, and cognitive processing as it relates to movement performance and analysis. A comparison of ideas from the original theory to current NDT theory and practice is presented in Table 1-1.

Table 1-1

NDT—Past and Present

Bobath Approach: Where We Began	*NDT Approach: Where We Are Now*
1. Analytic problem-solving approach based on reflex/hierarchical models	1. Analytic problem-solving approach based on a systems/selectionist model
2. Hierarchical model of CNS structure and function	2. Distributed model of CNS structures and function
3. CNS viewed as the "controller." Automatic postural control mechanism simplified the responsibility of the CNS in control of movement.	3. The CNS determines the pattern of neural activity based on input from the multiple intrinsic systems and extrinsic variables that establish the context for movement initiation and execution.
4. Skilled movement is determined by maturation of reflexive movement.	4. Skilled movement is determined by the specific functional goal.
5. Muscle and postural tone determine the quality of the patterns of posture and movement used in functional activities.	5. Task goal, experience, individual learning strategies, movement synergies, energy, and interest all affect the quality of the final action.
6. Sensory feedback is important for the correction of movement errors.	6. Sensory feed-forward and feedback are equally important for different aspects of movement control.
7. "Positive signs," including spasticity and abnormal coordination, are changeable, but limitations occur if abnormal movement patterns are repeated and practiced.	7. The "negative signs," including weakness, impaired postural control, and paucity of movement, are recognized as equally important as the "positive signs" in limitations of function.
8. The CNS is not "hard-wired." Spasticity and abnormal coordination are changeable, but limitations occur if abnormal movement patterns are repeated and practiced.	8. The CNS is capable of recovery and remains plastic throughout the lifetime. Functional changes are limited by structural damage to the CNS, secondary changes in the body systems, and the inability to adapt to environmental conditions.
9. Neurological and developmental aspects of the CNS pathology are the most important considerations during examination and treatment planning.	9. Interactions of neural and body systems and environmental context are part of examination and treatment planning.
10. Therapists must always ask "why" when examining and treating clients.	10. Therapists must always ask "why" when examining and treating clients.
11. Therapists can most strongly influence movement through the peripheral sensory system.	11. Therapists can use the body systems and the environment to influence movement outcome.
12. Treatment methods involve primarily inhibition and facilitation through "hands-on" control of the client.	12. Motor learning concepts, including changing the environment, verbal reinforcement, self-initiated movement, and trial and error, have expanded treatment options. NDT recognizes limitations in physical guidance as a treatment strategy.

(continued)

Table 1-1 *(continued)*

NDT—Past and Present

Bobath Approach: Where We Began	*NDT Approach: Where We Are Now*
13. Functional movement develops from automatic components of movements.	13. The need to teach and practice functions is as important as facilitating components of movement.
14. Family and others in programs ensure carryover in life settings.	14. Direct teaching of functional activities in community settings adds to carryover.
15. Successful outcomes are measured in subjective, descriptive terms based on the individual's response to intervention strategies.	15. Outcomes must include collecting clinical data to provide efficacy of NDT intervention.

Reprinted with permission from reference 42: Howle JM. Neurodevelopmental Treatment Approach: Theoretical Foundations and Principles of Clinical Practice. *Laguna Beach, Calif: North American Neuro-Developmental Treatment Association; 2002:363.*

The use of the NDT approach is recommended not only as an effective means of restoring normal motor function but also as a means of restoring a normal body scheme that ultimately assists in restoring higher level visual perceptual skills.

Bilateral activities used in the NDT approach stimulate body awareness, which in turn helps with unilateral neglect, and the approach has been found to be effective for improving perceptual motor skills.[46] Examples of the uses of neurodevelopmental treatment are described in the sections related to body scheme disorders.

CONSTRAINT-INDUCED THERAPY

One of the most promising therapeutic approaches developed in recent years is constraint-induced therapy (CIT). CIT is a functionally based intervention geared to improve motor control in individuals with upper extremity hemiplegia.[47] CIT is one of the few therapeutic interventions that has demonstrated efficacy in controlled experiments as well as demonstrating transfer of these effects into the client's real world environment.[48,49] In addition, research indicates these benefits are apparent even with chronic stroke clients (ie, greater than one year after the initial stroke).[48,50] Finally, research has also indicated that the benefits gained are still present at least 2 years after CIT is stopped.[51]

CIT consists of two main components: 1) constraining the movement of the unaffected upper extremity and 2) intensive, repetitive, and targeted training of the paretic arm.[48,52-55] Incorporated into the targeted training is the "shaping" technique. Shaping is a "...commonly used operant conditioning method in which a behavioral objective (in this case movement) is approached in small steps of progressively increasing difficulty."[48] Activities are designed to address the motor deficits the client exhibits, helping him or her to carry out parts of a movement sequence.[56] The therapist also provides explicit verbal feedback for small improvements in client performance. The client is rewarded with positive enthusiastic approval for even small gains and is never punished for failure.[48]

CIT is originally based on decades of animal studies during which a "learned nonuse" was observed.[47] The animals studied stopped using their affected extremity after just a short period of time because trying to use it was frustrating and unsuccessful.[47] The animals would use only the unaffected limb and "...when depression of neural activity had passed several months after surgery, the monkey never learned that the limb could be useful.[47] Research with these animals where they restrained the uninvolved limb for more than 3 days showed the monkeys could learn to use the involved limb.[47]

This learned nonuse is also present in adults with ABI, generally occurs in the initial postinjury period, and tends to persist.[48] CIT attempts to reverse this learned nonuse in the adult with ABI.[48] Recent efficacy research in the field is very encouraging. Blanton and Wolf treated a 61-year-old left cerebral vascular accident (CVA) client 4 months postinjury with CIT.[47] The client wore a mitt on her uninvolved hand during all waking hours (except water-based activities) for a 14 day treatment period. Improvement in the use of the affected upper extremity was noted pretreatment to post-treatment as well as on follow up on 16 evaluation tasks.[48] Miltner et al conducted a CIT study on 15 adult CVA clients with a postonset range of 0.5 to 17 years.[48] Treatment involved 1) restriction of movement of the unaffected upper extremity by placing it in a resting hand splint/sling ensemble 90% of walking hours for 12 days and 2) training of the affected arm by "shaping" for 7 hours per day on the 8-week days during that period. The results of this study indicated significant improvement at post-test and 6-month follow up. Miltner et al conclude that CIT is a powerful treatment tool for upper extremity rehabilitation in the chronic stroke client.[48]

Taub et al administered CIT to a CVA client who was 4 years postonset.[55] The client wore a sling on his unaffected arm 90% of waking hours for 14 days. On 10 of those days, the client received 6 hours of training the affected arm. Study results showed significant improvement in skill on quality of movement and greater real-world arm use, which was still present 2 years after the completion of treatment.[55] These authors theorize that improvements are the result of use dependent cortical reorganization, which would ensure that gains would remain long-term.[55] Recent functional magnetic resonance imaging (fMRI) research supports this theory of cortical reorganization associated with the therapeutic effect of CIT.[49]

One interesting and relevant finding of recent neuroimaging studies is that "...the size of cortical representation of a body part in adult humans depends on the amount of use of that part."[49] This finding has direct implication for the client with body neglect. Learned nonuse could in fact result in decreased cortical representation of the affected limb, which then perpetuates the body neglect. If this were the case, then theoretically, CIT could reverse this effect resulting in increased use and decreased neglect.

A study of 66 chronic CVA clients conducted by van der Lee et al appears to support this benefit of CIT with clients whom exhibit body hemineglect as well as those with sensory disorders.[57] The 66 clients were divided into two groups. The first group received 2 weeks of forced use training while the second group received equally intensive bimanual training based on neurodevelopmental theory (NDT). One week after the last training, a significant difference in effectiveness in favor of forced use was found compared to the bimanual group for dexterity of the affected arm as well as the use of the affected arm during ADLs.[57] Of particular interest is how the effect of forced use therapy was clinically relevant in the subgroups of clients with sensory disorders and hemineglect. These authors hypothesize that the positive results of forced use with this subgroup of clients is because clients "...with sensory disorders and hemineglect do not use the full motion potential of their hemiplegic arm and that their arm function may therefore be more amenable."[57]

In summary, research has shown that adding a specific targeted, meaningful intervention for the affected arm during the acute and chronic phase of recovery of the adult ABI client will result in a long-term positive effect on upper extremity function.[52] CIT appears to be a powerful tool for these clients and is thought to reverse the effects of "learned nonuse" through use-dependent cortical reorganization. It is of particular interest that CIT can have a significant effect on clients with hemineglect, body neglect, and sensory disorders. Some estimate that at least 50% of the total CVA population would be amenable to substantial improvement as a result of CIT.[48]

Brain Plasticity and Functional Reorganization

The term plasticity refers to the adaptive capacity to change, including the ability to learn and remember.[36] Brain plasticity provides a way for new learning and the means to compensate for loss.[36] It has been well known for years that the human brain is plastic; however, it is only recently that we have begun to understand the underlying mechanisms of this plasticity as well as the effect rehabilitation can have to enhance the process. Neural plasticity is being studied at many different levels from observing behavioral changes, viewing brain processing changes with neuroimaging, or studying the microscopic changes in cellular organization.[58] Research in the field of neuroscience has identified three mechanisms of brain recovery or plasticity and has shown that new neurons continually form in the brain throughout adulthood.[26,59,60] Structural brain changes in the elderly after environmental manipulation have in fact demonstrated that an enriched environment can reverse some of the consequences of aging.[36]

The first mechanism of brain plasticity is through a functional reorganization or reweighting of functional interactions within an existing network of brain regions.[60,61] Damaged axons can regenerate and form new terminals on the cells previously innervated, or axons from other neurons can sprout new terminals to form new synapses.[26] Research has shown that surviving neurons in a network maintain their function through increasing connectivity by creating additional dendrites to compensate for the loss of neurons.[62] Research has also demonstrated that these changes in dendritic growth after cortical injury are associated with a change in functional outcome.[61]

The second identified mechanism of neural plasticity is the creation of new circuits. This is accomplished either by forming new connections among remaining neurons or by generating new neurons.[61] Research has demonstrated that the brain utilizes both methods of repair.[60-62] The brain either recruits new areas into the affected network or uses an alternate network not normally used for a particular task performance.[60]

The third mechanism of neural plasticity involves the plasticity of the areas surrounding the damaged areas. During this mode of plasticity, there is a change in sensorimotor field representation, which results in these areas taking over the functions previously represented in the damaged area.[60] This reorganization ability may reflect an inherent plasticity of cortical cells and connections.[60]

Rehabilitation of the damaged brain can enhance or foster reconnection of damaged neural circuits.[62] It has been shown that active learning contributes to the enhancement of neuronal regeneration and brain reorganization.[61] It is now known that cortical structures can be altered and that this restructuring is influenced by various types of sensory and motor experiences.[61] There is strong evidence that "...the neural circuits underpinning high level cognitive functions are also amenable to both restitutive, reorganization as well as compensatory adjustment..."[62] Robertson and Murre have found that rehabilitation focused on improving sustained attention resulted both in increased sustained attention and an increase in activity of the right frontoparietal network, which is known to subserve this process.[62] These researchers believe the results support the theory of experience dependent restitution of brain function.[62]

Robertson and Murre provide the following theoretical assumptions related to observed rehabilitation induced plastic reorganization of damaged brain systems[62]:

1. Within the brain, there exists neural circuits or networks of synaptically connected neurons or sets of neurons which are functionally connected. These functionally connected networks become activated together when a particular cognitive activity occurs.

2. Brain damaged individuals can learn to do what they did before the damage more or less in similar ways. The basis of this is experience-dependent brain plasticity. This is supported by research showing experience dependent synaptic changes and axonal sprouting which has underpinned observable behavioral recovery.

3. The brain is capable of a large degree of self-repair through synaptic turnover. This synaptic turnover is an ongoing change in the dendritic branches of neurons with associated changes in the pattern of synaptic connectivity and is to some extent experience-dependent. This is a key mechanism underlying both learning and recovery of function following brain damage.

4. Recovery processes following brain damage share common mechanisms with normal learning and experience dependent plasticity processes.

5. Variations in the experience and inputs available to damaged neural circuits will shape synaptic interconnections and hence influence recovery.

It is important for the occupational therapist to have an understanding of neuralplasticity and brain recovery. This understanding of the structural changes in the brain after injury will help the therapist understand how to potentially stimulate functional recovery.[61] If the therapist can understand the structural changes associated with functional recovery, then he or she can begin to design interventions that will stimulate such plastic changes.[61]

It has become apparent that the human brain is shaped by behavior as much as behavior shapes the brain.[58] Brain stimulation through electrodes or intensive therapy has global effects on brain function that can cross modalities and functions.[58] Neuroscience research has now moved into examining what roles rehabilitative approaches have in fostering neural plasticity.[58] This exciting research trend has great potential as a way to measure the efficacy of occupational therapy practice with the adult with ABI.

NEUROIMAGING

One of the main contributions to advances in neuroscience and information about neural plasticity and functional reorganization is the development and refinement of neuroimaging techniques. As Burns points out, "… neuroimaging data with adult humans confirmed what animal researchers had been showing since the 1970s, namely that mature brains reorganize in important functional ways after injury."[58] More sophisticated functional imaging techniques have allowed researchers to objectively evaluate subtle cerebral pathology, and as previously described, to examine brain activity or plasticity as it occurs during specific task performance.[26,59-63] Some positron emission tomography (PET) scan studies have even supported neuropsychological findings when there was no other apparent evidence of brain damage from computed tomography (CT) scans.[63] New techniques such as PET scans and functional magnetic resonance imaging (fMRI) have allowed imaging of brain activity "in vivo" during sensory, motor, and cognitive behavior.[64] Neuroimaging has begun to uncover the routes or neural processing that occur during language, problem solving, and a multitude of other tasks.[19] These noninvasive techniques have only begun to uncover the neural networks that subserve complex functions.[56] For example, neuroimaging techniques have already demonstrated that the skills related to executive functions "…are subsumed by distributed circuitry rather than discrete structures."[65] Specifically, posterior cortical regions and subcortical structures collaborate with prefrontal cortex to mediate successful executive processing.[65] These results are confirmed by additional activation studies in normals, which pointed to circuitry related specific brain regions for particular components of supervisory processes.[56]

In an exciting study of clients with visual neglect, neuroimaging demonstrated that changes could be seen in the brain as a result of a specific rehabilitation program.[56,60] These client's brains were scanned before and after participation in visual scanning, reading, copying drawings, and verbal descriptions of pictures.

Functional neuroimaging represents an exciting tool in the study of functional brain recovery.[65] These studies potentially will provide data on the reorganizational plasticity potential in different forms of stroke.[65] They will help ascertain which of the previously described mechanisms of brain recovery is the most prominent within specific categories of stroke, which in turn will ultimately lead to better intervention strategies.[65]

As a result of neuroimaging data, neuroscientists have begun to regard sensorimotor and cognitive processing as the product of functional neural networks.[60] This is a shift from the traditional strict localization approach. Due to this change in philosophy, researchers are now focusing on the interactions among brain areas during specific types of cognitive or motor function activities and how these interactions change as the behavior changes.[60] This measurement of brain changes during the performance of activities can aid in the decision making and designing of specific rehabilitation programs as well as monitoring the effectiveness of such programs.[60] As Grady and Kapur state, neuroimaging can do the following[60]:

1. *Provide insight into alternative ways a particular cognitive (or motor) task can be accomplished.*

2. *Determine which brain areas are necessary for recover to happen, therefore, possibly identifying which clients have the most potential to benefit from rehabilitation.*

3. *Monitor the effectiveness of rehabilitation procedures during and after treatment is completed.*

In the world of rehabilitation, where the need to demonstrate the efficacy of our treatment is paramount, neuroimaging will likely develop into a crucial clinical research tool. It will help us understand how the brain adapts or recovers after damage with or without rehabilitation. The occupational therapist should begin to conceive of generating efficacy studies which incorporate neuroimaging techniques to support practice.

Frames of Reference Utilizing an Adaptive Conceptual Base: Top-Down Approaches

OCCUPATION-BASED MODELS

There are four models or frameworks related to occupational behavior described in the occupational therapy literature. These models include The Model of Human Occupation (MOHO), Occupational Adaptation (OA), The Ecology of Human Performance, and the Person-Environment Occupation Performance (PEO) model (Table 1-2). These models or frames of reference are at different stages of conceptual refinement as well as specific application to clinical practice. There are many shared concepts among each, and some concepts are also present in other models of practice. The following sections are summaries of each of these four models. This material presented was generated primarily from information provided in Willard and Spackman's Occupational Therapy.[70]

The Model of Human Occupation

The MOHO, which incorporates a systems view of the individual, is the result of an effort to create a theory to guide practice that would focus on occupation.[67] Under this model, it is assumed that behavior is both dynamic and context driven. More specifically, an individual's "... inner characteristics interact with the environment to create a network of conditions that influence a person's motivation, action, and performance."[67] A second assumption of the MOHO is that occupation is essential for self-organization. Therapy, therefore, is viewed as a process by which the client is helped to shape his or her abilities and identity.[67] The main mechanism for change during therapy relates to what the client thinks and feels about what he or she is doing.[67] Finally,

Table 1-2

Occupation-Based Theories

Theory	*Underlying Assumptions*
Model of Human Occupation	• Behavior is dynamic and context dependent. • Occupation is essential to self-organization. • Theory must be used to understand clients and decide the course of occupational therapy. • MOHO-based therapy is client-centered. • The human is composed of three elements: volition, habituation, and performance capacity.
Occupational Adaptation	• Competence in occupation is a life-long process of adaptation to internal and external demands to perform. • Demands to perform occur naturally as part of the person's occupational roles and the context in which they occur. • Dysfunction occurs when the person's ability to adapt has been challenged to the point where they cannot be met. • At any point in life, a person's adaptive ability can be impaired. • The greater the level of dysfunction, the greater the demand for changes in the person's adaptive processes. • Success in occupational performance is a direct result of the person's ability to adapt to the satisfaction of the self and others.
Ecology of Human Performance	• It is impossible to understand the person without understanding the person's context. • A person's performance range is determined by the interaction between the person and the context. • Contrived contexts are different from natural contexts. Contrived contexts may either facilitate or inhibit performance. • Assessment and intervention best approximate the person's true performance when carried out in natural environments. • Occupational therapy practice involves promotion of self determination and includes clients in all contexts. • Independence includes using contextual supports to meet the client's wants and needs.
Person-Environment-Occupation Model	• Behavior cannot be separated from environmental influences, temporal factors, and physical and psychological factors. • Environments are constantly changing, and as they change, the behavior necessary to accomplish a goal changes. • Environments can have an enabling or constraining effect on occupational performance. • The environment is more often amenable to change than the person. • Occupations are complex, pluralistic, and necessary for quality of life. • The relationship among the person, environment, and occupation is interwoven and difficult to separate. The outcome of this relationship is called occupational performance. • Occupational performance changes over a lifetime as an individual's roles change.

Adapted from references 1,66-69

the MOHO assumes that therapy should be client-centered and based on a collaborative approach with the client.[67]

The MOHO views the individual as being composed of three elements. Kielhofner et al define these elements as follows[67]:

- *Volition*—The process by which persons are motivated toward and choose what they do.

- *Habituation*—A process whereby people organize their actions into patterns and routines.

- *Performance capacity*—Refers both to people's underlying objective mental and physical abilities and to their lived experience that shapes performance.

The MOHO assumes that people and their environments are inseparable. The environment is viewed as encompassing both physical and social components. The values, interests, roles, habits, and performance capacities of an individual will determine how the environment will have an influence.[67]

The Occupational Adaptation Model

The OA model, as the name implies, deals with human adaptation and occupation. Shultz and Schkade outline six assumptions of the OA model as follows[68]:

1. Competence in occupation is a life-long process of adaptation to internal and external demands to perform.

2. Demands to perform occur naturally as part of the person's occupational roles and the context (person-occupational-environment interactions) in which they occur.

3. Dysfunction occurs because the person's ability to adapt has been challenged to the point that the demands for performance are not satisfactorily met.

4. At any stage of life, the person's adaptive capacity can be overwhelmed by impairment, physical or emotional disability, and stressful life events.

5. The greater the level of dysfunction, the greater the demand for changes in the person's adaptive processes.

6. Success in occupational performance is a direct result of the person's ability to adapt with sufficient mastery to satisfy the self and others.

The OA model describes the adaptation process as developing from an interaction between the person and occupational environment in response to occupational challenges.[68] These challenges occur within the context of performing occupational roles. The "…performance expectations from the occupational environment and from the person's own internal expectations influence the challenge experience."[68] The OA model views the therapist's role in intervention as to acknowledging and facilitating the client as an agent of therapeutic change, which is critical to the client's internal adaptation process.[68] OA is a client-centered approach with the ultimate goal of treatment being the client's ability to make his or her own adaptations to engage in relevant meaningful occupational activities.[68]

The Ecology of Human Performance Model

The Ecology of Human Performance model is a framework that was developed for considering context in occupational therapy practice.[66] The major assumption of this model is that "…ecology, or the interaction between a person and the context, affects human behavior and task performance."[66] This model assumes it is impossible to understand an individual without understanding his or her context. The individual's performance abilities are determined by the interaction between the individual and his or her context.[66] Dunn et al describe the following interventions, which would be used when applying the Ecology of Human Performance Model[66]:

1. *Establish or restore a person's abilities to perform in context.*

2. *Alter actual context or task in which people perform.*

3. *Modify (adapt) contextual features and task demands so they support performance in context.*

4. *Prevent the occurrence or evolution of performance problems in context*

5. *Create circumstances that promote more adaptable or complex performance in context.*

The Person-Environment-Occupation Model

The PEO model not only focuses on occupation, as the MOHO does, but also sets out to focus on the dynamic nature of occupational performance.[69] This is also a client-centered model that emphasizes occupations and performance.[16] The assumptions of this model relate to three elements and how they interact. As the model's name implies, these three elements are the person, the environment, and the occupation.

The PEO model assumes that the individual is naturally motivated to explore his or her world, to demonstrate mastery within it, and that situations in which the individual experiences success will help him or her feel good about him- or herself.[16]

The PEO model also assumes that the environment itself is constantly changing, can have either a facilitating or constraining effect on occupational performance, and is often more amenable to change than the individual.[69]

The PEO model defines the "person" element as a composite of mind, body, and spirit.[69] This model considers intrinsic factors of the individual, which can inhibit or facilitate occupational performance.[71] As Baum and Christiansen state "...this approach requires the practitioner to collect assessment information about the physiological, psychological, cognitive, neurobehavioral, and spiritual factors that may be interfering with or supporting their performance..."[71] The identification of person factors (body domain) are important to assess and understand as "...it is where we find the link between impairment, activities, and participation."[19]

Within the scope of the PEO model, occupation is defined to include all self-care, productive and, leisure pursuits.[69] It is assumed that occupations are "...complex, pluralistic, and necessary for quality of life and well-being."[69] Stewart et al describe the concepts of occupations, activities and tasks as follows[69]:

> *Activities are considered to be the basic units of tasks; tasks are sets of purposeful, related activities; and occupations are groups of self-directed, functional tasks and activities in which a person engages over a life span.*

The PEO model's key assumption is that "...the person, environment, and occupation interact continually across time and space in ways that increase or decrease their congruence: the closer the fit, the greater the overlap or occupational performance."[69] The model identifies which of these factors is relevant at a given time to occupational performance, which in turn provides a basis for intervention.[71] The occupational therapist works with the client to "...identify opportunities for building personal capabilities, modifying environments, or reconsidering occupational processes and goals."[71] As Baum and Christiansen state, under this model, the interaction of capacity, environment, and chosen activity lead to occupational performance and participation.[71] This participation and occupational performance changes over a lifetime, as an individual's roles and view of him or herself changes.[69]

FUNCTIONAL/OCCUPATION-BASED APPROACH

The functional approach is a top-down approach that works directly with actual occupations.[3,27,72] It uses functional or occupation-based tasks to maximize the client's independence. The functional approach emphasizes the client's strengths and can be domain specific (repetitive practice of a specific functional task) and/or involve specific adaptations or compensations.[27] The desired outcome of the functional approach is effective adaptation. Effective adaptation always occurs within an environmental context; therefore, a variety of functional activities are practiced in different environments. The functional approach utilizes two major categories of techniques: compensation and adaptation.

Compensation

In the compensation approach, the client is made aware of his or her problem and then taught to compensate or make allowance for it. For example, if the client neglects one-half of space because of unilateral neglect, the therapist would teach him to turn his head or scan with his eyes to the affected side. Alternatively, if he or she had dressing apraxia, the therapist would practice a particular dressing pattern with him or her daily.

Adaptation

Adaptation usually goes along with compensation. In this approach, the therapist makes changes in or adapts the environment of the client to compensate for his or her symptoms. For example, if he or she tends to neglect one-half of space, the therapist would put all of his or her food and utensils on the unaffected side to be sure that it is seen. If the client has figure-ground problems, the therapist would try to unclutter the environment to make it easier to locate objects. If the client has topographical disorientation, the therapist would mark the route to be followed every day. Informing the client's family about his or her problems so that they can make allowances for them, instead of thinking that the client is stubborn or crazy, is a more subtle form of adaptation. Adapting the client's "human" rather than his "nonhuman" environment is of major importance in many ways.

Summary

The functional approach is one of the most favored in the clinic today. Recent research has supported its use for improved self-care of clients with unilateral neglect or perceptual dysfunction.[72] Rubio and Van Deusen, however, found that for wheelchair mobility and driving, a combination of functional and restorative was the most effective approach.[72] An additional benefit of the functional approach is its relevance to the client. Clients often object to abstract perceptual and cognitive training, finding it childish, degrading, and not relevant to their problems.

One final benefit of utilizing a functional approach relates to the status or focus of today's health care. The trend for shorter hospital stays and the need for specific expedient measured outcomes necessitates the use of an approach that can meet these demands. Often, a restorative approach to treatment requires extended stays, which has become less and less an option.

DYNAMIC INTERACTIONAL APPROACH*

Central to the DIA is the concept that cognition is an ongoing production or outcome of the interaction among the individual, the task, and the environment.[24,73] The client's performance is analyzed by examining the underlying conditions and processing strategies that change

---

The DIA can be viewed as both a restorative and adaptive approach. In addition, a strong component of the approach considers the influence of context or environment on client performance. Some treatment alters the task or environment more than the person; however, ultimately the DIA is changing the person and how he or she performs the task (personal communication Joan Toglia, PhD, OTR, FAOTA). For the purposes of this book, the approach and related treatment ideas will be described under the adaptive approach.

performance, as well as the client's potential for learning.[24,74] Cognitive disability is framed in terms of deficiencies in processing strategies.[24] This model or framework views processing strategies and self-awareness as the fundamental aspects of cognitive function that interact dynamically with external factors such as the activity and environment as well as the internal variables such as structural capacity.[24,73] In some situations, the personal factors are important, and in some, it is the environmental factors. The DIA of evaluation and treatment assumes that by analyzing the demands of a particular activity, the conditions under which there is a breakdown of information processing can be identified. This is a contrast to the deficit specific approach, which assumes the deficit is defined by the task.[73]

As just mentioned, the DIA views processing strategies as a core element of cognition. It is assumed that the type of processing strategy the client uses will affect how well the information is processed as well as how well it is retained.[24] This approach assumes that modifying an individual's processing strategies can improve performance and that processing strategies cut across specific cognitive domains.[24,75] Attention to detail, for example, can subserve performance in attention, memory, and visual processing tasks.[24] Processing strategies can be either internal (self-reminders, mental, rehearsals etc) or external, as well as situational (effective in specific tasks or environments) or nonsituational (able to be used in a wide variety of tasks and environments.)[24]

The DIA assumes the client's social, physical, and cultural environment can influence his or her adaptation to environmental demands. The social environment can include those with whom the client interacts, and the physical can include the materials and objects that surround the client as well as visual or auditory distractions.[24,75] In addition to personal and environmental influence on performance, the DIA focuses on task or activity analysis and assumes that task characteristics will influence information processing and transfer of learning.[24] If the task or activity is too complex or above the client's processing abilities, then efficient processing strategies cannot be used. By changing task parameters, the conditions under which information processing and performance break down can be identified.[24] Toglia divides tasks into both surface and conceptual characteristics.[75] Surface characteristics are those characteristics that are readily observed. Conceptual characteristics, on the other hand, cannot be directly observed. These characteristics would include areas such as the strategies used to perform the task or what the task means to the client.

As previously mentioned, the DIA considers an individual's self-awareness as one of the core aspects of cognitive function. The evaluation and treatment of any deficits in the client's self-awareness are central to this approach. Toglia views self-awareness as multidimensional and defines these dimensions as follows[75]:

- *Self-knowledge*—includes the understanding of one's cognitive strengths and limitations that exist outside the context of a particular task.

- *On-line awareness*—includes metacognitive skills such as the ability to accurately judge task demands; anticipate the likelihood of problems; and monitor, regulate, and evaluate performance within the context of an activity.

Decreased self-awareness will affect speed of performance, effective strategy use, the ability to learn from mistakes, and the ability to use feedback to modify behavior.[75] As Toglia states, an individual's self-knowledge and perceptions influence strategy use, activity choices, and performance.[75]

The DIA utilizes dynamic assessment to evaluate the client's cognitive status. Toglia outlines assessment as consisting of 1) investigating self-perceptions of abilities prior to the task, 2) facilitating change in performance, and 3) investigating self-perceptions of performance and strategy use after the task.[75] Assessment focuses on the client's ability for change.[74] It includes task alteration and cues, strategy training, practice in a number of settings, and the examination of learner characteristics to facilitate learning transfer.[24] Assessment is focused on the client's ability to 1) evaluate the level of difficulty of a particular task, 2) plan ahead, 3) select appropriate strategies, 4) predict the consequences of the actions he or she takes, and 5) monitor performance.[24,75]

The previously listed skills are paramount to the generalization of new learning and are related to both motivation and experience. If a client believes he or she has some degree of control over his or her performance, his or her motivation will increase. This emotional state of mind will in turn influence how well information is processed and monitored.[76] Past experience guides how the client processes and organizes information.[24] When new information is processed by relating it to previous knowledge, understanding and retention improve.

In addition to examining the client's potential for change, assessment focuses on the client's best performance and what task and environmental criteria are needed to achieve this performance. This dynamic assessment process assumes that "…when activity demands or context changes, the type of cognitive strategies and self-monitoring skills required for efficient performance change as well."[77] If a client has difficulty, test procedures are changed and subsequent client response is examined. After the dynamic assessment, the client is not identified as having deficits in a specific cognitive domain, rather the assessment focuses on the common behaviors that influence task performance.[24,75]

Intervention-based on the DIA is performed in multiple contexts and has been termed the multi-context approach. The multi-context approach "…aims to change the person's use of strategies and self-monitoring skills within a just right challenge level."[77] By carrying out this treatment aim in a variety of contexts, the skills developed will not be associated with just one context.[74] This approach is best utilized with clients who have demonstrated during dynamic assessment that they can respond to cues or therapist mediation and they have at least some degree of self-awareness limitations.[77] The behaviors that have been observed in a large range of tasks as well as being the most responsive to cuing procedures are the ones addressed during treatment.[24]

In summary, the DIA to cognitive function is an individualized, process oriented approach that "…seeks to measure cognitive modifiability or the change that is possible under different conditions."[24] Tasks are analyzed and upgraded to place additional demands on the impaired processing system and the ability to transfer new learning.[24] A variety of activities, including tabletop, computer, functional, and gross motor tasks, can be used. Treatment begins at the level of breakdown, and the task is not upgraded until there is some evidence that generalization of learning has occurred at the highest level of transfer.[74] Task, strategy, and self awareness training are performed in a variety of settings with the ultimate goal of learning transfer.

The main limitations of this approach that have thus far been identified are: 1) the use of cues during assessment prevents it from being used as a measure of progress in performance over time, 2) most aspects of the DIA require the use of language skills, 3) it is difficult to generate empirical research when no two clients receive the same treatment in the same way, 4) it is time consuming, 5) it requires an experienced clinician, and 6) very little has been written about the approach.[24,77] Despite these limitations, this author believes continued theory development and refinement will generate continued data that supports that the DIA is a valid practical approach that can be used in the evaluation and treatment of the adult with ABI.

CONTEXTUAL INFLUENCE ON CLIENT PERFORMANCE

The traditional view of an individual with disabilities is that these disabilities stem solely from the individual. Recently, however, there has been a shift in thinking as to how disability is defined. No longer is the client disabled based on just individual capabilities, but rather the client's disability can also result from an environment that prevents or constrains performance.[78] The new International Classification of Functioning (ICF), which is the accepted international standard for describing and measuring health and disability, includes a mechanism to document the impact of the social and physical environment on an individual's performance.[78] The Occupational Therapy Practice Framework also supports this concept by identifying an individual's context as either a facilitator or constraint to occupational performance.[79,80]

A contextual approach supports the belief that "occupational performance is the result of complex interactions between the intrinsic person factors and extrinsic factors of the environment."[78] Environmental contexts include physical, social, cultural, and spiritual contexts.[79] As Stark and Sanford state, the environment "is the context for people's performance and includes everything that a person encounters during participation as a human being in society."[78] Spencer breaks down the domains of environment into four levels: 1) immediate scale contexts, which include the client's immediate surrounding in which he or she has direct contact, including direct personal interactions; 2) proximal scale contexts, which include surroundings at the level of a single behavior setting (eg, kitchen or clinic); 3) community scale contexts, which include geographic communities or neighborhoods; and 4) societal scale contexts, which include public policies or major social institutions.[79]

No matter what level or scale of contextual domain, a client's deficits will only become a disability when he or she interacts with an environment in which he or she cannot perform as needed. The occupational therapist, therefore, should evaluate the client as he or she engages in activities in a number of different contexts and note which contexts support or hinder change.[15]

Not only does environmental context have an important influence on overall occupational performance, but it is widely accepted to have a large or considerable influence on cognitive performance.[81] This influence ranges from basic perception to complex problem solving.[81] As described in the previous sections on plasticity and neuroimaging, enriching an individual's environment has direct consequences on brain functions and behavior.[81] As Woodruff-Pak and Hanson state, "... structural changes have been measured in the brain resulting from manipulations of the environment, and the brain plasticity for development of these changes is retained throughout life."[81] The results of extensive neuroimaging studies make the fact of experience dependent neuralplasticity impossible to refute.[63] Interventions that consider contextual or environmental influences on the client's level of disability will also influence the types of interventions that can be utilized.[25] As just described, context will influence the client's ability to learn and apply this learning to daily life performance. To compensate for contexts that impede occupational performance, the context or environment can be modified. This environmental modification can help prevent a deficit or impairment from becoming a disability.[82] Environmental modifications or alterations change factors that are external to the client without expectation of changing underlying performance components.[37] These adaptations or modifications can include strategies such as reducing clutter, simplifying a task, or reorganizing the client's kitchen.

Section II

ADDITIONAL FACTORS GUIDING EVALUATION AND TREATMENT

Client-Centered Practice

Although occupational therapists have traditionally viewed the client's needs and values as central to the therapeutic process, it is only in recent years that this concept has gained more focused attention and is now often referred to as "client-centered practice."

Client-centered practice is now viewed by some as a different model of service delivery where the therapist is engaged by the client to help him or her achieve identified goals in occupational performance.[83,84] It attempts to combine the experiential knowledge of the client and the academic and practical knowledge of the therapist.[85] One of the core assumptions of a client-centered model of intervention is that the therapist cannot actually promote change but can only create an environment that facilitates change.[84] Another core concept within client-centered occupational therapy is that clients are not separated from the environments and communities in which they live, work, and play.[86] The Occupational Performance models, described earlier in this chapter are therefore considered client-centered models of practice.[86]

In a client-centered approach, the client and therapist develop a collaborative relationship. They work together to "define the nature of the occupational performance problems, the focus and need for intervention, and the outcomes of therapy."[87] The therapist creates an environment of trust in which the client can use his or her own problem solving abilities to identify and reach therapeutic goals.[83] To help create this trusting environment, the therapist shows respect for the choices the client has made, the choices he or she will make, and his or her personal method of coping.[86] The client is viewed as an individual with unique values and needs.[88] When the therapist provides information about the client's occupational performance issues and potential solutions, he or she does so in an understandable manner so the client can make choices about the intervention process.[86] In a client-centered practice, the therapist provides the client with some intervention choices that are related to the client's stated interests and priorities. This process encourages client motivation and provides a means for the client to have some degree of control, which in turn supports self-efficacy.[25] Self-efficacy is central to a client-centered model of practice.[86,87]

A major goal of client-centered practice is that the therapeutic relationship between the therapist and his or her client is one of collaboration.[86] As Hammell states, "...collaborative goal setting by the client and occupational therapist ensures that the program of intervention is directed toward mastering skills that the client values and is likely to use."[85] In addition, in client-centered practice, the therapist not only collaborates with the client but, within the confines of client confidentiality, also collaborates with any individuals relevant to the client's environment.[87] This could include family members, teachers, neighbors, employers, or friends.

The evaluation process of a client-centered approach incorporates the concept that the client holds the most important information regarding his or her needs.[86] Additionally, the client should be encouraged by the therapist to choose the areas of occupational performance that are his or her priority for treatment. Client-centered assessment includes task performances that are meaningful to the client and evaluates the level of person-environment interaction.[6,87] Formal or informal interviews, client questionnaires, and tools such as the Canadian Occupational Performance Measure (COPM) are examples of evaluation tools that are client-centered.[84,87,89]

Client-centered evaluation can also include the evaluation of performance components. For example, a client has indicated that meal preparation is important to her and that because of a recent CVA, she is no longer able to prepare meals for her family. The occupational therapist would then initiate an evaluation of meal preparation, preferably in the client's home, to assess what is affecting performance. During the evaluation, the therapist observes several behaviors that could indicate a possible attention and/or problem solving deficit. At that point, additional performance component evaluations would be indicated. Findings from these performance component evaluations would then be incorporated into other information collected during the overall evaluation process. If the performance component evaluation indicated that there was an underlying attentional problem affecting the client's ability to prepare meals, this is then communicated to the client, and the information is then used in treatment planning. The client and therapist can decide together how to address the attentional problem during meal preparation (ie, a restorative, an adaptive approach, or both). Often times during this collaboration, once the client understands how a particular performance component (in this case decreased attention) is affecting a particular activity (in this case meal preparation), the client begins to understand and identify other contexts (eg, driving) that are being affected by the same performance component.

Before leaving the topic of a client-centered model of practice, it is important to understand both the advantages and disadvantages of its use. The major advantages of a client-centered practice are that it enhances self-esteem and self-efficacy and that it is an individualized approach.[83] Disadvantages may be that the client perceives the therapist as less skilled, the therapeutic relationship can become unclear, and there are a limited number of reliable, valid client-centered evaluation tools.[83,84] Client-centered practice can be difficult to practice in some organizations. Practical issues such as team philosophy, charting, and reporting requirements or length of stay can make it difficult for total incorporation of a client-centered practice.[83,84]

Another disadvantage of a "totally" client-centered approach relates to the ability to strictly apply it to the adult with ABI. These clients often have language deficits, such as aphasia, and are unable to communicate sufficiently. Cognitive deficits will also affect their ability to participate in planning their care. In these cases, Pollack and McColl suggest the therapist rethink who is actually the client and state it may be a close family member or caregiver.[83,84] These people might actually be making the change in therapy or the choices for the client. For these clients, it is the family or caregiver who should participate in the treatment planning.[87] Although this is a logical alternative, often times, especially with the CVA client, the family members, due to the tragic event (ie, CVA or TBI), are overwhelmed by the situation.

Despite these challenges to the application of a client-centered practice, in most situations, the client or the client's family member or caregiver should be encouraged to make some choices to the best of his or her ability. Law summarizes well client-centered practice as follows[86]:

> *With the client's information and the practitioners assessment of the client's capacity and constraints, a client-centered plan is constructed. The practitioner uses his or her skill to help the client understand what is possible and helps the client understand the issues involved in helping him or her meet his or her goals.*

Client and Family Education

An important outcome of the recent focus on client-centered practice is the increased attention being given to the importance and benefit of client, family, and/or caregiver education. In support of a client-centered practice, education, or the transfer of specific knowledge to the client, should relate to his or her needs and priorities.[25] Client education is an important element in involving clients in clinical decision making and requires them to be given appropriate information about the situation, principally through teaching.[90] In addition, an active family partnership should be fostered by the occupational therapist. This active partnership is essential, as families or caregivers are an important resource to providing information about the client's function in everyday life. The client's family can help to cue the therapist as to what he or she should look for in the assessment and intervention plans.[91] Families can also assist in promoting change and helping to modify habits and roles to deal more effectively with cognitive and other performance deficits.[91] A partnership with the client's family or caregiver is also important to help reduce the psychosocial issues, which are almost always associated with cognitive disorders.[91] It is also important for the occupational therapist to take care of the caregivers who will have their own needs for psychological support.[92]

The therapist should communicate a clear plan and purpose for the teaching or treatment session.[93] Individualized instruction rather than group instruction is often more appropriate with the ABI client due to both the nature of the deficits as well as the personal nature of the tasks that need to be learned (ie, dressing, hygiene).[7] In addition, individualized instruction enables the occupational therapist to get immediate feedback from the client as the session progresses and alter the amount and focus of learning as needed.[7] During family or caregiver education, specific cuing strategies utilized by the client are taught, whether they will be carried out in the client's home or a community setting.[7]

There are many ways to implement client or family education, from the use of written instructions, audio, or videotape to the internet.[7] The decision regarding what method or methods to use is based on the client's cognitive status as well as the learning style and capabilities of both the client and the family or caregiver. As Holm et al state, this is particularly true "...in situations which the person is new to the caregiver role, and time must be taken to assess the caregiver's capacity to understand and apply the information necessary for safe and effective management of the client's needs."[7] The motivation, skill level to be achieved, cognitive status, and available teaching time will all affect teaching outcomes.[93] No matter what method of teaching the therapist utilizes, it is important that he or she allow time for the client or family member to ask questions or seek clarification of instructions.[7]

Any client or family education program related to the adult with ABI must address and focus on the issue of safety. This can include covering topics of occupational performance such as stove usage, locking brakes, functional mobility crossing the street, or driving. In addition, the ultimate goal of client or family education is to teach the client how to manage his or her own occupational performance in a variety of environments.[20]

Proulx identifies the following questions related to cognitive rehabilitation for which family members or caregivers will likely need clarification[91]:

- *How do cognitive impairments relate to underlying brain functions?*
- *How do cognitive impairments translate to everyday activities?*
- *Do we remediate impairments or do we compensate for them?*
- *What are the spared cognitive functions and strengths that can be used to compensate for losses?*
- *What are the differences between remediation, compensation, and functional skills training?*
- *How do you accommodate to change and adjust interventions according to the natural history of the neurological condition?*
- *What are good educational references and lists of community support services?*

These questions can be easily applied to areas of visual and perceptual loss as well.

In summary, the occupational therapist should incorporate client, family, and/or caregiver teaching and education into the treatment plan and process of the adult with ABI. A client-centered practice requires the therapist not only to partner with the client but also with the family and/or caregiver. This partnership and education process facilitates rehabilitation, which can be viewed "…as teaching people with a disability to recalibrate their family life with the ultimate goal of generalizing …rehabilitation gains to the home setting."[91]

Proulx states as follows[91]:

> *Clear information and education regarding the impact of cognitive impairments on everyday behavior, better coping skills on the part of both patients and families, as well as assistance in finding appropriate community support services all reduce barriers to effective rehabilitation.*

The Client's Learning Capacity and Its Influence on Performance

The client's ability to learn is central to rehabilitation and his or her ultimate performance outcome. Learning, in fact, underpins or subserves much of the recovery that occurs after brain injury.[94] The physical, cognitive, and sensory deficits that occur as the result of ABI often limit many of the usual mechanisms of learning.[95] Clients with cognitive deficits such as decreased attention and memory will have an especially difficult time learning and following directions during intervention.[96] The rate at which the client is able to learn will affect how quickly rehabilitation goals are met. This in turn will affect the duration and cost of care.[95]

The client's learning capacity and potential must be evaluated. As Holm et al state, "…clients with a good capacity for learning and an openness to alternate methods may be able to address more task deficits because of increased intervention options and the reduced time required for learning."[7] In order to evaluate the client's learning potential, the therapist should have a basic understanding of specific types of learning and what may impede or facilitate the learning process. A basic overview of the components of learning that can guide evaluation and treatment follows. A comprehensive detailed review is not within the scope of this book and the reader is encouraged to refer to the references and seek out additional information on the topic.

There are three types of learning that require different types of information processing.[56,97] The first type of learning is association learning, which occurs when an individual makes an association between two events.[58] This is the ability to learn how two things are associated in the universe among many possible associations. Association learning occurs when the activity can be described as an "if this, then that" meaning. The individual must learn that when a certain "this" occurs, it only goes with a defined "that."[56] The most effective learning environment for the client for self-care and home management training whose only learning capacity is at the association level is in the home setting.

The second level of learning is representational learning. In representational learning, "…the individual forms an internal representation of events, which includes how events are organized and retrieved."[58] Clients who are functioning at the representational level of learning are able to tolerate changes in the set-up of an activity and can show near and intermediate levels of transfer of learning.[58] They are, however, unable to tolerate major changes in an activity presentation.

The third and highest level of learning capacity is the level of abstract learning.[56,58] The abstract learner is able to gain and store knowledge of rules that have been abstracted from events independently from the spatial and temporal contexts.[58] These learners are "…able to create alternative images for activity completion based on past experiences."[58] They are able to transfer what they have learned in the clinic to the home setting. This level of learning requires more complex information processing then the two previously described levels. Only some adults with ABI are able to function at this level.

There are many factors that can impede or facilitate the learning capacity of the adult ABI client. Medication use, mood, anxiety, and stress can all affect the client's learning potential.[95] The time of day the client is asked to perform will affect learning capacity. Toglia identifies six factors pertinent to the learning and generalization process: environmental context, nature of the task, learning criteria (external), metacognition, processing strategies, and learner characteristics (internal).[74,77] She further believes that performance is the result of the interaction among these factors.[74,77]

External factors that can affect learning include the external environment, nature of the task, and learning criteria. The physical environment can affect the client's attitude and ability to process and monitor information.[74] For example, crowded, unfamiliar environments are going to be more difficult than quiet, familiar environments.[74] The task parameters or nature of the task will also affect learning capacity. Task arrangement, familiarity, predictability, and number of items and steps required for task completion all affect information processing and learning ability.[77] For example, "...as the number of items increases, more demands are placed on the ability to select relevant stimuli, prioritize, screen out irrelevant details, and plan."[74] If the amount of information exceeds what the client is able to process, the client will have difficulty developing effective responses and may become frustrated or overwhelmed.[74]

The third external variable or factor related to learning is learning criteria. Learning criteria refers to the kinds of tasks that are used to measure the quantity of learning that is taking place.[75] Depending on the measures used, the results will vary.[75] Learner characteristics are internal factors that influence learning and are made up of previous knowledge, existing skills, attitudes, emotions, experiences, values, personality, motivation, and emotions.[74] Structural capacity is another internal factor affecting learning and refers to the inherent fixed abilities of the individual.[74] The individual's knowledge concerning his or her cognitive abilities as well as his or her ability to self-monitor are also internal factors that will affect learning.[75] Finally, the processing strategies employed by the individual, which are dependent on task familiarity and perceived difficulty, will affect learning capacity.[75]

One of the most recent and promising approaches being utilized in the rehabilitation of cognitive dysfunction that addresses the client's learning capacity is "errorless learning." During the utilization of the errorless learning approach, clients are cued as they learn a new skill to prevent them from making any errors.[98] The task is clearly defined, and if an error is made, it is corrected immediately.[98] Unlike the trial and error approach, errorless learning minimizes the exposure of the client to any high demand tasks or situations.[99] As the client becomes more competent, the depth and degree of cuing is reduced. Errorless learning is especially important for clients "...who rely on implicit memory processes to learn new information to avoid error early in the learning process."[56] If errors are made during the client's initial learning process, it may be difficult to eliminate these errors without access to explicit memory.[56] Giles also supports the use of errorless learning with clients with memory loss when he states the following[99]:

> *Errorless learning is the preferred method (versus trial and error) with memory loss. This is because the client with this deficit will not recognize a behavior as a failed strategy ...and the priming effect makes the last action the most available action and therefore increases the likelihood that it will be performed wrong again.*

In addition to using a theoretical model of learning to guide practice, the therapist should assess what type or style of learning the client utilized prior to the ABI, as well as previous education level or learning disabilities. For example, if the client was a visual learner prior to the ABI, if at all possible, visual learning should be utilized during treatment. Or if the client was dyslexic prior to the ABI, this would affect certain avenues of learning now during treatment.

Evidence-Based Practice

Any therapist involved in contemporary practice will be familiar with the term "evidence-based" practice. Evidence-based practice, or the translation and application of clinical research into practice, requires therapists to justify why they do what they do in addition to how they do it.[7,15,100,101] The implementation of an evidenced-based practice with concurrent use of best-practice guidelines can accomplish quality care outcomes while maintaining fiscal responsibility.[100] Policies, procedures, and competencies that reflect best evidence can be developed, which in turn will encourage changes in practice through providing supporting knowledge.[102]

The expectation of evidence-based practice is that the services delivered will result in expected outcomes.[20,71,102,103] Evidence-based practice, therefore, should be directly tied to outcomes assessment. Many therapists advocate that a systematic outcomes assessment is crucial to successful outcomes management.[98,102,104,105] Law and Philp state as follows[104]:

> _It is important for every therapist to employ outcome measurement strategies that will enable him or her to acquire evidence of whether or not occupational therapy intervention is effective as it is happening and whether it has made a difference overall for his or her clients._

Outcomes management requires continuous refinement of earlier clinical guidelines and practices as well as the development of new ones.[100] This evaluation and monitoring of outcomes is a final step to implementing and sustaining evidence-based practice.[102] Whereas evidence-based practice emphasizes the use of the best available evidence for each clinical situation, outcomes management emphasizes the continuous evaluation of the outcomes of the evidence-based practice.[100] Many health care organizations are now using a technique called "benchmarking" in analyzing outcomes. As DeLise and Leasure state, benchmarking compares outcomes from practice conditions with the more rigorously controlled experimental treatment and evaluation methods associated with a research study.[102] Benchmarking of client care against internal or external data from other health care providers or evidence from relevant studies identifies and facilitates quality care goals that can be routinely set and achieved.[103] Benchmarking or similar processes can validate the positive impact of the practice changes that are implemented.[102]

A major component of traditional evidence-based practice is the critical analysis of relevant research studies. The therapist need not confine the literature search to occupational therapy publications but can gain relevant information from studies published by other disciplines.[25] The general questions the therapist should be asking are as follows[101,106]:

- What are the study's findings?
- Is the study of sufficient quality?
- How similar were the study subjects to my clients?
- How convincing are the study results (ie, statistically or clinically significant)?
- How can the results help me care for my client?
- If it is a quantitative study, what are the reliability and validity measures?
- If it is a qualitative study, how rigorous is it?

Depending on the answers to these general questions, the therapist can choose to critically analyze the study in more detail or decide the study will not be helpful. There are many forms available to guide the therapist in a specific article review. Law and Philp provide comprehensive relevant forms that can be utilized for qualitative and quantitative research studies.[104] The therapist should also keep in mind that when considering the usefulness and validity of the evidence, most health care professionals subscribe to a "hierarchy of evidence." The highest level of evidence would be that which is least vulnerable to bias, more generalizable, and more likely to generate outcomes that can be attributed to the intervention studied.[92] This level could include meta-analytic studies, systematic reviews, or randomized controlled clinical studies using statistical analysis.[92] Evidence at the lower end of the hierarchy would include opinions of respected authorities, clinical evidence, single case studies, descriptive studies, reports of expert committees, and qualitative design studies.[92]

Evidence-based practice will improve the level of confidence in clinical decision making. It is important, however, that the therapist recognize that one solution is not appropriate for all situations and that the context into which the evidence is being implemented and the method of facilitating the change be considered.[102,107] Equally important, the therapist must always consider the client's individual needs.[100]

The evaluation and treatment recommendations presented in this book are based on extensive literature reviews, communication with experts in the field, and the author's 30 years of clinical research and teaching experience. Clinical research studies of all levels within the hierarchy of evidence were found and included when appropriate. All sources are referenced, and the reader is encouraged to seek out these references for more detailed information. In addition, the reader is encouraged to continue to develop research skills in order to analyze and interpret presented evidence.

Clinical Reasoning

Effective client care is accomplished through an ongoing, dynamic process during which the occupational therapist obtains and analyzes information about the client. This information pertains both to client capabilities as well as his or her particular situation in life. The knowledge of the client's life situation or context is crucial to this process, and one of the primary goals is to understand the meaning of the client's disability from his or her perspective.[108]

The occupational therapist analyzes the information gathered relating to the client's capabilities and life situation to define the client's problem areas, generate treatment goals, and outline the focus of treatment.[108] This thinking and decision making process that the therapist utilizes to plan, direct, perform, and reflect on client care is termed clinical reasoning.[109] Clinical reasoning is the thinking process therapists utilize no matter what the area of therapeutic practice and involves the use of many reasoning strategies throughout the various phases of client management and recovery.[108]

Clinical reasoning guides the decisions made relating to what theoretical frames of reference and techniques will be utilized during the treatment process. Table 1-3 illustrates a few examples of clinical reasoning questions the therapist might ask when deciding what theoretical frame of reference to use. A rapid, ongoing blending of different modes of reasoning occurs during which practical knowledge is integrated with theoretical knowledge.[49,108] These different modes of reasoning utilized by the therapist are subsequently reviewed.

Unsworth describes three main modes or categories of clinical reasoning: procedural, conditional and interactive.[49] During procedural reasoning, sometimes called diagnostic reasoning, strategies are utilized to determine what the client's problems might be and the appropriate

---

Table 1-3

Clinical Reasoning: Examples of Theory-Related Questions

Learning Theory	At what level if any can the client learn?
Occupational Behavior	What roles or occupations are affected by the visual, perceptual, or cognitive impairment?
Dynamic Interactional Approach	What changes to the activity, environment, or context can be made to change the client's processing strategies and self-awareness?
Neurodevelopmental Theory	What aspects of the client's impaired body scheme and visual perceptual processing are due to poor postural control and stability and/or abnormal movement patterns?
Constraint-Induced Therapy	Is any part of the client's visual body neglect the result of learned nonuse of the hemiplegic extremity?

---

interventions to address these problems. Procedural reasoning includes the consideration of environmental context in which a particular activity is occurring as well as what evidence supports the evaluation and interventions the therapist has selected.[49]

Conditional reasoning goes beyond the basic knowledge of the client's capabilities by examining and trying to understand how these capabilities affect his or her work, social situation, leisure, and overall self-concept.[49] The therapist considers the client's situation within a temporal context (ie, past, present, and future). He or she uses this form of reasoning to "...understand what is meaningful to clients in their world by imagining what their life was like before the illness or disability, what it is like now, and what it could be like in the future."[49]

The third mode of clinical reasoning described by Unsworth is interactive reasoning. Interactive reasoning occurs during the therapeutic process.[49] This mode of reasoning attempts to understand the client's interests, needs, values, and problems in order to understand the disability from the client's perspective. It is concerned with the best approach to communicate with the client as well as to understand the client as a person.[49] The therapist collaborating with the client is the means to interactive reasoning. Unlike procedural reasoning, which is factually based, interactive reasoning is intuitive.

Schell describes four modes or aspects of clinical reasoning: scientific, narrative, pragmatic, and ethical.[109] Similar to procedural reasoning described by Unsworth, scientific reasoning is concerned with problem definition, understanding the condition that is affecting the individual, and deciding which interventions are in the client's best interest. Narrative reasoning is concerned with understanding the meaning of the client's experience as a result of his or her disability and how it disrupts his or her life situation.[109] This parallels what Unsworth has described as conditional reasoning.

Pragmatic reasoning deals with "...the environmental influences that affect thinking and the therapist's personal context."[49] It is reasoning that is based on practice contexts such as organizational culture, resources, community services that are available, length of stay, and reimbursement issues.[109]

Ethical reasoning answers the question not of what can be done but of what should be done.[109] This is often challenging for the therapist due to consideration of all the pragmatic issues previously described. Scientific, narrative, and pragmatic reasoning all lead to an ethical reasoning process.[109]

To summarize, clinical reasoning involves the ongoing interaction of the modes of reasoning previously described. Therapists will monitor client evaluation and treatment (procedural) along with understanding the client's response and eliciting client cooperation (interactive). This monitoring and ongoing adjustment of treatment is done while also having to consider real world constraints such as length of stay or reimbursement for services (pragmatic). The blending and interaction of all these modes of clinical reasoning is the basis for effective decision making in clinical practice. When problems arise during the therapy process, it facilitates the therapist's ability to reason in order to reach a solution.[49] Not only are strong clinical reasoning skills a prerequisite for effective practice, but the therapist must also be able to communicate this reasoning in order to support practice.[49,110]

References

1. Christiansen C. Occupational therapy: intervention for life performance. In: Christiansen C, Baum C, eds. *Occupational Therapy: Overcoming Human Performance Deficits*. Thorofare, NJ: SLACK Incorporated; 1991.
2. Mosey AC. The paper focus of scientific inquiry in occupational therapy: frames of reference. *Occup Ther J Res*. 1995;9(4):195-201.
3. Abreu B, Duval M, Gerber D, Wood W. Occupational performance and the functional approach. *AOTA Self Study Series: Cognitive Rehabilitation*. Bethesda, Md: The American Occupational Therapy Association, Inc; 1994.
4. Mcdonald B, Flashman LA, Saykin AJ. Executive dysfunction following traumatic brain injury: neural substrates and treatment strategies. *Neurorehabilitation*. 2000;17(4):333-344.
5. Taub E, Uswatte G, Elbert T. New treatments in neurorehabilitation founded on basic research. *Nat Rev Neurosci*. 2002;3(3):228-236.
6. Fisher AG. Uniting practice and theory in an occupational framework. *Am J Occup Ther*. 1998;52(7):509-521.
7. Holm M, Rogers JC, James AB. Interventions for daily living. In: Crepeau E, Cohn ES, Schell BAB, eds. *Willard and Spackman's Occupational Therapy*. Philadelphia, Pa: Lippincott, Williams and Wilkins; 2003.
8. Oddy M, McMillan TM. Future directions: brain injury services in 2010. In: Wood RL, McMillan TM, eds. *Neurobehavioral Disability and Social Handicap Following Traumatic Brain Injury*. Philadelphia, Pa: Psychology Press; 2001.
9. Abreu B, Toglia J. Cognitive rehabilitation: a model for occupational therapy. *Am J Occup Ther*. 1987;41(7):439-448.
10. Butler RW, Namerow NS. Cognitive retraining in brain-injury rehabilitation: a critical review. *J Neuro Rehab*. 1988;2:97-101.
11. Trombly C. Anticipating the future: assessment of occupational function. *Am J Occup Ther*. 1993;47(3):253-257.
12. Ben-Yishay Y, Diller L. Cognitive deficits. In: Griffith E, Bond M, Miller J, eds. *Rehabilitation of the Head Injured Adult*. Philadelphia, Pa: FA Davis; 1983.
13. Farrell W, Schultz-Krohn WA. A computer program for enhancing visuomotor skills. *Am J Occup Ther*. 1990;44(6):557-559.
14. Weinstock-Zlotnick G, Hinojosa J. Bottom-up or top-down evaluation: is one better than the other? *Am J Occup Ther*. 2004;58(5):594-599.
15. World Health Organization. International Classification of Functioning, Disability and Health (ICF). 2001. Available at: http://www3.who.int/icf/icftemplate.cfm.
16. Baum C, Christiansen C. Person-environment-occupation-performance: an occupation-based framework for practice. In: Christiansen C, Baum C, eds. *Occupational Therapy: Performance, Participation, and Well-Being*. Thorofare, NJ: SLACK Incorporated; 2005.
17. Weiller C. Imaging recovery from stroke. *Exp Brain Res*. 1998;123(1-2):17.
18. Arnadottir G. *The Brain and Behavior: Assessing Cortical Dysfunction Through Activities of Daily Living*. St. Louis, Mo: CV Mosby; 1990.
19. Law M, Baum C, Dunn W. Occupational performance assessment. In: Christiansen C, Baum C, eds. *Occupational Therapy: Performance, Participation, and Well-Being*. 3rd ed. Thorofare, NJ: SLACK Incorporated; 2005.
20. Moyers P. The guide to occupational therapy practice. *Am J Occup Ther*. 1999;53(3):247-322.

21. Wolf SL, Lecraw DE, Barton LA, Jann BB. Forced use of hemiplegic upper extremities to reverse the effect of learned nonuse among chronic stroke and head-injured patients. *Exper Neurol.* 1989;104:125-132.
22. Neistadt ME. Assessing learning capabilities during cognitive and perceptual evaluations for adults with traumatic brain injury. *Occup Ther Health Care.* 1995;9(1):3-16.
23. Fordyce DJ. Neuropsychologic assessment and cognitive rehabilitation: issues of psychologic validity. In: Finlayson MAJ, Garner SH, eds. *Brain Injury Rehabilitation: Clinical Considerations.* Baltimore, Md: Williams and Wilkins; 1994.
24. Toglia JP. A dynamic interactional approach to cognitive rehabilitation. In: Katz N, ed. *Cognitive Rehabilitation: Models for Intervention in Occupational Therapy.* Boston, Mass: Andover Med Pub; 1992.
25. Youngstrom MJ, Brown C. Categories and principles of interventions. In: Christiansen C, Baum C, eds. *Occupational Therapy: Performance, Participation, and Well-Being.* Thorofare, NJ: SLACK Incorporated; 2005.
26. Constantinidou F, Thomas RD, Best PJ. Principles of cognitive rehabilitation: an integrative approach. In: Ashley MJ, ed. *Traumatic Brain Injury: Rehabilitative Treatment and Case Management.* 2nd ed. Boca Raton, Fla: CRC Press; 2004.
27. Neistadt ME. A critical analysis of occupational therapy approaches for perceptual deficits in adults with brain injury. *Am J Occup Ther.* 1990;44(4):299-303.
28. Dougherty PM, Radomski MV. *A Dynamic Assessment Approach for Adults with Brain Injury: The Cognitive Rehabilitation Workbook.* Gaithersburg, Md: Aspen Publishers; 1993.
29. Neistadt ME. A meal preparation treatment protocol for adults with brain injury. *Am J Occup Ther.* 1994;48(5):431-438.
30. Kramer P, Hinojosa J. Activity synthesis. In: Hinojosa J, Blount ML, eds. *The Texture of Life: Purposeful Activities in Occupational Therapy.* Bethesda, Md: The American Occupational Therapy Association, Inc; 2000.
31. Radomski MV, Dougherty PM, Fine SB, Baum C. Case studies in cognitive rehabilitation. In: Royee CB, ed. *AOTA Self Study Series: Cognitive Rehabilitation.* Bethesda, Md: The American Occupational Therapy Association, Inc; 1994.
32. Dixon RA, Backman L. Concepts of compensation: integrated, differentiated and janus faced. In: Dixon RA, Backman L, eds. *Compensating for Psychological Deficits and Declines.* Mahwah, NJ: Lawrence Erlbaum Assoc; 1995.
33. White B. Neurodevelopmental theory. In: Crepeau E, Cohn ES, Schell BAB, eds. *Willard and Spackman's Occupational Therapy.* Philadelphia, Pa: Lippincott, Williams and Wilkins; 2003.
34. Allen CK. Treatment plans in cognitive rehabilitation. *Occup Ther Pract.* 1989;1(1):1-8.
35. Salthouse TA. Refining the concept of psychological compensation. In: Dixon RA, Backman L, eds. *Compensating For Psychological Deficits and Decline.* Mahwah, NJ: Lawrence Erlbaum Assoc; 1995.
36. Wood RL. A neurobehavioral approach to brain injury rehabilitation. In: von Steinbuchel N, von Cramon DY, Poppel E, eds. *Neuropsychological Rehabilitation.* Berlin: Springer-Verlag; 1992.
37. Mateer CA. The rehabilitation of executive disorders. In: Stuss DT, Robertson IH, eds. *Cognitive Neurorehabilitation.* New York, NY: Cambridge University Press; 1999.
38. Bruce MAG. Cognitive rehabilitation: intelligence, insight, and knowledge. In: Royeen CB, ed. *AOTA Self Study Series: Cognitive Rehabilitation.* Bethesda, Md: The American Occupational Therapy Association, Inc; 1994.
39. Carstenson LL, et al. Selection and compensation in adulthood. In: Dixon RA, Backman L, eds. *Compensating for Psychological Deficits and Decline.* Mahwah, NJ: Lawrence Erlbaum Assoc; 1995.
40. DeGangi GA, Royeen CB. Current practice among neurodevelopmental treatment association members. *Am J Occup Ther.* 1994;48(9):803-809.
41. Bobath B. *Adult Hemiplegia: Evaluation and Treatment.* London: William Hennemann Medical Books Ltd; 1978.
42. Howle JM. *Neurodevelopmental Treatment Approach: Theoretical Foundations and Principles of Clinical Practice.* Laguna Beach, Calif: North American Neuro-Developmental Treatment Association; 2002.
43. Davies PM. *Steps to Follow—A Guide to the Treatment of Adult Hemiplegia.* Berlin: Springer Verlag; 1985.
44. Meltzer M. Poor memory: a case report. *J Clin Psychol.* 1983;39(1):3-10.
45. Jarus T. Motor learning and occupational therapy: the organization of practice. *Am J Occup Ther.* 1994;48(9):810-816.
46. Bryan V. Management of residual physical deficits. In: Ashley MJ, Krych DK, eds. *Traumatic Brain Injury Rehabilitation.* Boca Raton, Fla: CRC Press; 2004.
47. Blanton S, Wolf SL. An application of upper-extremity constraint-induced movement therapy in a patient with subacute stroke. *Phys Ther.* 1999;79:847-853.
48. Miltner WH, Bauder H, Sommer M, Dettmers C, Taub E. Effects of constraint-induced movement therapy on patients with chronic motor deficits after stroke: a replication. *Stroke.* 1999;30(3):586-592.

49. Unsworth C. How therapists think: exploring therapists' reasoning when working with patients who have cognitive and perceptual problems following stroke. In: Gillen G, Burkhardt A, eds. *Stroke Rehabilitation: A Function-Based Approach.* St. Louis, Mo: Mosby; 2004.

50. Platz T, Winter T, Muller N, et al. Arm ability training for stroke and traumatic brain injury patients with mild arm paresis: a single-blind, randomized, controlled trial. *Arch Phys Med Rehabil.* 2001;82:961-968.

51. Tankle RS. Application of neuropsychological test results to interdisciplinary cognitive rehabilitation with head-injured adults. *J Head Trauma Rehabil.* 1988;3(1):24-32.

52. Feys H, De Weerdt W, Verbeke G, et al. Early and repetitive stimulation of the arm can substantially improve the long-term outcome after stroke: a 5-year follow-up study of a randomized trial. *Stroke.* 2004;35(4):924-929.

53. Liepert J, Miltner WH, Bauder H, et al. Motor cortex plasticity during constraint-induced movement therapy in stroke patients. *Neurosci Lett.* 1998;250(1):5-8.

54. Nelles G, Jentzen W, Jueptner M, et al. Arm training induced brain plasticity in stroke studied with serial positron emission tomography. *Neuroimage.* 2001;13(6[Pt 1]):1146-1154.

55. Taub E, Crago JE, Uswatte G. Constraint-induced movement therapy: a new approach to treatment in physical rehabilitation. *Rehab Psychol.* 1998;43:152-170.

56. Stuss DT, Winocur G, Robertson IH, eds. *Cognitive Neurorehabilitation.* Cambridge, Mass: Cambridge University Press; 1999.

57. van der Lee JH, Wagenaar RC, Lankhorst GJ, et al. Forced use of the upper extremity in chronic stroke patients: results from a single-blind randomized clinical trial. *Stroke.* 1999;30(11):2369-2375.

58. Burns MS. A whole-brain approach to adult and pediatric rehabilitation. *Adv Occup Ther Practition.* 2005;21(2):48.

59. Eriksson PS, Perfilieva E, Bjork-Eriksson T, et al. Neurogenesis in the adult human hippocampus. *Nat Med.* 1998;4:1313-1317.

60. Grady C, Kapur S. The use of neuroimaging in neurorehabilitative research. In: Stuss D, Winocur G, Robertson IH, eds. *Cognitive Neurorehabilitation.* New York, NY: Cambridge University Press; 1999.

61. Kolb B, Gibbs R. Frontal lobe plasticity and behavior. In: Stuss D, Knight R. *Principles of Frontal Lobe Function.* New York, NY: Oxford University Press; 2002.

62. Robertson IH, Murre JM. Rehabilitation on brain damage: brain plasticity and principles of guided recovery. *Psychological Bulletin.* 1999;125:544-575.

63. Mateer C. Attention. In: Raskin SA, Mateer CA, eds. *Neuropsychological Management of Mild Traumatic Brain Injury.* New York, NY: Oxford University Press; 2000.

64. Corbetta M. Functional anatomy of visual attention in the human brain: studies with positron emission tomography. In: Parasuraman R, ed. *The Attentive Brain.* MIT Press; 1998.

65. Elliot R. Executive functions and their disorders. *Brit Med Bulletin.* 2003;65:49-59.

66. Dunn W, McClain LH, Brown C, et al. The ecology of human performance. In: Crepeau E, Cohn ES, Schell BAB, eds. *Willard and Spackman's Occupational Therapy.* Philadelphia, Pa: Lippincott Williams and Wilkins; 2003.

67. Kielhofner, Forsyth K, Barrett L. The model of human occupation. In: Crepeau E, Cohn ES, Schell BAB, eds. *Willard and Spackman's Occupational Therapy.* Philadelphia, Pa: Lippincott Williams and Wilkins; 2003.

68. Schultz S, Schkade J. Occupational adaptation. In: Crepeau E, Cohn ES, Schell BAB, eds. *Willard and Spackman's Occupational Therapy.* Philadelphia, Pa: Lippincott Williams and Wilkins; 2003.

69. Stewart D, Letts L, Law M, et al. The person-environment-occupation model. In: Crepeau E, Cohn ES, Schell BAB, eds. *Willard and Spackman's Occupational Therapy.* Philadelphia, Pa: Lippincott, Williams and Wilkins; 2003.

70. Crepeau E. Analyzing occupation and activity: a way of thinking about occupational performance. In: Crepeau E, Cohn ES, Schell BAB, eds. *Willard and Spackman's Occupational Therapy.* Philadelphia, Pa: Lippincott Williams and Wilkins; 2003.

71. Baum C, Christiansen C. Outcomes: the results of interventions in occupational therapy practice. In: Christiansen C, Baum C, eds. *Occupational Therapy: Performance, Participation, and Well-Being.* Thorofare, NJ: SLACK Incorporated; 2005.

72. Rubio KB, van Deusen J. Relation of perceptual and body image dysfunction to activities of daily living of persons after stroke. *Am J Occup Ther.* 1995;49(6):551-559.

73. Titus MLD, Gall NG, Yerxa EJ, Roberston TA, Mack W. Correlation of perceptual performance and activities of daily living in stroke patients. *Am J Occup Ther.* 1991;45(5):410-417.

74. Toglia J. Generalization of treatment: a multicontext approach to cognitive perceptual impairment in adults with brain injury. *Am J Occup Ther.* 1991;45:505-516.

75. Toglia JP. A Dynamic interactional approach to cognitive rehabilitation. In: Katz N, ed. *Cognition and Occupation Across The Life Span.* 2nd ed. Bethesda, Md: The American Occupational Therapy Association, Inc; 2005.

76. Brown AL. Motivation to learn and understand: on taking charge of one's own learning. _Cognition and Instruction._ 1988;5:311-321.

77. Toglia J. Multicontext treatment approach. In: Crepeau E, Cohn ES, Schell BAB, eds. _Willard and Spackman's Occupational Therapy._ Philadelphia, Pa: Lippincott, Williams and Wilkins; 2003.

78. Stark SL, Sanford JA. Environmental enablers and their impact on occupational performance. In: Christiansen C, Baum C, eds. _Occupational Therapy: Performance, Participation, and Well-Being._ Thorofare, NJ: SLACK Incorporated; 2005.

79. Spencer JC. Evaluation of performance contexts. In: Crepeau E, Cohn ES, Schell BAB, eds. _Willard and Spackman's Occupational Therapy._ Philadelphia, Pa: Lippincott, Williams and Wilkins; 2003.

80. Occupational therapy practice framework: domain and process. _Am J Occup Ther._ 2002;56(6):609-629.

81. Woodruff-Pak DS, Hanson C. Plasticity and compensation in brain memory systems in aging. In: Dixon RA, Backman L, eds. _Compensating For Psychological Deficits and Declines._ Mahwah, NJ: Lawrence Erlbaum Assoc; 1995.

82. Charness N, Bosman EA. Compensation through environmental modification. In: Dixon RA, Backman L, eds. _Compensating For Psychological Deficits and Decline._ Mahwah, NJ: Lawrence Erlbaum Assoc; 1995.

83. McColl MA. Occupational therapy interventions in a rehabilitation context. In: Christiansen C, Baum C, eds. _Occupational Therapy: Performance, Participation, and Well-Being._ Thorofare, NJ: SLACK Incorporated; 2005.

84. Pollack N, McColl MA. Assessment in client-centered occupational therapy. In: Law M, ed. _Client-centered Occupational Therapy._ SLACK Incorporated; 1998.

85. Hammell KW. Client-centered occupational therapy: collaborative planning, accountable intervention. In: Law M, ed. _Client-centered Occupational Therapy._ Thorofare, NJ: SLACK Incorporated; 1998.

86. Law M. _Client-centered Occupational Therapy._ Thorofare, NJ: SLACK Incorporated; 1998.

87. Baum C. Client-centered practice in a changing health care system. In: Law M, ed. _Client-centered Occupational Therapy._ Thorofare, NJ: SLACK Incorporated; 1998.

88. Barth R. Stroke survivors share insight into rehabilitation. _OT Practice._ 2004:23-24.

89. Simmons DC, Crepeau EB, White BP. The predictive power of narrative data in occupational therapy evaluation. _Am J Occup Ther._ 2000;54(5):471-476.

90. Ersser S, Atkins S. Clinical reasoning and patient-centered care. In: Higgs J, Jones M, eds. _Clinical Reasoning in the Health Professions._ Oxford: Butterworth Heinemann; 2000.

91. Proulx GB. Family education and family partnership in cognitive rehabilitation. In: Stuss DT, Robertson IH, eds. _Cognitive Neurorehabilitation._ New York, NY: Cambridge University Press; 1999.

92. Holm MB. Our mandate for the new millennium: evidence-based practice; the 2000 Eleanor Clarke Slagle lecture. _Am J Occup Ther._ 2000;54:575-585.

93. Culler K. Home management. In: Crepeau E, Cohn ES, Schell BAB, eds. _Willard and Spackman's Occupational Therapy._ Philadelphia, Pa: Lippincott, Williams and Wilkins; 2003.

94. Robertson IH. The rehabilitation of attention. In: Stuss DT, Robertson IH, eds. _Cognitive Neurorehabilitation._ New York, NY: Cambridge University Press; 1999.

95. Fuhrer MJ, Keith RA. Facilitating patient learning during medical rehabilitation: a research agenda. _Am J Phys Med Rehabil._ 1998;77:557-561.

96. Kong KH, Chua KS, Tow AP. Clinical characteristics and functional outcome of stroke patients 75 years old and older. _Arch Phys Med Rehabil._ 1998;79(12):1535-1538.

97. Giuffrida Cl, Neistadt M. Overview of learning theory. In: Crepeau E, Cohn ES, Schell BAB, eds. _Willard and Spackman's Occupational Therapy._ Philadelphia, Pa: Lippincott Williams and Wilkins; 2003.

98. Berkeland R, Flinn N. Therapy as learning. In: Christiansen C, Baum C, eds. _Occupational Therapy: Performance, Participation, and Well-Being._ Thorofare, NJ: SLACK Incorporated; 2005.

99. Guiles G, Clark-Wilson J. _Rehabilitation of the Severely Brain-Injured Adult._ 2nd ed. United Kingdom: Gray Publishing; 1991.

100. Bondoc S, Burkhardt A. Evidence-based practice and outcomes management in occupational therapy. _OT Practice._ 2004;9:CE1-CE8.

101. Dunn W. Measurement issues and practices. In: Law M, Baum CM, Dunn W, eds. _Measuring Occupational Performance: Supporting Best Practice in Occupational Therapy._ 2nd ed. Thorofare, NJ: SLACK Incorporated; 2005:21-32.

102. DeLise D, Leasure R. Benchmarking: measuring the outcomes of evidence-based practice. _Outcomes Manage Nurs Pract._ 2001;5(2):70-74.

103. Luquire R, Houston S. Linking outcomes management and practice improvement. The link between outcomes management and JCAHO functions. _Outcomes Manag Nurs Pract._ 1998;2(4):143-146.

104. Law M, Philp I. Evaluating the evidence. In: Law M, ed. _Evidence-Based Rehabilitation: A Guide to Practice._ Thorofare, NJ: SLACK Incorporated; 2002:97-109

105. Law M, Baum C, Dunn W. *Measuring Occupational Performance: Supporting Best Practice in Occupational Therapy*. 2nd ed. Thorofare, NJ: SLACK Incorporated; 2005.

106. Kellegrew DH. The evolution of evidence-based practice. *OT Practice*. 2005;10(12):11-16.

107. Kitson A, Harvey G, McCormack B. Enabling the implementation of evidence-based practice: a conceptual framework. *Qual Health Care*. 1998;7(3):149-158.

108. Chappero C, Ranka J. Clinical reasoning in occupational therapy. In: Higgs J, Jones M, eds. *Clinical Reasoning in the Health Professions*. Oxford: Butterworth Heinemann; 2000.

109. Schell BAB. Clinical reasoning: the basis of practice. In: Crepeau E, Cohn ES, Schell BAB, eds. *Willard and Spackman's Occupational Therapy*. Philadelphia, Pa: Lippincott Williams and Wilkins; 2003.

110. Rosenfeld M. From OT theory to practice: a bridge too far? *OT Practice*. 2004;9(13):14-19.

Resources

Backman L, Dixon RA. Psychological compensation: a theoretical framework. *Psychological Bulletin*. 1992;112:259-283.

Burbaud P, Degreze P, Lafon P, et al. Lateralization of prefrontal activation during internal mental calculation: a functional magnetic resonance imaging study. *J Neurophysiol*. 1995;74(5):2194-2200.

Chi MTH, de Leeuw N, Chiu MH, LaVancher C. Eliciting self-explanations improves understanding. *Cognitive Science*. 1994;18:439-477.

Cicerone KD, Dahlberg C, Kalmar K, et al. Evidence-based cognitive rehabilitation: recommendations for clinical practice. *Arch Phys Med Rehabil*. 2000;81(12):1596-1611.

Davis ES, Radomski MV. Domain-specific training to reinstate habit sequences. *Occup Ther Pract*. 1989;1(1):79-88.

Fernandez-Ballesteros R, Zamarrón MD, Tárraga L, et al. Cognitive plasticity in healthy, mild cognitive impairment (MCI) subjects and Alzheimer's disease patients: a research project in Spain. *Eur Psychol*. 2003;8(3):148-159.

Feys H, De Weerdt W, Verbeke G, et al. Early and repetitive stimulation of the arm can substantially improve the long-term outcome after stroke: a 5-year follow-up study of a randomized trial. *Stroke*. 2004;35(4):924-929.

Fisher B, Yakura J. Movement analysis: a different perspective. *Ortho Phys Ther Clin N Am*. 1993;2(1):1-14.

Furphy KA. Community reentry options for stroke survivors. *OT Practice*. 2005;10:10-14.

Gutman SA. *Quick Reference Neuroscience for Rehabilitation Professionals*. Thorofare, NJ: SLACK Incorporated; 2001.

Katz DI, Mills VM. Traumatic brain injury: natural history and efficacy of cognitive rehabilitation. In: Stuss DT, Robertson IH, eds. *Cognitive Neurorehabilitation*. New York, NY: Cambridge University Press; 1999.

Kellegrew, DH. The evolution of evidence-based practice: strategies and resources for busy practitioners. *OT Practice*. 2005;10:11-15.

Kemick DP. Evidence-based medicine and treatment choices. *The Lancet*. 1997;349:570.

Larin H. Motor learning: theories and strategies for the practitioner. In: Campbell SK, Vander Linden DW, eds. *Physical Therapy For Children*. Philadelphia, Pa: WB Saunders; 2000.

Lyons A, Phipps SC, Berro M. Using occupation in the clinic. *OT Practice*. 2004;9(13):11-16.

Mathiowetz V. Role of physical performance component evaluations in occupational therapy functional assessment. *Am J Occup Ther*. 1993;47(3):225-230.

Melville LL, Baltic TA, Bettcher TW, Nelson DL. Patients' perspectives on the self-identified goals assessment. *Am J Occup Ther*. 2002;56(6):650-659.

Osman DC, Smet IC, Winegarden B, Gandhavadi B. Neurobehavioral cognitive status examination: its use with unilateral stroke patients in a rehabilitation setting. *Arch Phys Med Rehabil*. 1992;73(5):414-418.

Parker RS. *Concussive Brain Trauma: Neurobehavioral Impairment and Maladaptation*. Boca Raton, Fla: CRC Press; 2001.

Rijntjes M, Weiller C. Recovery of motor and language abilities after stroke: the contribution of functional imaging. *Prog Neurobiol*. 2002;66:109-22.

Schell BAB, Crepeau E, Cohn ES. Overview of intervention. In: Crepeau E, Cohn ES, Schell BAB, eds. *Willard and Spackman's Occupational Therapy*. Philadelphia, Pa: Lippincott, Williams and Wilkins; 2003.

Schlund MW, Pace G. Relations between traumatic brain injury and the environment: feedback reduces maladaptive behavior exhibited by three persons with traumatic brain injury. *Brain Injury*. 1999;13:889-897.

Seidel A. Rehabilitative frame of reference. In: Crepeau E, Cohn ES, Schell BAB, eds. *Willard and Spackman's Occupational Therapy*. Philadelphia, Pa: Lippincott Williams and Wilkins; 2003.

Uswatte G, Taub E. Constraint-induced movement therapy: new approaches to outcome measurement in rehabilitation. In: Stuss DT, Winocur G, Robertson IH, eds. _Cognitive Neurorehabilitation._ New York, NY: Cambridge University Press; 1999:215-229.

Wilson BA. Compensating for cognitive deficits following brain injury. _Neuropsychol Rev._ 2000;10(4):233-243.

Winstein CJ, Rose DK, Tan SM, et al. A randomized controlled comparison of upper-extremity rehabilitation strategies in acute stroke: a pilot study of immediate and long-term outcomes. _Arch Phys Med Rehabil._ 2004;85(4):620-628.

Zemke R. Task skills, problem solving, and social interaction. In: Royeen CB, ed. _AOTA Self Study Series: Cognitive Rehabilitation._ Bethesda, Md: The American Occupational Therapy Association, Inc: 1994.

CHAPTER 2

GENERAL EVALUATION ISSUES

Before the evaluation of visual, perceptual, and cognitive processing abilities can be initiated, several general evaluation issues must be taken into consideration. There are many types of assessment techniques available to the therapist, ranging from informal interviews to rigorous standardized testing. In addition, assessment can be dynamic or static, qualitative or quantitative, and constructed around a particular theoretical base. Also, evaluations can be designed from a top-down or bottom-up perspective. The decision the therapist makes pertaining to evaluation choices ultimately determines the direction of treatment.[1] Different testing methods can be used in isolation or in combination depending on the ultimate purpose.[2] The client's stage of recovery will also affect assessment procedures and choice of evaluation. The therapist must also consider outside issues such as reimbursement and the treatment facility's mission.[3] Finally, environmental conditions and context should be considered in evaluation choice as well as interpretation of performance difficulties.[3-5]

Clinical decision making pertaining to treatment is based on evaluation results. It is, therefore, crucial for the therapist to understand why he or she has chosen a certain evaluation approach or instrument. The therapist must critique an instrument relative to issues such as reliability, validity, focus, and usability before choosing it as appropriate for his or her client.[6] Information pertaining to these key issues related to the process of evaluation are subsequently described.

Top-Down and Bottom-Up Assessments

Traditionally, visual, perceptual, and cognitive evaluations have included both top-down and bottom-up assessment procedures. Bottom-up assessments are specific tests designed to measure component skills such as attention or constructional praxis. Research has shown, for example, that constructional praxis abilities correlated with dressing; therefore, the client with constructional apraxia would likely have an associated problem with dressing.[7] A top-down assessment, on the other hand, would examine the client's performance in a particular occupational performance task as a means to understand possible underlying causes of poor performance.

The decision to administer top-down or bottom-up assessments or a combination of the two is dependent on all areas of the therapist's clinical reasoning process, as described in Chapter 1, as well as the specific purpose of the evaluation. For example, in some settings, it may be appropriate to first assess the client's occupational performance status; identify where the breakdown in performance occurs and the potential visual, perceptual, and cognitive performance components affecting occupational performance; and then proceed with selected bottom-up tests of these performance components.[8] On the other hand, in certain cases, an initial bottom-up approach to testing may be more appropriate. For example, a client may be referred to occupational therapy because he is having difficulty in his job as an accountant. During the initial interview, it becomes apparent to the therapist that the problems he is describing relate primarily to attentional and calculation difficulties. The therapist can then evaluate these specific performance components to determine the presence and level of severity of these problems. In this instance, it is more appropriate and efficient to zero in on the specific performance components that are affecting job performance. If the therapist can ascertain at what level this client's calculation abilities are breaking down, for example, the appropriate level and type of treatment can be established.

Occupation-Based Evaluations

Some therapists now believe that interventions that are directed at improving visual, perceptual, and cognitive function so that acquired brain injury (ABI) clients can function better in their daily life performance require instruments that measure these skills in real life situations.[5,9-11] In answer to this philosophy, in recent years, there has been some development of occupation-based evaluations of visual, perceptual, and cognitive dysfunction. These evaluations purport to measure underlying deficits through specific occupational performance tasks. The difference between these and previous top-down evaluation techniques is that these are formal, structured evaluations that contain established administration and scoring procedures as well as validity and reliability measures. These evaluations attempt to address both the need for occupation-based evaluations as well as the need for reliable and valid measurement instruments, which can be utilized by the occupational therapist. These evaluations are described in the appropriate chapters throughout the book.

Quantitative (Static) Assessment

Static evaluations provide quantitative measurements of developed abilities.[12] These evaluations do not allow any active intervention on the part of the therapist during the evaluation process in order to improve performance.[8,13,14] Static assessments are concerned with the products of learning rather than the learning process itself.[15] Quantitative evaluations quantify the measured parameters through numbers.[16] Specific quantitative measures include accuracy measures (number of errors, percentage correct, number correct), time (speed of performance, rate of responding), and cuing (amount of cuing, type of cuing used, number of self corrects, etc).[17]

A standardized quantitative evaluation can compare the client's performance with established norms. Results will tell the therapist how severe the impairment is as well as provide a baseline with which to measure progress over time.[2,8] As Toglia states, "…static evaluations are important for diagnosis, monitoring progress, discharge planning, and client or caregiver education regarding expected behaviors."[2] Standardized static evaluations can also be utilized for clinical research to provide evidence-based practice.

Qualitative Assessment

Unlike quantitative evaluation, qualitative assessment provides non-numerical data.[18] This non-numerical data can highlight a problematic performance component and provide in-depth detailed information about that performance.[18,19] During qualitative evaluation, important characteristics of the client's activity performance are described.[16] The therapist observes the process of how a client goes about performing a particular task or activity.[2] This type evaluation will yield information about "why" a client has failed to perform.[20] Qualitative assessment, through subjective rating scales, can provide documentation of the experience of the ABI client.[21] These measures can include internal factors such as depression, level of confidence or distraction, and external factors such as noise or interruptions. Distinctive error patterns such as errors grouped at the beginning, throughout, or the end of therapy, can also be measured.[19] Sohlberg and Mateer provide the following information pertaining to common error patterns[22]:

- *Increased errors over time*—Inadequate sustained attention, fatigue factor
- *Increased errors at the beginning of a task*—Difficulty picking up a new task or poor mental flexibility
- *Many errors throughout the task*—Inability to understand the directions or simply cannot do the task.

There are three main methods of qualitative evaluation: clinical observation, interviews, and visual data (ie, medical records such as evaluations and discharge summaries). Information pertaining to clinical observation and interviewing is contained in the subsequent sections.

Qualitative analysis of the client's performance goes beyond specific performance data and should be collected along with quantitative information.[22] In addition there may be situations where standardized quantitative assessments are unavailable or inappropriate.[23]

No matter whether a quantitative or qualitative evaluation or a combination of the two is used, the therapist should choose assessments that will likely generate the greatest yield across a variety of individuals.[24]

Clinical Observation

Clinical observations can be used for initial assessment, assessment of progress, motivation, or response to therapy.[18] This direct observation of occupational performance should be guided by the client's former occupations and expected roles and routines.[8] During clinical observation, the therapist should note motor, visual, perceptual, and cognitive factors that appear to be impeding the client's performance. This qualitative information can guide the therapist towards any quantitative evaluation of component skills that should be more formally assessed. For example, qualitative observation of why the client is unable to complete bed to wheelchair transfers brings out the fact that he appears to over-reach, under-reach, or hesitate when reaching for the armrest of the wheelchair. The therapist must decipher the underlying reason for this behavior. Assuming the therapist has ruled out a primary motor deficit, he or she can ask, is the problem due to decreased visual acuity? A motor planning problem? Decreased depth perception? The therapist hypothesizes potential underlying causes of what he or she has observed clinically and subsequently can move from this qualitative assessment to a more formal quantitative assessment of, in this case, the client's visual processing, visual discrimination, and motor planning skills.

In conjunction with the qualitative clinical observation and analysis of the client's internal factors that may be impeding performance, the therapist observes for external factors such as the environment or context. Using the same example, does altering the set-up of the transfer by placing the wheelchair closer to the client alter performance?

In addition to individual, informal clinical observation, there are now more formal standardized directed observation assessments available for clinical use. Examples of these are the Functional Independence Measure (FIM), Rapideau Kitchen Evaluation (RKE-R), A-One, Assessment of Motor and Process Skills (AMPS), and the Cognitive Performance Test (CPT).[8] Several of these evaluations are described in subsequent chapters.

Interviewing

Interviewing not only helps the therapist understand the client but also helps build rapport and establish a client-centered intervention. During an initial client interview, an informal assessment through observation of the client's behavior can begin.[25] Therapists can begin to understand how this client came to them, what his or her typical day was like, what was important to the client, where the client hopes to go after he or she leaves, and the direction he or she sees life going after the intervention.[26]

There are many elements to a successful interview. An interview requires preparation (ie, chart review, preparing the client, getting his or her permission, and deciding where the interview will take place).[18,26] The successful interview also requires good questioning techniques. Questions can range from open-ended questions with probes (questions that ask for clarification, similarities [ie, what other situations make that happen], dissimilarities [ie, how it is different from other times], and description [ie, examples of when it happens]), to a more concrete structured approach.[18,26] Recent research has indicated that specific, behaviorally anchored questions appear to be most effective for client interviewing.[27] The therapist should verbally and nonverbally attend and listen to the client throughout the interview.[26] Finally, the therapist should summarize what information was gathered and discuss with the client plans for setting goals together.[26]

Many ABI clients, especially those with cognitive deficits, may feel threatened or intimidated by an extensive, probing face-to-face interview. In these instances, a shorter interview process can be used in conjunction with self-report questionnaires. Questionnaires have the advantage of providing information on attributes or deficits not immediately apparent from an interview.[27] A questionnaire can be completed prior to the client interview; in addition to the client completing it, a family member or caregiver can complete one as well. This process is especially helpful in discerning the client's self-awareness of occupational performance by comparison of results between his or her answers with those of the family member or caregiver. This is especially important with ABI clients with cognitive deficits.[8]

Dynamic Assessment

Unlike static assessment, which aims to quantify developed abilities, dynamic assessment examines an individual's latent capacity and aims to quantify his or her learning potential.[12] It is an interactional approach to evaluating the client's learning potential and seeks to access the weakened skills which lie beneath the surface but have potential to function.[2,12,15] The inherent assumption of dynamic assessment is that through cognitive plasticity, cognitive abilities are modifiable.[28] The approach assumes that changes and learning takes place with task experience.[2] One of its major goals is to evaluate thinking processes that are themselves constantly changing and to ascertain to what degree these processes can change or be modified.[13] Dynamic assessment examines the learning process as well as its products.[12] It tries to ascertain the existence, appropriateness, and flexible use of strategies.[15]

Dynamic assessment attempts to modify performance through the assistance of the examiner.[29] As Toglia states, "…learning and the ability to transfer information flexibly across task boundaries are seen as integral components of cognition. Therefore, learning potential and learning transfer are directly addressed in assessment."[2] Dynamic assessment includes deliberate and planned teaching or intervention and the evaluation of how that intervention affects the client's performance.[12,13] Rather than just observing client performance, it evaluates the conditions that facilitate the client's learning.[8] Dynamic assessment asks the question "what is the client's ability to master, apply, and reapply knowledge he or she has been taught?"[12] It evaluates the client's thinking, perception, learning, and problem solving by an active teaching process aimed at modifying functioning.[13]

Dynamic assessment can range from providing simple feedback to taking the form of targeted intervention.[12,30] It can use both guided assistance and task alterations to determine the amount or degree of cognitive modifiability.[2] Assessment procedures can differ in the standardization of procedures, nature of the tasks used, and/or the type of assistance given.[2] As Toglia states, "…it provides an in-depth look at self-perceptions of abilities and strategies as well as changes in self-perceptions and strategy use that may occur with mediation or alterations in activity parameters."[2]

In recent years, there has been a growing interest in the use of dynamic assessment with adults who have sustained brain damage. Some feel it can provide clinically helpful diagnostic information as individual differences in performance can be analyzed in response to different interventions.[30] Others advocate the dynamic assessment process over static assessment because they feel it mirrors the learning process.[31] Most therapists, however, believe that dynamic assessment can function to supplement static evaluation rather than replace it.[8,14,29]

Toglia believes dynamic assessment is relevant to occupational therapy practice, as it assumes that learning and change can take place during activity experiences.[2] Because the aim of dynamic assessment is to understand what the client is capable of doing with help, it can help to predict the client's response to treatment.[8] Cognition is viewed in global terms, and in order to understand the client's true cognitive status, the therapist must analyze the interaction among the task parameters, the context, and the person.[2,8] The therapist goes beyond a basic qualitative analysis by using methods that attempt to change the client's performance.[2] Treatment is based on the individual client's response, and there is no predetermined or prescribed sequence of treatment activities.[2] Common underlying behaviors are identified that cause difficulty on a number of tasks.[2]

Toglia has begun to operationalize a dynamic interactional approach to the evaluation and treatment of visual, perceptual, and cognitive deficits, which is applicable to occupational therapy practice. These evaluations and related information are included in subsequent chapters of this book. In addition, Table 2-1 describes key differentiating factors between static and dynamic assessment.

Test Reliability

A test's reliability refers to its consistency and accuracy.[6,23,25,32] Reliability can be measured in several ways, and the goal of the specific evaluation will direct which types of reliability measures are important.[3] Reliability measures include test-retest, intra-rater and inter-rater, and measures of internal consistency.

Test-retest reliability measures the test's stability over time.[32,33] The test or evaluation is administered to an individual several times. If the score is approximately the same over repeated examinations, the test-retest reliability is said to be good.

By repeating this procedure with a large group of people, one can perform a statistical analysis and derive a coefficient of correlation r for the test. A test's test-retest correlation r can range from 0 to 1.0. The higher the r, the better the test-retest reliability. A reliability coefficient of 0.90 or

---

Table 2-1

Static Versus Dynamic Assessment

Static	*Dynamic*
Concerned with products formed as a result of pre-existing skills	Emphasis on quantifying the psychological processes involved in learning and change
Examiner presents a graded sequence of problems, and the test-taker responds to each of these problems	Examiner presents a graded sequence of problems, but after the presentation of each task, the examiner gives the test-taker feedback and continues the feedback until test-taker succeeds or gives up.
No feedback to the test-taker regarding quality of performance	Feedback is given
One-way relationship between examiner and test-taker	Two-way interactive relationship between examiner and test-taker; tester-testee interaction is individualized for each client

Adapted from reference 12: Grigorenko EL, Sternberg RJ. Dynamic testing. Psychological Bulletin. *1998;124:75-111.*

---

above is considered high[6] by some, whereas other therapists state a reliability coefficient of 0.80 or above to be excellent.[23] It is generally accepted that a correlation coefficient less than 0.60 is unacceptable for clinical use.[6,23,32] The therapist should be sure that a test has a fairly high test-retest correlation if he or she intends to use the test as a measure of improvement following treatment.

The next type of reliability measurement examines the reliability or consistency of the rater or raters of the test. Intra-rater reliability measures the variation that occurs within a rater as a result of multiple exposures to the same stimulus.[3] Inter-rater reliability examines whether different raters can independently assign similar ratings to the client performing the evaluation.[23,33,34] For inter-rater reliability, the scores of two or more raters are compared. The closer the sets of scores are to each other, the better the test's scorer reliability. Again, the range of the coefficient of correlation r is from 0 to 1.0, and the closer it is to 1.0, the better.

It is important to note that correlation coefficients for inter-rater reliability are not always the strongest statistical procedure for measuring inter-rater reliability. Items rated on scales with few response alternatives, where there is the likelihood of agreement by chance, provide inflated inter-rater reliability statistics unless chance is factored out.[33] This is accomplished by the Kappa coefficient.

Unless the criteria for making the judgment for score assignment is explicit on a subjective test, the scorer reliability of the test is likely to be low. Therefore, it is difficult to compare results between clients or between testings of the same client if the test is scored by different examiners. However, since anyone giving an objective test should get the same results as anyone else, the scorer reliability is likely to be high. It still may not be a reliable or consistent test; its test-retest reliability may be low.

The internal consistency of an instrument measures the "sameness" of test items to the attribute being measured and is measured at one point in time.[3] It examines whether all parts of the evaluation are highly inter-correlated so that the measured skill is being measured by all items.[33]

Common reliability statistical procedures include Cronbach's coefficient alpha, Kappa coefficient, Pearson correlation, and intra-class correlation. The definition of these procedures as well as those related to validity and measurement appear in Appendix A.

Test Validity

A test's validity refers to how well the test measures what it purports to measure.[25,34,35] There are several types of validity. The three major types of validity usually considered are content, construct, and criterion validity.[6,23,32,33,36] Content validity is established by "…judging the comprehensiveness of the assessment and whether it includes all aspects of the particular attributes that are important to measure."[23] It describes how well the test represents the total universe of the content of the property being measured.[6,33,37] As Polgar states, content validity requires that 1) all aspects of the domain are adequately covered, 2) the content is relevant to the construct, and 3) underlying processes necessary for satisfactory interpretation of test items and response are relevant.[6] In addition to the actual content of a particular test, components such as wording, guidelines for procedures, or scoring are relevant to content validity.[6] Expert opinion, evaluating how clients arrive at a response (which addresses the validity of underlying processes), and empirical studies (which compare a particular instrument with others that measure the same domain) are all methods of establishing content validity.[6]

Construct validity measures how much test scores conform to previous theoretical relationships or formulations.[23,32,33] As Polgar states, "…evidence of validity as it provides support for the underlying construct is necessary to justify a particular evaluation with a specific population in a given context."[6] A given instrument is considered to have excellent construct validity if more than two well designed studies have shown that the test conforms to prior theoretical relationships, and adequate construct validity would have one or two studies.[32]

Criterion validity measures how much a particular instrument agrees with another established accurate measure of some trait.[23,32,36] Criterion validity can be concurrent, predictive (ie, the ability of the test to predict future performance), or both.[25,32] A test is considered to have excellent criterion validity if more than two well designed studies show agreement and adequate criterion validity if one or two studies show agreement. The value of correlation coefficients is used to indicate the strength of the criterion validity.[3]

Only a few studies have been done to correlate results of tests of perception and cognition with actual functional abilities and disabilities. This is part of examining the test's validity. For example, an adult client may do very poorly on Ayres' Figure-Ground Test yet have no observable functional deficit in that area. Any perceptual or cognitive tests that have been shown to correlate with functional performance will be specified when each specific deficit is described. The problem of lack of research to correlate test scores and functional performance has led some occupational therapists to rely solely on functional tests (eg, can a client dress himself) rather than on formal perceptual or cognitive tests. The problem that functional tests present is that one cannot always discern why the client is having trouble doing the task. One can hypothesize reasons and then test them with the more discrete formal visual, perceptual, and/or cognitive test. In this way, a combination of functional and perceptual or cognitive tasks can be most useful.

The definitions of statistical procedures that can be used to establish validity are contained in Appendix A. The therapist should note that if validity has not been statistically established, a low score on any one test is not conclusive evidence that the client has that particular deficit. A low score on one test should signal the need for follow-up with additional similar tests.

Standardization

Not all objective visual, perceptual, or cognitive tests have been standardized for adult populations, although some have been standardized for children. A standardized test is defined as any test that has been administered to a large sample of the population one wishes to test so that the examiner knows how the average person in this population scores on this test. Standardized tests generate norms, which are statistics generated from a well-defined group that has been evaluated using a test in a standardized manner.[6] Randomized sampling should be used to establish norms, and the sample size should be large enough to reduce the possibility of measurement error.[6] Polgar provides the following guidelines for evaluating the usefulness of a set of norms in interpreting the client's score[6]:

- What is the information given about the characteristics of the sample used to create the norms?
- What was the method of recruiting the sample?
- To what degree does the sample represent the test's target population?

When tests have not been standardized, interpretation of scores is tenuous, since there are no norms for comparison.[38,39] In such instances, it is suggested that if one is unfamiliar with the test and with how the normal adult will perform, it should first be administered to several normal adults, preferably of the same age, sex, and occupational or educational level as the client. In this way, one can develop skill in test administration and gain some idea of how well a normal adult should score on the test.

Test Scoring

If the test has been standardized, it is important to administer it exactly according to the accompanying directions in order to use the test's norms. Any standardized objective test can, however, also give subjective or qualitative information depending on how data are collected. For example, the standardized procedures may be utilized but the client's approach to the task, and client verbalizations may be recorded.[40]

Three categories of tests are examined in this book:

1. *Standardized*—Scored objectively, standardized with adults.
2. *Nonstandardized*—Scored objectively, not standardized with adults.
3. *Subjective*—Scored subjectively, not standardized.

In scoring subjective and nonstandardized tests, a client's performance is usually labeled intact, impaired, severely impaired, or absent. An intact performance is defined as a normal adult performance on the test. A severely impaired/absent performance is defined as one in which the client is making many errors, taking longer than normal to do the test, and/or having trouble completing the test. An impaired performance is between severely impaired and intact performance. The client completes the test but makes one or two errors or does not perform the task quite right. In the following chapters, intact performance will be described on those tests scored subjectively or nonstandardized. If the client's performance is not intact, the labeling of his performance as "impaired" or "severely impaired" will at times be left up to the examiner, since the difference between the two is one of degree of impairment.

When some tests are used to evaluate more than one deficit, a description of impaired performance will be included to distinguish qualitative differences of performance among clients with different deficits. For example, a Copy Flower, House Test, in which the client is asked to copy a drawing of a house and a flower, is used to test for both unilateral neglect and constructional apraxia. In order to differentiate between the two deficits, when the test is examined during evaluations for unilateral neglect, a description of how a client with unilateral neglect would perform is included.

Administration of Tests

In administering the tests described in the following chapters, one should be aware of several additional problems. First, none of these tests measure completely discrete functions. They may emphasize one main function, but most overlap into other areas. To use these tests with greater validity, one must first rule out other deficits the client may have. For example, in testing tactile agnosia (ie, the inability to recognize objects by touch although sensation is intact) one must first test to be sure that the client has intact tactile sensation. Throughout the test descriptions, under the heading "To Improve Validity," those deficits that may interfere with performance on a particular test should be tested first. Unfortunately, other deficits may be an inherent part of the test and thus be impossible to completely rule out. For example, a client with right hemiplegia and a client with left hemiplegia may perform equally poorly on a constructional praxis test but for entirely different reasons. The client with right hemiplegia tends to have trouble initiating or carrying through the construction, which is more an execution problem; the client with left hemiplegia tends to pick up and move blocks around randomly, which is more a spatial relations problem.[41] Therefore, the examiner must be aware of the different causes of poor performance on a given test and look closely at the qualitative performance by the client for clues to the reason for his or her failure.

Second, all the tests require comprehension of the directions, and some require verbal responses. Thus, their use with aphasic clients must take this into account. These tests may not be valid for clients with aphasia; the tests may measure language rather than perceptual or cognitive skills. There are, however, some tests that have been adapted for use with aphasic clients, which are presented in various sections of the book.

Third, many of the tests require some motor act as part of the response. Clients should first be tested for apraxia and primary motor skills to rule out problems in the areas in the test for which a motor response is required.

Fourth, although the client appears to be mentally alert, he or she may do poorly on these tests because he or she is inattentive or easily distracted. This may be the result of brain damage. Certain lesions or damage affect a client's ability to form intentions or goals, to attend and concentrate. The client may be inattentive because the task is too abstract for him or her. Hague showed that clients with left hemiplegia have a definite impairment of complex abstract behavior and should be tested on the concrete level.[42] Moreover, a client may have a very short immediate visual memory, making it difficult for him or her to attend to the task.

Vision is also a factor in many of these tests. Often, clients who have sustained a CVA are elderly and have poor eyesight that is not always corrected well by their glasses. This should be checked before administering tests for which visual acuity is important. Information about aging, vision, and visual evaluation and treatment are covered in detail in Chapters 3 and 12.

A client's pre-ABI level of intelligence, perceptual and cognitive skills, and educational and cultural background can also affect performance. For example, if a client was developmentally delayed before the ABI, he or she will have difficulty with some abstract concepts in the tests even if there are no perceptual or cognitive problems as a result of the insult or trauma. Likewise, if the client's background is such that he never learned to write or draw, paper and pencil tests may not be valid. Additionally, if for various reasons, he or she never developed perceptual or cognitive skills to the fullest capacity, low scores on the tests would not necessarily be the result of an ABI.

Lastly, one may get poor results because the client reacts negatively to this type of testing. He or she may find the tasks childish and refuse to do them. Clients may think that they are intelligence tests and become very anxious about performance. For this reason, the therapist must be careful in explaining the purpose of all tests.

Evaluation Choice

There are many factors to consider in deciding which evaluation to utilize. This book contains descriptions of multiple evaluation tools for each area described and it is not intended for the therapist to administer all evaluations! Factors such as aphasia, motor and visual ability, client setting, and occupational performance status will all play into the ultimate decision. Outside pressures such as reimbursement, cost of materials, and therapist time will also have to be considered. Client response, the theoretical support for the technique, and the therapist's ability to administer the test adequately should also be considered.[43]

Unsworth provides the following questions to consider when choosing an evaluation[25]:

Client-Related Questions

- *Is the client ready to participate in formal assessment?*
- *What is the age and diagnosis of the client?*
- *What further information do I want to know about this client?*

Assessment-Related Questions

- *What model guides my practice, and does it favor a restorative or adaptive orientation?*
- *What population was this assessment developed for?*
- *Am I qualified to use this assessment?*
- *Am I satisfied that I can interpret the data and that the assessment has acceptable reliability and validity?*
- *What domains of cognitive and perceptual areas does this assessment cover? Do I want to target these domains?*
- *Is the assessment sensitive to change in client status?*
- *Can the assessment be used before and after intervention to measure change?*

References

1. Weinstock-Zlotnick A, Hinojosa J. Bottom-up or top-down evaluation: is one better than the other? *Am J Occup Ther.* 2004;58(5):594-599.
2. Toglia J. A dynamic interactional approach to cognitive rehabilitation. In: Katz N, ed. *Cognition and Occupation Across The Life Span.* Bethesda, Md: The American Occupational Therapy Association, Inc; 2005.
3. Law M, Baum C, Dunn W, eds. *Measuring Occupational Performance: Supporting Best Practice in Occupational Therapy.* 2nd ed. Thorofare, NJ: SLACK Incorporated; 2001.
4. Spencer J. Evaluation of performance contexts. In: Crepeau E, Cohn ES, Schell BAB, eds. *Willard and Spackman's Occupational Therapy.* Philadelphia, Pa: Lippincott, Williams and Wilkins; 2003.
5. Uswatte G, Taub E. Constraint-induced movement therapy: new approaches to outcome measurement in rehabilitation. In: Stuss D, Winocur G, Robertson IH, eds. *Cognitive Neurorehabilitation.* New York, NY: Cambridge University Press; 1999.
6. Polgar J. Critiquing assessments. In: Crepeau E, Cohn ES, Schell BAB, eds. *Willard and Spackman's Occupational Therapy.* Philadelphia, Pa: Lippincott, Williams and Wilkins; 2003.
7. Baum B, Hall K. Relationship between constructional praxis and dressing in the head injured adult. *Am J Occup Ther.* 1981;35(7):438-442.
8. Golisz K, Toglia J. Perception and cognition. In: Crepeau E, Cohn ES, Schell BAB, eds. *Willard and Spackman's Occupational Therapy.* Philadelphia, Pa: Lippincott Williams and Wilkins; 2003.

9. Arnadottir G. Evaluation and intervention with complex perceptual impairment. In: Unsworth C, ed. *Cognitive and Perceptual Dysfunction*. Philadelphia, Pa: FA Davis; 1999.

10. Fisher A. Uniting practice and theory in an occupational framework. *Am J Occup Ther*. 1998;52:509-521.

11. Kreutzer JS, Marwitz JH, Seel R, Serio CD. Validation of a neurobehavioral functioning inventory for adults with traumatic brain injury. *Arch Phys Med Rehabil*. 1996;77(2):116-124.

12. Grigorenko EL, Sternberg RJ. Dynamic testing. *Psychological Bulletin*. 1998;124:75-111.

13. Haywood CH, Tzuriel D. Applications and challenges in dynamic assessment. *Peabody J Edu*. 2002;77(2):40-63.

14. Tzuriel D. Dynamic assessment of young children: educational and intervention perspectives. *Edu Psychol Rev*. 2000;12:385-435.

15. Lidz C. *Dynamic Assessment: An Interactional Approach to Evaluating Learning Potential*. New York, NY: Guilford Press; 1987.

16. Rogers J, Holm M. Activities and daily living and instrumental activities of daily living. In: Crepeau E, Cohn ES, Schell BAB, eds. *Willard and Spackman's Occupational Therapy*. Philadelphia, Pa: Lippincott, Williams and Wilkins; 2003.

17. Sohlberg M, Mateer CA. *Introduction To Cognitive Rehabilitation: Theory and Practice*. New York, NY: The Guilford Press; 1989.

18. Corcoran M. Using qualitative measurement methods to understand occupational performance. In: Law M, Baum C, Dunn W, eds. *Measuring Occupational Performance: Supporting Best Practice in Occupational Therapy*. 2nd ed. Thorofare, NJ: SLACK Incorporated; 2001.

19. McNeny R. Activities of daily living. In: Rosenthal M, Griffith ER, Kreutzer JS, Pentland B, eds. *Rehabilitation of the Adult and Child With Traumatic Brain Injury*. 3rd ed. Philadelphia, Pa: FA Davis; 1999.

20. Ratcliff G. Perception and complex visual process. In: Meir MJ, Benton AL, Diller L, eds. *Neuropsychological Rehabilitation*. New York, NY: Guilford University Press; 1987.

21. Raskin S. Executive functions. In: Raskin S, Mateer C, eds. *Neuropsychological Management of Mild Traumatic Brain Injury*. New York, NY: Oxford University Press; 2000.

22. Sohlberg M, Mateer CA. Effectiveness of an attention-training program. *J Clin Exper Neuropsych*. 1987;9(2):117-130.

23. Law M, Baum C, Dunn W. Occupational performance assessment. In: Christiansen C, Baum C, eds. *Occupational Therapy: Performance, Participation and Well-Being*. Thorofare, NJ: SLACK Incorporated; 2001.

24. Cohn ES, Schell BAB, Neistadt ME. Overview of evaluation. In: Crepeau E, Cohn ES, Schell BAB, eds. *Willard and Spackman's Occupational Therapy*. Philadelphia, Pa: Lippincott, Williams and Wilkins; 2003.

25. Unsworth C. *Cognitive and Perceptual Dysfunction*. Philadelphia, Pa: FA Davis; 1999.

26. Henry A. The interview process in occupational therapy. In: Crepeau E, Cohn ES, Schell BAB, eds. *Willard and Spackman's Occupational Therapy*. Philadelphia, Pa: Lippincott, Williams and Wilkins; 2003.

27. Whyte J, Laborde A, DiPasquale MC. Assessment and treatment of the vegetative and minimally conscious patient. In: Rosenthal M, Griffith ER, Kreutzer JS, Pentland B, eds. *Rehabilitation of the Adult and Child With Traumatic Brain Injury*. 3rd ed. Philadelphia, Pa: FA Davis; 1999.

28. Hesseks-Schlatter C. A dynamic test to assess learning capacity in people with severe impairments. *Am J Ment Retard*. 2002;107(5):340-351.

29. Swanson HL, Lussier CM. A selective synthesis of the experimental literature on dynamic assessment. *Rev Edu Res*. 2001;71:321-363.

30. Wiedl KH. Cognitive modifiability as a measure of readiness for rehabilitation. *Psychiatr Serv*. 1999;50:1411-1413.

31. Embretson S. Toward development of a psychometric approach. In: Schneider C, ed. *Dynamic Assessment: Interactional Approach to Evaluating Learning Potential*. New York, NY: The Guilford Press; 1987.

32. Law M, Philp I. Evaluating the evidence. In: Law M, ed. *Evidenced-Based Rehabilitation: A Guide to Practice*. Thorofare, NJ: SLACK Incorporated; 2002.

33. Hall K. Functional assessment in traumatic brain injury. In: Rosenthal M, Griffith ER, Kreutzer JS, Pentland B, eds. *Rehabilitation of the Adult and Child With Traumatic Brain Injury*. 3rd ed. Philadelphia, Pa: FA Davis; 1999.

34. Lincoln N. Outcome measurement in cognitive neurorehabilitation. In: Stuss D, Winocur G, Robertson IH, eds. *Cognitive Neurorehabilitation*. New York, NY: Cambridge University Press; 1999.

35. Dunn W, Foreman J. Development of evidence-based knowledge. In: Law M, ed. *Evidence-Based Rehabilitation: A Guide to Practice*. Thorofare, NJ: SLACK Incorporated; 2002.

36. Portney L, Watkins M. *Foundations of Clinical Research: Applications to Practice*. 2nd ed. Upper Saddle River, NJ: Prentice Hall Health; 2000.

37. Luria AR. Functional organization of the brain. *Sci Am*. 1970;222:66-72.

38. Boys M, Fisher P, Holzberg C, Reid DW. The OSOT perceptual evaluation: a research perspective. *Am J Occup Ther.* 1988;42(2):92-98.
39. van Deusen-Fox J, Harlowe D. Construct validation of occupational therapy measures used in CVA evaluation: a beginning. *Am J Occup Ther.* 1984;38(2):101-106.
40. Milberg WP, Herben N, Kaplan E. The Boston process approach to neuropsychological assessment. In: Grant I, Adams KM, eds. *Neuropsychological Assessment of Neuropsychiatric Disorders.* New York, NY: Oxford University Press; 1986.
41. Harrington DO. *The Visual Fields: A Textbook and Atlas of Clinical Perimetry.* 4th ed. St. Louis, Mo: CV Mosby; 1976.
42. Hague HR. An investigation of abstract behavior in patients with cerebral vascular accidents. *Am J Occup Ther.* 1959;13:83-87.
43. Okkema K. *Cognition and Perception in the Stroke Patient.* Gaithersburg, Md: Aspen Publishers; 1993.

Resources

Falik LH, Feuerstein R. Cognitive modifiability: a needed perspective on learning for the 21st century. Dynamic Cognitive Assessment. Available at: http://www.icelp.org/asp/Dynamic_Cognitive_Assessment.shtm.
Law M. *Client-Centered Occupational Therapy.* Thorofare, NJ: SLACK Incorporated; 2001.
van Deusen-Fox J, Harlowe D. Continued construct validation of the St. Mary's CVA evaluation: bilateral awareness scale. *Am J Occup Ther.* April 1987;41(4):242-245.

CHAPTER 3

VISUAL PROCESSING SKILLS

Vision plays a major role in our ability to adapt to the environment. It serves as a primary receptor for motor, cognitive, communicative, and emotive functions.[1] Visual processing allows for the rapid assimilation of details from the environment, which helps to enable quick decision making.[2] Visual impairment can change the client's ability to interact with all aspects of the environment including the people and objects within it.[3] A large portion of our daily life requires effective visual processing and visual-motor performance.[4] It is an important prerequisite to perception and cognition and influences both motor planning and postural control. In conjunction with the proprioceptive and vestibular systems, it is the basis for normal upright stance.[5] It allows us to anticipate information, which is necessary for successful adaptation to the environment.[6] Visual deficits can have a significant effect on activities of daily living (ADLs), reading, driving, and eye-hand coordination.[7] Visual skills "…are the most basic functional skills necessary for the development and management of all visual perception and visual motor activities, and they must be intact for a person to receive, process, interpret, and respond appropriately to input from the environment."[8] Without an efficient level of visual function, the rehabilitation process is adversely affected.[9] An undiagnosed visual defect can undermine the rehabilitation effort.[10] Visual system disorders and their rehabilitation should, therefore, be viewed as an integral part of the rehabilitation program.

The occurrence of visual dysfunction following traumatic brain injury (TBI) is high.[11,12] The acquired brain injury (ABI) client may experience asthenopia, headaches, diplopia, dizziness, inability to focus, movement of print when reading, and difficulty tracking and fixating.[13] There may be a reduction in acuity, binocular dysfunction, accommodative dysfunction, and/or oculomotor dysfunction.[13] Physical damage as a result of TBI can affect any of the brain structures related to the visual system, and the areas of the brain that are associated with visual function are very vulnerable to injury.[14,15]

Although there is not a high occurrence of specific injury to the ocular structures of the eye with cerebral vascular accident (CVA), most clients who have sustained a CVA are elderly and will likely display some degree of retinal and crystalline lens pathology from associated diabetes and hypertension. In addition, the CVA itself often causes visual system deficits. Since normal vision depends on trouble free brain flow, occlusion, hemorrhage, or any interruption to oxygen flow in any of the arteries in the brain's blood circulation system can result in vision or visually related deficits.[16] Since efficient visual processing depends on contributions from each cortical hemisphere and vision is represented in approximately thirty visual cortical areas, it is inevitable that the CVA client will have some degree of visual system impairment.[17,18]

Primary visual deficits as a result of CVA or TBI can include decreased near and distant acuity, accommodation, convergence, quality of saccade, pursuit, fixation and functional scanning, color perception, stereopsis, central blindness, and strabismus.[8,19] Suchoff et al note common visual deficits associated with ABI to include visual field loss (eg, central, congruous, and incongruous homonymous hemianopsia and quadrantanopsias), neglect, eye movement disorders (eg, fixation, pursuit, saccade, and nystagmus), ocular muscle dysfunctions (eg, strabismus, anisocoria, lagophthalmus, and ptosis), and binocular dysfunctions (eg, exophoria, convergence insufficiency, vertical phorias, and fusional instabilities), accommodative dysfunctions (eg, amplitude, flexibility, and sustainability), perceptual dysfunction (eg, contrast sensitivity and color vision), and visually involved vestibular dysfunction (eg, vertigo and loss of balance).[15] Suchoff et al, in a separate study of 62 TBI clients, also report external eye pathology in 23% of their clients, which is twice that which is found in the general population.[15]

O'Dell et al classify common visual problems subsequent to TBI as "post-trauma vision syndrome."[19] Deficits of the syndrome include exotropia or high exophoria, accommodative dysfunction, convergence insufficiency, low blink rates, spatial disorientation, poor fixations and pursuits, and diplopia. In addition, the TBI client can have an injury to the eye itself. The therapist, therefore, should have at least a basic understanding of the components of the eye itself. The major components of the eye and their function are summarized in Table 3-1. For additional information on the structure and anatomy of the eye, the reader is referred to the references.

Visual processing occurs through two modes: focal control or attentive vision and ambient, peripheral, or preattentive vision.[9,13,22,23] Focal vision provides attention to important features of an object for perception and discrimination. Ambient vision works in connection with proprioceptive, kinesthetic, tactual, and vestibular systems and acts as a feed-forward system.[13] In order for the focal visual process to function effectively, the ambient process must initially organize and stabilize the visual field. Peripheral or ambient vision detects events in the environment and their location in space and distance from the individual.[6,13] It monitors verticality of objects and body alignment with them. Ambient vision is also the mode of vision that ties into functional mobility.[24]

Visual deficits sustained subsequent to ABI may be due to a "dysfunction of the ambient process in its ability to organize spatial information with other sensory-motor systems."[13] This inability, in turn, will cause a compromise to the focal process. Successful adaptation requires that both the ambient and focal systems work together and that the visual system as a whole be integrated with other sensory input.

As previously mentioned in Chapter 1, it is crucial for the occupational therapist to have a theoretical framework or model to guide evaluation and treatment. This is definitely the case when considering visual processing dysfunction. For example, applying treatment techniques without a model of visual processing in mind "...may encourage attempts to rehabilitate splinter skills such as convergence in cases where a more holistic approach is necessary to get the client reading again or reoriented in space."[25] With this is mind, the following two models for intervention are briefly described. The first (utilized by many therapy-oriented optometrists) is a modification of general information processing theory. The second is a hierarchal theory of visual processing described by Warren that has gained popularity with many occupational therapists.[23,24]

Table 3-1

Major Components of the Eye and Their Functions

Component	Function
Orbit of the eye	Bony recess in the skull that contains the eye ball, optic nerve, eye muscles, and their nerves and vessels.
Eyelids	Protects the eyes from injury and excessive light; keeps the cornea moist.
Cornea	Transparent tissue that covers the anterior surface of the eye; primary refractive component of the eye.
Conjunctiva	Peripheral to the cornea and surrounds the remainder of the anterior surface as well as lining the inner surface of the eyelid; has mechanical, protective, and nutrient features.
Aqueous humor	Fills the space between the cornea and iris and crystalline lens; provides nutrients for the avascular cornea and lens.
Crystalline lens	Secondary refractive component of the eye; changes shape to accommodate or focus on objects.
Vitreous humor	Located behind the lens; transmits light, holds the retina in place, and provides support for the lens.
Sclera	External lining of the eye; white portion of the eye; covers the posterior five-sixths of the eye; has mechanical and protective functions.
Choroid	Intermediate lining of the eye; has nutritional function.
Iris	Controls the amount of light entering the eye by the variable diameter, circular pupil.
Fovea	Part of the retina; to look at an object, the eye must be aimed so that the image is focused on the fovea; smooth pursuits and saccades enable the individual to always use the fovea.
Retina	Light sensitive inner lining of the eye; composed of optic disc (blind spot) and fovea; contains two types of photoreceptors: cones (detect fine detail and color and controls focusing function of the eye) and rods (detect low level of light as well as object motion).

Adapted from references 5, 20, and 21

Modified Information Processing Theory

INPUT/RECEPTION

The first, or *input*, stage of processing is affected by the integrity of the optical system or eye health, a clear optical image, the intact functioning of the accommodative and convergence systems, good fusional ability, and efficient oculomotor control.[4] These systems are important for progressing visual input to the visual cortex accurately.

Ocular motor skills are required for visual reception or input.[12] Basic ocular motor skills "...are dependent on feedback from areas that monitor head and body orientation and movement as well as those areas that monitor feedback from the ocular-motor driver."[12] At the primary visual cortex, binocular vision occurs and visual input is processed as color, contour, contrast, and depth.[27]

PERCEPTION/INTEGRATION

During the second, or *integrative*, stage of processing, sensory and proprioceptive information are mixed. This blending or combination of information results in a concept or plan that will serve as a guide to an action or response. Organization of space and motion, form perception, object recognition, and visual awareness are developed at this stage.[12] Visual integration is dependent on "…intact communication within visual processing areas and pathways between these processing areas, as well as intact reception."[12] In addition, pathways mediating other sensory and motor areas aid in the integration of visual input. It is important, therefore, "…to maintain a holistic model of the functions of this stage of processing so that one can test and address functional loss with some guidance from available topographic details of the injury."[27]

MOTOR OUTPUT/BEHAVIOR

Visual input and integration influence and ultimately guide behavior. This includes visually guided motor behavior such as mobility or eye-hand coordination.[25] As Suter states, "…these visual percepts and the resultant thought processes dependent on them are the foundations for much of the everyday behavior of a sighted person."[25]

Warren's Hierarchal Model of Visual Processing

An alternative view to visual processing that has recently gained popularity with therapists involves the concepts of a hierarchy of visual processing and a view of visual processing as a process of adaptation.[6] Visual information processing is viewed as an interactive product of both bottom-up and top-down processing.[28] Vision and visual processing are viewed holistically as a "single, unified process used by the central nervous system (CNS) to adapt."[6] Visual processing occurs within a hierarchy of skills rather than a series of independent skills. Skills at the bottom of the hierarchy form the foundation for each level above it. Higher-level skills "…evolve from the foundation skills and depend on complete integration of the lower-level skills for their development."[26]

The top of the hierarchy is visual cognition. It is the end product of all preceding skills and is the highest level of visual skills integration within the nervous system. It can be defined as "…the ability to mentally manipulate visual information and integrate it with other sensory information to solve problems, formulate plans, and make decisions."[26] Visual cognition fosters complex visual analysis and serves as the basis or foundation of academic activities.[3] Disorders of visual cognition can include agnosia, alexia, decreased visual closure, disorders of spatial analysis, decreased figure-ground, and decreased position in space.[29]

The next level down in the hierarchy from visual cognition is visual memory. Visual memory is "…the mental manipulation of visual stimuli and requires the ability to create a picture of the object in the mind's eye while the visual analysis is being completed."[3] Below visual memory is pattern recognition. This involves the ability to identify shape, contour, and general and specific features of an object, such as color and texture, which are all required for object recognition.[26] Pattern recognition is at a lower-level than visual memory because "…before a visual image can be stored in memory, an individual must recognize the pattern making up the image."[3]

At the most basic level of the hierarchy is the registration of visual input through oculomotor control, visual fields, and acuity. These three primary skills control visual attention and the higher-level skills in the hierarchy. For example, pattern recognition is dependent on organized scanning of the visual environment.[18,26] Oculomotor control, for instance, through quick and accurate eye movements, enables perceptual stability.[3] In conjunction with visual fields and acuity, they control the quality and quantity of visual input.

A disruption of any level of the hierarchy will affect the total structure of the hierarchy. Warren states, "...each skill level depends on the integration of those before it and cannot function effectively without the assistance of its predecessors. Thus, visual cognition cannot maintain its integrity without the support provided by visual memory, scanning, attention and so on."[29]

The evaluation and treatment of the client's visual ability should incorporate both the component skills and how the system as a whole is working. The therapist should examine where in the visual hierarchy the breakdown of performance is occurring, evaluate what conditions cause a breakdown in the adaptation process, and determine what changes can be made within the task and environment to improve performance. For example, "...what appears to be a deficit in a visual cognitive skill, such as decreased figure-ground ability, may actually be due to inaccurate pattern recognition caused by an asymmetrical scanning pattern that results from visual inattention compounded by a visual field deficit."[26] Treatment of the figure-ground deficit will not be effective without addressing the deficits at the lower-level first.

Evaluation and Treatment of Visual Skills

Vision and visual processing skills are often evaluated by several team members. Some members of the rehabilitation team who may administer a vision screening or evaluation are a neurologist, ophthalmologist, neuro-ophthalmologist, occupational therapist, and rehabilitative or functional optometrist.[8] The ophthalmologist is a medical doctor who specializes in diseases of the eyes. His or her evaluation is conducted with the goal of identifying the need for eye surgery or medication. The optometrist evaluates the visual system with an emphasis of how the status of the system relates to the environment and how the individual uses his or her eyes.[21] The treatment emphasis of the optometrist is vision therapy to rehabilitate a wide variety of visual disorders.[21] Optometrists accomplish this through a variety of techniques. Table 3-2 describes some of these techniques and how they work. Occupational therapists should be familiar with and have a basic understanding of these techniques. Although it is the optometrist's role to prescribe lenses or prisms, the client will often use these aids during occupational therapy. It is important for the occupational therapist to communicate to the rehabilitative optometrist how the aid is helping the client in ADLs, if the client is resistant to its use or if there are any problems related to the aid and its use during functional tasks.

Unlike the ophthalmologist or optometrist, the occupational therapist evaluates for visual or visual processing dysfunction as a means to explain functional limitations.[2,3] As Bryan states, "the purpose of the screening is not to diagnose but to detect potentially unrecognized visual deficits which may be impacting daily life."[11] The visual screening will also identify visual strengths that can aid functional independence. Warren outlines the three purposes of the occupational therapy visual assessment as 1) to identify the functional impairment, 2) to link the presence of the functional impairment to the presence of a visual impairment, and 3) to determine appropriate treatment intervention based on the results of the assessment.[3]

The clinical evaluation of the component skills within the hierarchy of visual processing and how they affect functional adaptation is well within the occupational therapist's role. Included in the evaluation are pupillary response, ocular alignment, acuity, visual fields, oculomotor control (saccadic eye movements, smooth pursuit movements), convergence, visual attention/scanning, visual memory, and visual cognition. In addition, due to the close connection of the two systems, the client's visual vestibular processing should be evaluated and incorporated into the occupational therapy program. Finally, prior to and during screening, the occupational therapist should observe the client in areas as listed below in general guidelines for visual evaluation. The occupational therapist should also interview the client, family, and/or caregiver prior to screening regarding

Table 3-2

Summary of Optometric Treatment
Used With Brain Injury Patients

Technique	*Use*
Lenses	Improve clarity and sight, reduce or eliminate double vision, reduce visual discomfort or stress
Compensatory Prism	Eliminate a strabismus condition, alleviate double vision, reduce head tilt or turn
Yoked Prism	Alter a client's spatial awareness, modify a client's midline perception, change weight shifting, may benefit field loss clients
Filters or "Tints"	Decrease light sensitivity
Total Occlusion	Double vision; used when double vision is constant and no other treatment is successful
Partial Occlusion	Intermittent double vision; useful for noncomitant strabismus with double vision in just certain gazes

Adapted from reference 30: Hellerstein L. Visual problems associated with brain injury. In: Scheiman M, ed. Understanding and Managing Vision Deficits. *Thorofare, NJ: SLACK Incorporated; 1997.*

their perceptions of any visual problems the client may be having. A sample of an interview is presented in Figure 3-1.[11]

General Guidelines for Visual Processing
Skills Evaluation

CLINICAL OBSERVATIONS

Observe for possible indications of visual stress such as shutting an eye, squinting, increased muscle tone in head and jaw, turning or cocking the head, changing head position during ambulation, complaints of headaches or fatigue, or sudden agitation when a task is presented. Observe for any sensitivity to light.[31]

Examine the face for lacerations. Check the eye lid position, and check skin sensation to evaluate if there is cranial nerve damage.[1] Ask the client and/or the family or caregiver if the client had any premorbid conditions such as strabismus, amblyopia, glaucoma, ocular trauma, or retinopathy associated with diabetes mellitus and hypertension.[3] In addition, the therapist should observe the following:

1. Do the eyes work together?
2. How well do the eyes work together?
3. Where is the visual control most and least efficient?
4. What kinds of eye movements are the most and least efficient?
5. How does altering the environment or task alter performance?

Visual Symptoms Checklist

Prescription glasses: Yes _____   No _____

If yes: Were glasses worn prior to injury?_____

Since the injury only? _____

Last vision examination?_____

New prescription? _____   Date: _____

Answer yes or no to the following questions: **Yes**   **No**

1.   Do you have blurred or double vision?   _____   _____
2.   Do you tilt you head to see more clearly?   _____   _____
3.   Do you squint or close an eye to see?   _____   _____
4.   Do you get a headache while reading, watching television, or riding in or driving a car? Other?_____   _____   _____
5.   Do your eyes feel "tired?"   _____   _____
6.   Do you lose your place while reading?   _____   _____
7.   Do you hold objects or reading material close to see?   _____   _____
8.   Do you avoid reading or not read as often as you did before the injury?   _____   _____
9.   Do you miss words, letters, or numbers while reading?   _____   _____
10. Do you have difficulty distinguishing colors?   _____   _____
11. Do you avoid dark areas or avoid driving after dark?   _____   _____
12. Do you sometimes confuse which direction is right or left?   _____   _____
13. Do you reverse letters, numbers, or words?   _____   _____
14. Do you have difficulty recognizing road or street signs before it is too late to turn?   _____   _____
15. While you are standing still, do objects seem to jump or move?   _____   _____
16. While you are walking, do objects seem to jump or move?   _____   _____
17. Do you bump into objects on one side or the other?   _____   _____

Figure 3-1. Visual symptoms checklist.[1] (Reprinted with permission from Morton RL. Visual dysfunction following traumatic brain injury. In: Ashley MJ, ed. *Traumatic Brain Injury Rehabilitative Treatment and Case Management.* Boca Raton, Fla: CRC Press; 2004.)

Pupillary Response

The pupils are normally circular and smooth, approximately equal in size and centered within the iris.[2,32] They constrict rapidly in response to light and near vision and redilate equally fast to their offset.[32] At rest, "...the diameter is largest at the age of 15 to 20 years (7.5 mm in darkness) and thereafter diminishes progressively at a rate of 0.05 mm/year, and at the age of 70 years, the average darkness diameter is 5.0 mm, but normal pupils will range from 3.5 mm to 6.5 mm in size.[32]

Normal pupillary function is crucial to accurate focusing of an image on the retina and, therefore, should be assessed before acuity.[2] An abnormal pupillary response can result in anything from blurred vision to light sensitivity. Brainstem injury can result in the client having "...difficulty regulating the speed and efficiency of the pupillary response, causing them to be hypersensitive to light (photophobia) and have a slowness to adapt to changes in illumination."[2] TBI or CVA can cause impairment of pupil size, responsiveness to light, and responsiveness to accommodation.

Screening of Pupillary Response[33]

Pupil Size

In a dimly illuminated room, the client is asked to look at a distant object. A dim light source is directed into the face from below so that pupil size can be assessed.

Response to Light

A bright light is then shone into one eye. The speed of constriction is noted as well as the eventual size of the pupil. The consensual pupil response is then observed by shining the light into the other eye while still observing the same pupil. The direct reaction should equal the consensual one.

Response to Accommodation – biVABA*[2]

Bilateral pupillary constriction accompanies convergence of the eyes when an object is brought into near focus.

Test Materials

- Basic Visual Function Assessment test form
- Distant target (large enough to be seen easily at 6 plus feet without eyeglasses)
- Near target (large enough to be seen at 16 inches without eyeglasses)

Environment

Well lighted room; ensure that the light source is not shining directly into the client's eyes.

Procedure

1. The client is seated comfortably with eyeglasses off, if worn.
2. Instruct the client to focus on the distant target; observe pupil size.
3. Then instruct the client to focus on the near target; observe pupil size. The pupils should constrict as the client changes focus from the distance target to the near target.
4. Record the client's performance on the test form.

Instructions to the Client

"I am going to check to see how well you are able to switch from looking at this (point to distance target), which is far away, to looking at this (show near target). Please look from one target to the other when I tell you to do so."

Treatment of Impaired Pupillary Response

Possible impaired pupillary responses and their potential associated functional impact are outlined in Table 3-3.

If any impairment or abnormal response is noted, the therapist should refer the client to an ophthalmologist, neuro-ophthalmologist, or neurologist to assess what is causing the abnormality.

---

*Reprinted with permission from VisAbilities Rehab Services, Inc (http://www.visabilities.com), reference 2: Warren M. Brain Injury Visual Assessment Battery For Adults: Test Manual. Birmingham, Ala: VisAbilities Rehab Services Inc; 1998.

Table 3-3

Impaired Pupillary Response

Response	*Possible Functional Impact*
↓d pupil size on observation	Blurred vision when focusing at near distance; light sensitivity
Dilated pupil on observation (if client has vision and pupil remains dilated during accommodation)	Blurred vision in the eye when focusing at a near distance; difficulty with reading and completing near vision tasks. Possible ↓d sensitivity to light
Sluggish pupillary response during direct light stimulation	Difficulty adapting to changes in light conditions
Nonstimulated pupil reacts sluggishly or is unable to maintain constriction and begins to dilate during direct stimulation of the other	Light sensitivity to bright light. Difficulty maintaining a clear focus during sustained near viewing
Pupil does not constrict to direct stimulation but constricts consensually with stimulation of the other eye	No impact as the amaurotic (blind) eye reacts to stimulation of the other eye; with both eyes open it will constrict consensually during accommodation
↓d pupillary constriction during accommodation	Reduced quality of retinal image with near viewing. May have blurred vision
No pupillary response to direct light stimulation, but constriction with accommodation	Light sensitivity but should not have blurred vision with near vision

Adapted from reference 2: Warren M. Brain Injury Visual Assessment Battery For Adults: Test Manual. *Birmingham, Ala: VisAbilities Rehab Services Inc; 1998.*

Visual Acuity

Visual acuity, or the resolution power of the eye, is the product of the integration of the optical systems of the eye and CNS processing.[21,34] It affects the quality of what reaches the CNS and contributes to the CNS's ability for object recognition.[3,26,35] Decreased acuity will result in blurred vision, visual fatigue, and eye strain.[8] Acuity, which begins with the focusing of light onto the retina, can be affected by TBI, CVA, and/or the process of aging or age related disease. The retina can be directly damaged by disease, or injury. TBI can cause shearing or tearing of the optic nerve.[3] Corneal scarring from direct trauma to the eye in TBI may occur.[3] Trauma to the eye can result in bleeding into the vitreous humor, which prevents light from passing through.[3] Trauma "...to the crystalline lens may cause displacement or result in the subsequent development of a cataract that clouds the lens and reduces acuity."[3] In other words, as Warren describes, clients with ABI most often have acuity deficits as a result of 1) decreased focus of light onto the retina, 2) decreased ability of the retina to process an image, or 3) decreased ability of the optic nerve to transmit information to the CNS.[2]

Visual acuity can be divided into near vision visual acuity and distance acuity. Near vision acuity can be defined as "...the ability to see, inspect, identify, and understand objects clearly at near distances, within an arms length."[8] Distance acuity consists of the same skills but performed at a distance. Distance acuity deficits will affect the client functionally in areas such as depth perception, spatial judgments, and facial recognition. Near vision deficits will affect reading, writing, and any other functional activities requiring "close work." In addition, acuity can be viewed as central, (macular) or peripheral. Central acuity loss, which affects the ability to distinguish small details, contrast, and color, results in impaired writing, reading, and fine motor coordination.[3] Functional activities that may be affected are reading labels, writing checks, putting on make up, or dialing a phone.[3] Peripheral acuity or visual field loss, on the other hand, will affect overall mobility (ie, use of landmarks, seeing obstacles, driving, shopping).[3] Visual acuity is described by the testing distance at which the individual recognizes the test stimulus and the distance at which the test stimulus being viewed could be identified by an individual with normal visual acuity.[21] For example, as Scheiman describes, "…20/100 suggests that a client with normal visual acuity could identify the letter presented at a distance of 100 feet. The actual individual being tested could only see this letter at 20 feet, indicating that the visual acuity is reduced relative to the normal finding."[21]

Impaired visual acuity can be the result of myopia, hyperopia, astigmatism accommodative disorders, binocular vision disorders, amblyopia, or eye disease.[21] As previously stated, it is not the role of the occupational therapist to discern the underlying cause of a detected visual acuity deficit during visual screening. If a deficit is detected, the occupational therapist should refer the client to the appropriate eye specialist. When the therapist refers the client to the eye specialist, it is extremely helpful for him or her to verbally or in writing describe how the deficit is affecting the client's performance during functional activities.

GENERAL GUIDELINES FOR EVALUATION

1. Distance acuity is tested initially at 20 feet. Near acuity is tested at 4 cm or 16 inches.[10]

2. The client should wear glasses during the evaluation if he or she normally does so.

3. A Tumbling E chart, Landolt C chart, Lighthouse Picture Symbols test, or Lea Symbols test is especially useful with the aphasic and TBI client.[21]

4. For the client with severe visual perceptual problems, modify the testing by presenting one visual stimulus at a time, and direct the client's eye to the stimulus by pointing.

5. Evaluate high contrast, low contrast, distance, and near acuity.[3]

6. Perform testing in a well-lit room with full and even illumination of the test chart. Eliminate any sources of glare.[2] Adequate illumination is important because when illumination decreases, so does acuity.[3]

7. Slowness of response from the client with language, cognitive, and/or perceptual problems does not necessarily mean the client lacks the visual acuity to identify the test stimulus. If the client struggles with identifying the test stimulus on each line but does so accurately, then continue the test until the client reaches a line for which he or she can no longer identify the majority of items on that line.[3]

8. When testing the ABI client with cognitive and perceptual problems, test at near before at distance. It is easier to teach the test procedure and maintain the client's attention at near than at far.[21]

VISUAL ACUITY SCREENING

Test 1 – Near Visual Acuity*[7]

Purpose

To test clearness of vision at near (within arm's length)

*Reprinted with permission from Lynn Hellerstein, OD, Homestead Park Vision Clinic, PC, 6967 S. Holly Circle, Suite 105, Englewood, CO 80112

Vision Problems Detected

Vision loss, reduced vision due to uncorrected refractive error, accommodation dysfunction, etc

Control

Habitual glasses for near, if worn. Make sure lighting is adequate.

Equipment

Near visual acuity card (letter, picture, etc)

Procedure

Hold card at appropriate distance (as noted by each card, usually 13 or 16 inches). Test right eye first. Procedure is the same as for distance visual acuity.

Retest/Referral

Client should be able to read 20/20 or better with each eye. 20/40 or worse is a referral.

Test 2 – Near Acuity: The Warren Text Card*[2]

Description

The Warren Text Card test is a subtest of the Brain Injury Visual Assessment Battery for Adults (biVABA). The client reads down the lines of text on the Warren Test Card as far as he or she can, and the acuity is recorded for the last line read accurately. The Warren Text Card is designed so the sentences can be read at the fifth grade level of reading.

Scoring

Snellen fraction equivalents are given for each line.

Test 3 – Pepper Visual Skills for Reading Test[36]

Description

The Pepper Visual Skills for Reading Test (VSRT) provides an accurate and reliable estimate of the client's ability in the visual components of the reading process. It is primarily designed for use with clients with macular disease, which creates central scotomas, which inhibits reading ability. The VSRT measures the following components skills:

1. Visual word recognition ability
2. Saccadic and return sweep eye movement control
3. How well the client can position the central scotoma so that it does not obscure the field of view necessary for reading

The test is arranged in order of difficulty, timed, and individually administered in approximately 10 to 15 minutes. It contains 15 rigid cards printed in size 5 prints. The cards have unrelated letters and words on them.

Scoring

The VSRT provides both accuracy (mean percentage corrected for each completed line) and rate (correct words per minute) measures. The types of errors made are also recorded.

---

*The results of this test can be used 1) to make sure all written materials used by the client (ie, instructions, home programs, etc) will be at the right size of print and 2) to determine if magnification is needed and, if so, how much.[2]

Validity

Correlation measures between the VSRT and Gray Oral Reading Test were taken. Pearson-product moment correlation for the reading rates of both tests was 0.82 (p < 0.05).

Reliability

Pearson-product moment correlation for accuracy measures was 0.90 (p < 0.01). Pearson-product moment correlation for rate scores was 0.97 (p < 0.01).

Test 4 – Distance Visual Acuity*[7]

Purpose

To test clearness of vision at distance

Vision Problems Detected

Loss of vision, reduced vision due to uncorrected refractive condition (myopia, hyperopia, astigmatism), amblyopia (lazy eye), etc

Control

Habitual glasses for distance, if worn by client. Client may be seated or standing at the appropriate distance from the chart (varies with each other). Make sure lighting is adequate.

Equipment

Distance acuity chart (Snellen, pictures, tumbling E, Broken Wheel) occluded

Procedure

Test the right eye first; occlude the left eye. Ask the client to read the smallest letters (or picture). If the client reads the line correctly, proceed to the next smaller line. Do not allow the client to squint. Encourage "guessing." If the client has difficulty, isolate letters. Continue until the client misses a letter. Once completed, switch occluder to right eye and test left eye, then both eyes. Always watch the client, not the chart.

Recording

Write down the ratio listed next to the smallest line read. If the client missed any letters on that line, record the ratio minus the number of letters missed (eg, if the client read four of six letters on the 20/20 line, record as 20/20-2). If the client must move to ten feet to read off a chart meant to be used at 20 feet, record as test distance/smallest line read (eg, if client could see the 20/100 letters at 10 feet, record as 10/100).

Retest/Referral

Client should be able to read at least 20/30 with each eye. 20/40 acuity or worse is a referral.

Test 5 – Dynamic Visual Acuity

Information on Dynamic Visual Acuity evaluation is contained in the section on Visual Vestibular Processing.

TREATMENT OF IMPAIRED VISUAL ACUITY

If screening indicates impairment, initiate a referral to an ophthalmologist or optometrist for continued evaluation, prescription lens, or additional treatment, as needed.

Utilizing an Adaptive Approach

If acuity cannot be corrected with lenses, utilize enlarged print, control the density of presented stimuli, and utilize contrast and lighting. Adapt the environment or functional task as needed to increase the client's independence and create a safe environment in which he or she can function.

Adaptations

1. For example, suggest to the client that he or she could use prechopped or premeasured food ingredients, wrinkle free clothing, computerized banking, etc.[3]

2. Enlarge objects whenever possible. For instance, transfer small packages of foods (eg, macaroni, cereal, etc) to large, clear storage containers, and relabel with large print.

3. Utilize larger print watches, calculators, cards, etc.[3] Utilize low vision magnifiers, magnifying mirrors, etc.[19]

4. When deciding how much to enlarge print for the client, "...the last line that is easily read on the reading acuity test card indicates the minimum size for which to enlarge print for the client."[3] Provide a copy of this card to the client, family, and/or caregiver to use as a guide for future adaptations to printed material the client will be using at home. This is especially important if a home visit is not possible.

5. If the client appears to have difficulty processing visually under conditions of low illumination, provide environmental adaptation as follows[3]: Increase light with minimum glare through halogen or fluorescent lighting. Reduce shadows by avoiding single bulb or recessed lighting. Filters or absorptive lenses can be incorporated into prescription lenses. Nonglare paper or a sheet of yellow acetate can be placed over a page of print. Visors and side shields can also be used if glare is a problem. For near tasks, the light should be placed on the side of the best eye or opposite the working hand. Place the light to provide full, even illumination without areas of surface shadow.

6. Elderly clients require more light to see, and often TBI clients are light sensitive. Therefore, use a light that can be adjusted.[21]

7. Motion lights that turn on automatically when someone enters a room or dark hallway can help prevent falls.

8. When the client is utilizing a computer, use software that has zoom lens capabilities to magnify text or graphics.[37]

9. To compensate for visual loss, utilize the remaining sensory systems (hearing, tactile discrimination, kinesthesia, proprioception) to assist in increased function.[29] Also, have the client rely on language to interpret form and space.[38]

10. Provide treatment in a variety of contextually relevant environments.

11. Applying an occupational performance frame of reference, identify the areas of occupational performance which are affected by the changes in visual performance. Warren outlines five key areas that are addressed in the treatment plan[29]:

a) Efficient and effective use of optical devices to read materials needed for daily living

b) Ability to write legibly to complete communications needed for daily living

c) Ability to complete financial transactions and manage financial affairs independently

d) Ability to complete self-care and homemaking activities with optimum efficiency, independence, and safety

e) Ability to engage in leisure and community activities

Contrast Sensitivity

Reduced contrast sensitivity can affect both the client's independence and performance of ADLs. Contrast sensitivity, which is also sometimes referred to as low contrast acuity, contributes to the CNS's ability to detect and recognize objects.[3] Impaired contrast sensitivity can often result in impairment in the ability to recognize faces and objects.[21] Contrast can be defined as "...the degree of blackness to whiteness of a target or the luminance level of an object when compared with the luminance of its surrounding background."[5] The normal eye has a maximum contrast sensitivity at midrange spatial frequencies and is less sensitive to higher and lower spatial frequencies.[33]

Contrast sensitivity can be impaired despite normal performance on traditional acuity tests, such as the Snellen Acuity test.[5] Often, the client who tests normally on traditional acuity tests may complain of a feeling that his or her vision is not quite right.[39] Decreased contrast sensitivity can occur in conjunction with other visual impairments.[2] Testing it tells us about the quality of the client's available vision and has become recognized as an important tool for measuring functional visual changes.[5,21] Its testing helps determine the client's ability to distinguish borders, as for example seeing coffee in a dark cup.[40] As Warren states, "...by measuring acuity over a range of frequencies, contrast sensitivity function testing provides a more comprehensive assessment of the person's visual capacity."[26]

Contrast sensitivity testing uses targets made up of sine-wave gratings, and the client's ability to detect these gratings at different degrees of contrast is assessed.[5,33] The gratings may be computer generated or specially designed charts such as the Lea Numbers and Lea Symbols Low Contrast Chart or the Pelli-Robson Chart.[3] The Pelli-Robson chart was designed "...to discriminate normal from abnormal peak contrast sensitivity and has been found to be highly effective in detecting pathology without the need to test contrast sensitivity at individual spatial frequencies."[33]

EVALUATION OF CONTRAST SENSITIVITY

Test 1 – Lea Numbers and Lea Symbols, Low Contrast Tests[21,41]

Description

The client is asked to match pictures or numbers at each contrast level. Testing can be done at both distance and near.

Test 2 – Functional Acuity Contrast Test[21]

Description

The tester shows the client sample gratings at the bottom of a chart, which are labeled left, right, up, and blank. The client starts at the top of the chart and, with one eye occluded, identifies the orientation of the test stimuli from left to right in each of the five rows.

TREATMENT OF IMPAIRED CONTRAST SENSITIVITY

Utilizing an Adaptive Approach

If the client appears to have difficulty with visual processing under conditions of low contrast, provide environmental adaptations as follows.[3,6,42-44]

1. Use different colors for better contrast (ie, no white napkins on a white tablecloth).

2. Black on white or white on black print is better than any other combination.

3. Change background color to contrast with an object (ie, black mug for milk).

4. Utilize solid colors for rugs, bedspreads, dishes, countertops, etc. Patterns can blend with the background and cause decreased object identification.

5. Decrease clutter in the environment (ie, cabinets, closets, countertops, etc). Self-threading needles and magnetic padlocks that do not require a combination can also help.

6. For writing, bold tip pens or markers can be used to make large letters. Bold line paper, stand magnifiers, closed circuit televisions that provide magnification of the writing area, typewriters, and computers can all be used as needed.

7. Use bright tape on stairs, bright paint on doors and cabinets, and bright labels on prescriptions, canned goods, etc. Use light walls with dark furniture, light switch plugs, and electrical outlets. Vertical blinds and shades can help control the amount of light in the room.

Ocular Alignment

Ocular alignment is crucial to the coordinated function of both eyes and visual processing in general. Normal alignment of the eyes is guaranteed by a normally functioning sensory and motor fusion system.[45] The motor system that moves the eye is accomplished by six muscles and controlled by three cranial nerves. Therefore, for both eyes together, there are 12 muscles and six cranial nerves.[1] Injury to any of these muscles or nerves can affect ocular alignment. These 12 extraocular muscles are responsible for aligning the eyes, allowing them to be pointed at the same object, and moving the eyes to different positions of gaze.[1] This allows for ongoing perception of a single image.

As just described, damage to the six cranial nerves associated with the oculomotor system can cause ocular deviation. Deviation from cranial nerve palsies "…is often initially noncomitant or variable in different directions of gaze."[1] Often, more deviation is present when looking to the side of the affected muscle.[1] In addition to lesions affecting the individual cranial nerves and muscles, brainstem lesions affecting the medial longitudinal fasciculus (MLF) can cause ocular misalignment.[1]

The term used for the condition in which the eyes are misaligned is called strabismus. The three most common types of strabismus are esotropia (eyes turning in) exotropia (eyes turn out) and hypertropia (one eye turns up).[21] A strabismus is "comitant" if the eye of the strabismus remains relatively constant in all nine positions of gaze.[8,21] The size of the strabismus is not compared from one distance to another. It is compared from one position of gaze to another at the same distance. If the strabismus is intermittent, then at least a portion of the time, the client has binocular vision.[21] With intermittent strabismus, the client alternately switches use to the right or left eye or suppresses just the right or left eye.[8] Newly acquired strabismus as the result of ABI is usually noncomitant (ie, eye turn changes depend on the direction in which the eyes are looking).[8] When ocular deviation is relatively even in primary and reading gaze, prisms can be used to move the image to compensate for misalignment.[1]

If both eyes are not aligned, the client may close one eye, ask for a patch, or develop an awkward head turn to reduce symptoms. The awkward head position compensates so that the client does not have to use the action of the paralyzed muscle.[2,21] The client may experience double vision (diplopia), vertigo, confusion, clumsiness, motion sickness, and/or poor spatial judgment.[8,49]

EVALUATION OF OCULAR ALIGNMENT

Test 1 – Hirschberg Technique[46]

Procedure

Client fixates on a penlight held directly in front of him. Observe the reflection of the light on the corneas of both eyes.

Scoring

If the eyes are evenly aligned, the reflection will appear in the same location in each pupil.

> *Esotropia*—One eye is deviated inward; the reflection will occur on the lateral aspect of the pupil in that eye
>
> *Exotropia*—The reflection will be observed on the medial side of the pupil

Test 2 – Scheiman Alignment Screening*[21]

Equipment Needed

1. Eye alignment Near Card (Figure 3-2)
2. Disposable penlight
3. Red Maddox Rod

Setup and Testing Strategy

As with acuity testing for adults with cognitive and perceptual problems, it is wise to test at near before distance. It is easier to hold the client's attention and teach the procedure at near than at far. Positioning is important, and the occupational therapist should try to find the positioning that best permits the client to attend and concentrate on the task. For binocular vision testing, the client's head ideally will be vertically erect.

Procedure

1. Hold the Maddox Rod, a lens with striations, in front of the right eye with the lines oriented horizontally, and ask the client to look at a penlight and tell you what he or she sees. He or she should see a vertical line passing directly through the light. If the client cannot see this, the test cannot be used.
2. Hold the eye Alignment Near Card at 16 inches.
3. Hold the penlight behind the card, and direct the light through the hole in the center of the card.
4. Ask the client to tell you which number the vertical line is passing through, or the client can simply point to the number through which the line is passing. This measures the horizontal alignment of the eye. For example, if a client reports that the vertical line is seen three spaces to the left of the center, it represents a 3-prism diopter exophoria.
5. Now orient the Maddox Rod with the vertical lines.

*Reprinted with permission from Scheiman M. Understanding and Managing Vision Deficits. Thorofare, NJ: SLACK Incorporated; 1997:96. Equipment needed may be purchased from the Bernell Corp, 750 Lincolnway East, PO Box 4637, Southbend IN 46634; 1-800-348-2225, www.bernell.com

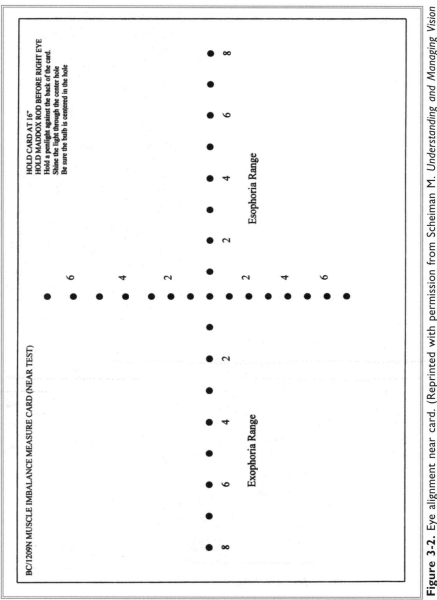
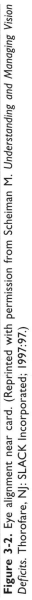

Figure 3-2. Eye alignment near card. (Reprinted with permission from Scheiman M. *Understanding and Managing Vision Deficits*. Thorofare, NJ: SLACK Incorporated; 1997:97.)

6. Ask the client to tell you which number the horizontal line is passing through, or have the client simply point to the number through which the line is passing. This measures the vertical alignment of the eyes. For example, if a client reports that the horizontal line is seen three spaces above the center, it represents a 3-prism diopter right hyperphoria.

Expected Findings and Possible Responses

An acceptable response at near is any number between 0 and 7 exophoria and 0 and 3 esophoria. If the amount of exophoria or esophoria is greater than these amounts, a referral is indicated. Any vertical phoria is significant.

TREATMENT OF DEFICITS IN EYE ALIGNMENT

There are numerous underlying causes of decreased eye alignment. If the screening indicated a problem, a referral should be made to an optometrist, ophthalmologist, or vision specialist.

Utilizing a Restorative Approach

1. If it is established by the optometrist, ophthalmologist, or vision specialist that the problem is due to a muscle imbalance, then eye exercises can be initiated. Active range of motion exercises should be done in the direction of the paresis (Warren, personal communication).

2. If the client is experiencing double vision, provide a) occlusion and b) activities to obtain fusion. For example, provide a control target at the distance the client can obtain fusion. Gradually move the target away to have the client maintain fusion at a further distance.

3. Integrate the techniques from numbers 1 and 2 into ADLs. When you have established the distance the client can maintain fusion, place clock, menus, etc at that distance and alter as the client improves.

Visual Fields

An individual's visual field is the area of the visual system that allows him or her to orient to specific spatial areas.[8] It is the field of view of the external world that is viewed by both eyes without turning the head.[19,47] The visual fields ensure that the CNS receives complete information and, in essence, reflects the underlying function of the receptor cells in the retina.[2,3] Intact visual fields are dependent on first, the distribution and integrity of the retinal receptors, and second, the integrity of the visual pathway from the optic nerve to the occipital area.[5] Kelly describes the visual fields as follows[47]:

> *The axons from the retina exit toward the optic disc, which is the region where they become myelinated and join other axons to form the optic nerve. The optic nerves from each eye join at the optic chiasm. There, fibers destined for particular regions in the brain stem are sorted out. This sorting process can best be understood in terms of the visual fields, or the way in which the visual world is projected on the retina.*

The fovea, or area of greatest acuity, is surrounded by the macular area of the field. This area is referred to as the central visual field.[2,48]

The fovea is the area most sensitive to illumination and can perceive small dimly lit targets.[2] On the other hand, "...as an object in space is positioned so that it falls on points further and further from the fovea (more peripherally on the retina), it must become either larger and/or brighter in order to be discerned."[48] The central field area is thought to extend about 5 degrees around the point of fixation.[48] This area is strongly involved in reading and other close work. The area of space beyond the central or perifoveal field is defined as the peripheral field.[48] The peripheral field is highly responsive to motion, while the central field has a low responsiveness to motion.[48]

Peripheral and central vision are both required for a full field of vision. Impaired peripheral field vision will affect safety for ambulation, awareness of the environment, and safe driving.[11] An impairment of the central visual field, especially the fovea, may cause the client to poorly identify visual details and can affect functional performance for areas such as reading.[26] An inferior field loss has been linked to decreased balance, decreased mobility, difficulty seeing steps or curbs, short strides, walking near walls and using them for balance, and difficulty identifying visual land-marks.[8] A superior visual field cut has been associated with problems seeing signs, decreased reading and writing ability, and decreased check writing.[8] If the visual field loss is on the same side as the client's dominant hand, then he or she may have problems guiding the hand in fine motor activities.[3] This can manifest functionally in a reduction of writing legibility.[3] Additional common behavioral changes associated with visual field deficits are a narrowing of the scope of scanning, slow scanning towards the blind side, and decreased visual monitoring of the hand.[2] Visual search into the blind field is usually slow and delayed.[3] The client, in fact, often "…turns the head very little and limits visual search to areas immediately adjacent to the seeing side of the body."[3]

Functional deficits associated with visual field loss are numerous and diverse. Warren identifies the following four factors, which will influence whether field loss will affect overall function[6]:

1. *Whether the field cut is homonymous or congruous in each eye*

2. *The contour of the boundary between the sound and scoptic field (ie, if the boundary is abrupt, the client has more difficulty compensating)*

3. *The presence of a central field cut*

4. *Client's awareness of the field cut*

The types of common visual field deficits and associated lesion sites are illustrated in Figure 3-3.

EVALUATION OF VISUAL FIELDS

An individual's visual field is measured in degrees with the center of fixation serving as the zero referent.[1] The normal monocular field of vision is approximately 60 degrees upward, 60 degrees inward, 70 to 75 degrees downward, and 100 to 110 degrees outward. The type of deficit the client sustains depends on location and size of the lesion. Deficits may include homonymous hemianopias, quadrantanopias, and/or scotomas (areas of decreased sensitivity).[149] Visual fields deficits may be seen in clients with or without associated visual neglect. Clients do generally exhibit small saccadic eye movements, decreased speed of scanning (particularly with saccades toward the impaired field), and a narrower scope of scanning.[6,31]

Visual fields may be evaluated by confrontation testing, which is a gross measure, or perimetry, which is a more refined method. The major advantage of confrontation testing is that it requires no elaborate device.[1] Perimetry testing can require two different types of devices depending on the type of perimetry evaluation being performed. For kinetic perimetry evaluation, the stimulus presented to the client is a spot of light of a specific size and intensity that is moved towards the center of fixation until the client indicates that he or she sees it.[1] Static perimetry testing utilizes a static device that measures the client's visual fields by increasing the brightness of a spot at a fixed location until the client indicates that he or she sees it.[1] Whether perimetry testing is static or dynamic, it involves three parameters. As outlined by Warren, these are 1) fixation on a central target by the client while the testing is completed, 2) presentation of a target of a specific size in a designated area of the visual field, and 3) acknowledgement of the target by the client.[2]

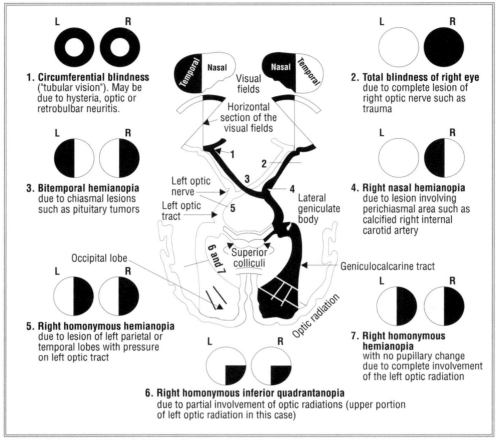

Figure 3-3. Visual field deficits and associated lesion sites.

As previously mentioned, confrontation testing is considered to be a gross measurement of the client's visual fields. Some clinicians, however, feel that confrontation testing is a readily available technique that can detect significant defects such as central scotomas, altitudinal defects, and hemianopias.[33] However, some neurologists, optometrists, and ophthalmologists may reject confrontation testing results because they consider them to be insensitive.[21] The therapist should keep this in mind when utilizing confrontation testing and use the results as a way to "rule in" a visual field problem but not completely rule one out.[21] Findings should be reported as "visual fields are grossly intact on confrontation testing." In addition, the therapist should evaluate and report any indications of potential field loss picked up through clinical observations of the client during functional activities. For example, the client changing head position when asked to look at something placed in a certain visual plane, the client consistently bumping into objects on one side, misplacing objects in one field, or consistent errors in reading.[3] As Warren states, "...consistent paralexic reading errors, such as missing or misreading the beginning or ends of words or misreading numbers, may indicate the presence of a central field scotoma."[2]

In response to the concern that confrontation testing can be insensitive, some clinicians have switched from testing with a single examiner to having two examiners.[2,21] These clinicians believe the client will truly be responding to the perception of the target versus the examiner's arm movements during testing.[21] With this method, one examiner presents the targets from behind the client while the other monitors the client's fixation.[21]

Test 1 – Confrontation Testing*[21]

Set-Up and Testing Strategy

The client must be seated opposite the examiner, and it is important to position the client so that the head is vertical. Confrontation field testing is not necessary in children who have not experienced head trauma. It is suggested that it be reserved for adults and children with ABI. Although this is a significant test to attempt when dealing with such clients, it is important to remember that good fixation ability and a high level of concentration and attention are necessary. If these skills are not present, this testing will not be possible.

The underlying concept when doing confrontation field testing is that you compare your own visual field to the client's visual field. Specifically, if you can see the target that you are presenting, then the client should be able to see it.

Equipment Needed

1. Two eye patches

2. A target (white sphere, 3 mm or less in diameter, mounted on a nonglossy wand)

Procedure

Step I

1. Place an eye patch over the client's left eye and an eye patch over your right eye.

2. Sit opposite the client so that your left eye is directly opposite the client's right eye. You should be about 20 inches from the client. It is preferable that the background for the client be dark and uniform.

3. Explain that you will be moving the target from the side, and the client should report as soon as he or she sees it while looking directly at your left eye.

4. Begin at the 12 o'clock position, and slowly move the target down until the client first reports seeing it. Compare the client's response to yours. If the client cannot see the target as soon as you can, it is an indication of a possible problem.

5. Move clockwise to the 2, 4, 6, 8, and 10 o'clock positions, and repeat step 4.

6. Record approximately where the client reports seeing the target in each orientation tested.

7. Place the eye patch over the client's right eye and an eye patch over your left eye.

8. Sit opposite the client so that your right eye is directly opposite the client's left eye and repeat steps 3 through 6.

Step II

9. Place an eye patch over the client's left eye and an eye patch over your right eye. Sit opposite the client so that your left eye is directly opposite the client's right eye.

10. Now extend both your right and left hands in the 3 and 9 o'clock positions simultaneously. Place your fingers so that you can just see them from your open eye. Ask the client to tell you how many fingers you are holding up with each hand.

11. Place the eye patch over the client's right eye and an eye patch over your left eye. Sit opposite the client so that your right eye is directly opposite the client's left eye, and repeat step 10.

Reprinted with permission from Scheiman M. Understanding and Managing Vision Deficits. *Thorofare, NJ: SLACK Incorporated; 1997:110-111.*

Expected Findings and Possible Responses

In step I, the client should be able to see the target at approximately the same point at which you can see it. If there appears to be a significant discrepancy, a visual field deficit may be present, and a referral is necessary for a more precise measurement of the client's visual field.

In step II, you are testing the client's ability to see two objects simultaneously. Clients with visual neglect will have problems with this task even if they do well in step I.

Test 2 – Damato 30-Point Multifixation Campimeter

Description

This test was developed by Bertil Damato MD, PhD and is incorporated as a subtest of the biV-ABA.* The test uses a series of numbered fixation targets to move the client's eye in a controlled manner, which places the test stimulus at known points in the visual field.[2]

TREATMENT OF VISUAL FIELDS DEFICITS

Treatment of visual field deficits should be undertaken if it has been established that the field cut impacts the client's performance with ADLs. Although the primary method of treatment falls under the adaptive realm, restorative methods can also be effective, especially when used in conjunction with the adaptive approach.** For example, utilizing scanning worksheets at the beginning of a treatment session as a "warm up" followed by scanning activities that involve functional tasks can be very effective. Oftentimes, this can be a useful way for the client to begin to make the connection of how his or her visual field cut is affecting functional performance.

For the client with severe cognitive impairments, it is crucial to educate the family and/or caregiver about the client's visual field deficit and how it affects function. Be sure to discuss how it will affect safety issues at home and in the community. In addition, low functioning cognitive clients may not be able to benefit from traditional methods and may have to rely on optometric techniques such as mirrors and yoked prisms.

Utilizing a Restorative Approach

1. Work with the client on establishing an effective search strategy.[3] Warren outlines the following components of an effective search strategy[3]:

   ◆ Initiation of a wide head turn towards the blind field

   ◆ An increase in the number of head and eye movements toward the blind field

   ◆ Execution of an organized and efficient search pattern that begins on the blind side

   ◆ Attention to and detection of visual detail on the blind side

   ◆ Ability to quickly shift attention and search between the central visual field and the peripheral visual field on the blind side

2. Have the client start his or her search strategy in the hemianopic field and then carry it out in a circular fashion into the general environment.[3] Scheiman applies this concept in the following activity[21]:

   Place 15 to 20 numbers, letters, or other targets randomly on the side of a full-size chalkboard corresponding to the client's field defect. The client is centrally positioned in front of and at least 10 feet from the board and locates targets with a

---

*The biVABA is published and distributed by VisAbilities Inc, Hoover, Ala (http://www.visabilities.com).
**Recent research has demonstrated that Vision Restitution Therapy (VRT) induced visual field enlargement as well as having an effect on color and pattern recognition.[50] In addition, the use of a visuospatial cue to focus attention at areas of residual vision showed even greater restoration of vision.[44]

flashlight that are called out by another person. As the client gains mastery of this task, the board is erased and new targets are written, still mainly in the affected hemifield but with some on the unaffected side. The client is first instructed to scan the board in a circular manner as Warren recommends and then to "pay more attention" to the affected side during the task. Gradually, the targets are evenly distributed between the two sides. The same type of activity can be accomplished at near with targets linearly arranged and the clients locating specified numbers or letters with a pencil in the same manner (ie, with targets first being contained on the side of the compromised field and gradually distributing them so that an equal number appear in both fields).

3. Reinforce strategy search with games such as concentration or checkers.[3]

4. Place a bedside table, comb, newspaper, and any commonly used objects on the side of poor vision, forcing the client to look to that side.

5. Provide verbal, auditory (bell, finger snapping), and tactile cuing to encourage the client to look to the affected field of vision.

6. Practice worksheets as described in the treatment of visual scanning and unilateral neglect. Warren's prereading and writing exercises for clients with macular scotomas can also be used.[3]

7. Provide the client with computer retraining, utilizing software specifically designed for the remediation of visual field deficits.*

8. Work on increased speed and accuracy of eye movements. Utilize walking during scanning tasks, or other forms of movement to integrate vision, movement, and perception.[8] Aloisio states, "...planning routes verbally and visually assists the client in alert thinking and 'going into' the deficit area."[8]

Utilizing an Adaptive Approach

1. In order to adapt or compensate for his or her impaired field of vision, the client must be aware of the problem and how it is affecting function. The therapist can assist the client in developing this awareness through prompting or cuing during functional activities. Initial prompting questions might be "What part of this activity gave you the most problems?" As the client progresses, provide cues such as "Where would I be telling you to look if I were to do so?"[21]

2. Place all necessary items for functional independence within the client's field of vision.

3. Educate the client and his or her family about the client's field loss and how it will potentially affect function. Situations where safety may be a problem should be covered.

4. If possible, have the client identify his or her own compensation strategies and provide a variety of tasks that allow the client to apply these strategies. Carry out the tasks in a variety of contexts or environments.

5. For reading, utilize anchoring techniques and a ruler or straight edge under each line of text. An L shaped marker with Velcro can also be used so the client can feel where the boundaries are.[21] For writing, have the client watch the tip of the pen and maintain that fixation as his or her hand moves across the page.[3]

6. Add color and contrast to door frames and furniture to help the client be able to locate them.[3]

---

* The use of computer retraining for visual field deficits remains controversial and should be used in conjunction with other approaches. Its effectiveness with the client should be monitored closely.

Oculomotor Control

Oculomotor control is crucial to the efficient processing of visual information. The underlying neural system for oculomotor function is extensive and, therefore, vulnerable to trauma.[34] The parts of the brain that control eye movement is called the oculomotor system. This system places the fovea on target and keeps it there long enough for the individual to process what he or she sees.[51] This is accomplished by five separate neural control centers, which include saccadic eye movements, smooth pursuit movement, optokinetic movement, vestibulo-oculomotor reflex, and vergence movement.[8,51] All these systems have different neural controls but have a common final path.[45]

As just described, oculomotor function brings images of an object onto the fovea and keeps the image there for visual processing. This is accomplished by two different types of eye movements. The first group includes saccadic eye movements, quick phases of nystagmus, rapid eye movements that are used to change the line of sight quickly, and vergence.[52] Although vergence movements are slower, they do bring the images of a single object onto the foveae of both eyes at the same time, which allows for stereopsis.[52]

The second group of eye movements are those that keep the image on the fovea for a sufficient amount of time for visual processing. The image must be "…kept there quietly for enough time (perhaps 100 ms or so) for the visual system to be able to analyze the new information and to determine the nature of the object of interest and its depth and motion."[52] The group of eye movements that performs this function includes 1) vestibular and optokinetic movements, which compensate for head movements; 2) pursuit movements, which allows the individual to keep objects that are moving in the environment on the fovea; and 3) vergence, which keeps images on both foveae at the same time.[55]

Binocular vision is also accomplished through the functioning of the oculomotor system. Binocular vision "…ensures perception of a single image even though the CNS is receiving two separate visual images (one from each eye)."[3] Oculomotor control allows for efficient conjugate movements. Conjugate movements are those movements when both eyes move together in the same direction.[53] Disjunctive movements are those eye movements that move in opposite directions, such as convergence or divergence.[53] All five oculomotor control systems must move the eyes precisely together to accomplish and maintain binocular vision.[53]

Oculomotor deficits are common after brain damage and can vary depending on the size and location of the lesion or injury. There may be the presence of a dynamic abnormality such as nystagmus or strabismus.[34]

Decreased oculomotor control results in slower speed, control, and coordination of eye movements with a subsequent disruption of visual scanning and attention.[3,6] Deficits can severely impair the client's ability to effectively scan his environment and, in turn, devastate him functionally. During activities, the client may squint, tilt his or her head, shut one eye and complain of headaches, or fatigue, or become agitated during certain tasks.[26] Deficits in eye movement are termed ocular motility disorders or eye movement disorders. Oculomotor control disorders can be divided into three areas: fixation stability, saccadic function, and pursuit function.[21]

Additional deficits that commonly occur with ABI are diplopia, or double vision, and nystagmus, or involuntary rhythmic oscillations of one or both eyes. The evaluation and treatment of diplopia is covered in this section, and information related to nystagmus is covered in the section titled Visual Vestibular Processing.

Visual Fixation

The ability to visually attend is present in elementary form at birth and matures by 4 weeks. For the normal adult, visual fixation is a voluntary act. The normal adult has no difficulty in selecting objects within his environment and focusing his gaze upon them. Steady fixation is the result of a complex motor act for which several movements contribute.[45] During fixation "...afferent sensory input from the retina is used to elicit appropriate efferent signals to the extraocular muscles to maintain eye position."[45] Fixation is maintained presumably by suppressing any conscious saccadic eye movements; however, during steady fixation on a target, there are continuous, unconscious small movements of the eyes, characterized as slow drifts and quick flicks. Gouras states as follows[53]:

> *The drifts move the fovea over a target of interest; the flicks are small saccades that return the fovea to a target, as often a drift carries it too far away. Because of the flicks, there is no net displacement of the target. We are able to continue seeing objects only if their edges are continuously moving on the retina.*

The "field of fixation" can be defined as the area within which central fixation can be accomplished by moving the eye but not the head.[45] The practical field of fixation, on the other hand, is the field of fixation that can be accomplished by moving both the eyes and the head as in "casual seeing."[45]

The adult ABI client may have difficulty in visually attending to objects within the environment. The deficit may be an inability to obtain fixation or the inability to sustain it. It may be associated with or occur separately from spatial or body neglect or inattention. Poor fixation will result in off task behavior that can give the impression that the client is inattentive or impulsive.[8]

EVALUATION FOR VISUAL FIXATION

Test 1 – Warren[6]

Procedure

Evaluate the client's ability to locate and fixate on a target in various locations within the visual fields as follows. Present target first at midline and then to the right and left of midline at near (16 to 20 inches) and middle (21 to 36 inches) focal distances.

Scoring

Client should be able to locate the target, fixate on it, and maintain fixation for several seconds.

TREATMENT FOR VISUAL FIXATION

1. Treatment for visual fixation is generally addressed with scanning due to their close connection (Warren, personal communication). Tasks can include letter recognition through reading, progressing to more difficult tasks such as paragraph reading.

2. If the client cannot fixate and do other activities such as walking at the same time, work on fixation while the client is sitting or laying down and progress to walking.[21]

Saccadic Eye Movements

Saccadic eye movements are sequenced rapid eye movements that change the line of sight. The saccadic eye movement system is responsible for rapidly directing the fovea to a target of interest in visual space.[53] Saccades keep the CNS updated on all objects within the visual field.[2] They are "...the movements that take us from word to word in reading and from object to object in driving."[12] In fact, as Abrams surmises, if we could understand the process involved in planning and controlling saccadic eye movements, then maybe it would help us understand the process related to reading and scanning the environment.[54] Saccades allow the individual to inspect some previously uninspected part of the environment.[54] Visual stimuli that reach the periphery of the retina and attract our attention will elicit saccadic eye movements.[55] The saccade will place the image on the fovea and keep it there as long as the image attracts our attention. The importance of saccadic eye movements can be summarized as follows[56]:

> *When we move our eyes, the image of the visual world shifts on our retina, yet we are nevertheless able to maintain a stable percept of visual space. This spatial constancy across saccadic eye movements is a basic function of visuospatial perception and a prerequisite for an accurate localization of visual targets in space.*

Saccades are extremely fast, occurring several times a second and, once initiated, are extremely difficult to correct.[53,54] The duration of a small saccadic is about 20 ms and increases to about 100 ms for very large movements.[57] Saccadic eye movements are largely controlled by the pontine gaze center.[53] In addition, frontal areas are involved with the temporal aspects of saccades, and the posterior parietal cortex is involved in the spatial programming.[56] Reflex saccades are associated with parietal lobe function, and voluntary saccades are associated with frontal structure.[52] Saccadic accuracy is often impaired with cerebellar disorders, with the main deficit of overshooting.[58,59] Clients with parietal lobe damage sometimes are unable to break fixation and look away from what they are looking at.[57] In other words, they are unable to generate saccades. Frontal lobe damage, on the other hand, can cause an inability for the client to suppress saccades even when instructed to look to the opposite side of a suddenly appearing visual stimulus.[40] Bilateral frontal lesions can result in the client having difficulty with rapidly alternating his or her gaze between two stationary targets.[50] Damage to oculomotor neurons, oculomotor nerves, and oculomotor muscles causes slowing of saccades "...when the paretic muscle is the agonist required to generate the sudden force necessary to move the globe rapidly."[59] Slowing of saccadic eye movements can actually be caused by lesions anywhere in the central pathways involved in their generation.[58]

EVALUATION OF SACCADIC EYE MOVEMENT

The quality, speed, and accuracy of saccadic eye movements should all be assessed.[21] Tests of saccadic eye movements can include direct observation by the therapist, timed or standardized tests involving a visual verbal procedure, and objective eye movement recording using electro-oculographic instruments.[21] The primary methods appropriate for saccadic screening by the occupational therapist are direct observation and/or timed tests. Following are descriptions of these methods.

Test 1 – Northeastern State University College of Optometry[8,21]

Description

Two penpal fixators are held 16 inches from the client's face, 4 inches from his or her midline and separated horizontally about 8 inches. The examiner states, "When I say red, look at the red target. When I say green, look at the green target. Remember, do not look until I tell you." The client is asked to look from one target to another for five round trips for a total of 10 fixations.[21]

Scoring

Clinical observation of accuracy, head or body movement, and overall ability are scored. For example, does it take one eye movement to reach the target or more than one? Can the client complete five round trips? Specific scoring criteria for this screening as well as a minimum score to pass for ability, accuracy, and head movement have been established by Northeastern State University College of Optometry (NSUCO).

For further information on this test and scoring, the reader is referred to the references.

Test 2 – Developmental Eye Movement Test[23]

Description

This test consists of three subtests (subtests A and B are considered together for the vertical component and subtest C in the horizontal component). For subtests A and B, the client is asked to read numbers down two columns as quickly as possible, and for subtest C, he or she is asked to read the numbers across the rows as quickly as possible. Figure 3-4 shows the test stimulus used for subtest C of the Developmental Eye Movement Test (DEM).

Scoring

The vertical time score is generated by adding completion times of subtests A and B. Horizontal time score is calculated with a formula of the time and the omission and/or transposition errors. These numbers are compared to normative data, which was generated from a sample of children ages 6 to 13. Even though normative data is only available up to age 13, the test can be used with adults with ABI because only limited additional improvement is expected in performance on this test with increased age.[21] The adult with ABI should perform at least as well as the top level norms.[21]

Validity

1. Raw scores indicated a variation in scores as a function of age (ie, increased age with increased time and errors).

2. Internal consistency—Correlation coefficients between the components of the DEM (significant at $p < 0.001$)

3. Correlation coefficients between the subcomponents of the DEM and the Wide Range Achievement Test (WRAT) administered to 58 randomly selected children ($p < 0.001$)

4. Comparison of scores of performance between normal and learning disabled children (40 of each)

Reliability

1. Test-retest reliability was established by performing the DEM on two occasions 1 week apart with 40 subjects: vertical time $r = 0.89$ ($p < 0.001$), horizontal time $r = 0.86$ ($p < 0.001$) ratio $r = 0.57$ ($p < 0.01$).

Test C

3		7	5			9			8
2	5			7		4			6
1			4		7		6		3
7		9		3		9			2
4	5				2			1	7
5			3		7		4		8
7	4		6	5					2
9		2			3		6		4
6	3	2		9					1
7				4		6	5		2
5		3	7			4			8
4			5		2			1	7
7	9	3			9				2
1			4			7		6	3
2		5		7			4		6
3	7		5			9			8

Figure 3-4. Developmental Eye Movement (DEM) test.[23] (Reprinted with permission from Richman J, Garzia P. *Developmental Eye Movement Test.* Test booklet. South Bend, Ind: Bernell Corporation; 1987.)

2. Inter-rater reliability—two raters, 40 subjects: horizontal time $r = 0.91$ ($p < 0.001$), vertical time $r = 0.81$ ($p < 0.001$), ratio $r = 0.57$ ($p < 0.01$).

Test 3 – Pepper Visual Skills for Reading Test[36]

The Pepper Visual Skills for Reading Test (VRST) test is described in the section for the Evaluation of Visual Acuity on page 56.

TREATMENT OF SACCADIC EYE MOVEMENT DEFICITS

Utilizing a Restorative Approach

1. Have the client perform activities such as calling out or pointing to letters from two columns printed on either side of a page (Figure 3-5). To progress with the activity, the column of printed letters should be printed closer to the center of the page (Figure 3-6). This activity can be adapted further by placing the columns on a blackboard and changing the distance between the columns as the client progresses.

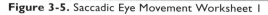

IF	TI
2N	U2
3P	P3
4V	X4
5R	A5
6M	W6
7H	F7
8O	B8
9S	Z9
10T	L10
11K	E11

Figure 3-5. Saccadic Eye Movement Worksheet 1

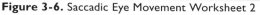

IX	CI
2M	T2
3A	W3
4F	B4
5O	L5
6Z	H6
7P	N7
8W	S8
9C	X9
10G	R10
11N	V11

Figure 3-6. Saccadic Eye Movement Worksheet 2

2. Provide vestibular-based movement activities in conjunction with demands for saccadic skills. For instance, have the client roll one-quarter turn and identify a number or letter that has been randomly placed on a suspended ball. Repeat the activity with a half turn, a three-quarter turn, and so on.

3. Provide computer retraining utilizing software designed specifically for the restoration of basic oculomotor deficits.

> *Utilizing an Adaptive Approach*
> 1. Provide anchoring during reading tasks.
> 2. Control the density of the visual information being presented.

Smooth Pursuit Eye Movements

Smooth pursuit eye movements are those movements that keep an image steady on the retina. They are limited in speed to 30 degrees per second and are complementary to the vestibulo-ocular reflex (VOR) in holding images stationary on the retina when an individual is moving.[12] This system works for stationary as well as moving objects and uses different processes for each kind of target.[53] Smooth pursuit movements or scanning allows us to follow a moving image or object across the visual field without compensatory head movement.[60] Whereas saccadic eye movements are utilized for activities such as reading, smooth pursuit movements are the type of eye movements used in activities such as watching a football in the air.[16]

Smooth pursuit movements are the motor expression of attention and require voluntary involvement or participation of the cerebral cortex.[59] Clients with temporal-occipital lesions or trauma are often unable to make accurate smooth pursuits, generally as a result of selective deficits in the detection of motion.[52] Clients with smooth pursuit deficits will also require the help of corrective saccadic eye movements to keep up with the target they are trying to maintain on the retina.[49,59] This jerky interruption of smooth pursuits is considered abnormal.

Warren describes well the overall function and mechanism of the smooth pursuit system as follows[2]:

> *The smooth pursuit system ensures that the target is maintained on the fovea during fixation and when the object is moving. If the eyes and the target are both stationary, the smooth pursuit system supplies continuous unconscious small eye movement, which move back and forth over the boundaries of the target to ensure that the target stays fresh on the retina and does not fade. If a target moves away and the viewer remains stationary, the target eventually will slip off of the retina and go out of focus. To prevent this, the smooth pursuit system initiates eye movement in the direction of the target's movement, the velocity of the target movement ensuring that the image stays focused on the fovea.*

EVALUATION OF SMOOTH PURSUIT MOVEMENTS

Test 1 – Direction of Gaze

Description

All six muscles that move each eye (the four rectus muscles—superior, inferior, lateral, and medial—and the two oblique muscles—superior and inferior) are tested. The therapist asks the client to "look first to one side and then to the other" to test the medial and lateral rectus muscles. While looking to the one side, the subject is instructed to look up and down; in this position, the adducted eye is elevated by the superior rectus muscle and depressed by the inferior muscle. The abducted eye is elevated by the inferior oblique muscle. Repeat the procedure with the opposite side to test the opposite muscles.

Scoring

Nonstandardized

> *Intact*—The client is able to direct his gaze in all directions as requested.

Impaired—The client is unable to direct his gaze in one or more directions requested. (Specify which movements are impaired.)

Unable to perform—The client is unable to direct his gaze in any direction as requested.

Validity

To improve validity, rule out aphasia and poor visual attentiveness as causes of poor performance.

Test 2 – Pursuits: Direct Observation Method—NSUCO Test[21]

Setup and Testing Strategy

If possible, the client should be standing with feet shoulder-width apart directly in front of the examiner. If the client cannot stand, try to position the client so that the head is erect and not supported in any way. If this is not possible, it is best to position the head vertically erect with support. The test is performed binocularly and is appropriate for clients who are at least 5 years of age.

Equipment Needed

One Pen-Pal Target

Procedure

1. Hold one Pen-Pal Target or another small, interesting target 16 inches from the client's face.

2. No instructions are given to the client to move or not to move his or her head.

3. Use the following instructional set: "Watch the ball as it goes around. Don't take your eyes off the ball."

4. Move the target clockwise for two rotations and counter-clockwise for two rotations.

5. Determine if the client can keep his or her attention under control to complete four rotations. Assign a score of 1 through 5 based on the scoring criteria in Table 3-4.

6. Observe the accuracy of the pursuit eye movements. Assign a score of 1 through 5 based on the scoring criteria in Table 3-4.

7. Observe if the client moves his or her head or body. Assign a score of 1 through 4 based on the scoring criteria in Table 3-4.

Expected Findings and Possible Responses

Table 3-4 lists the scoring criteria for direct observation of pursuits, and Table 3-5 lists the failure criteria findings.

Organized Scanning

EVALUATION OF ORGANIZED SCANNING

Test 1 – Scanboard Test*[2]

Description

This test was developed by Mary Warren MS, OTR in collaboration with members of the Occupational Therapy Department, Eye Foundation of Kansas City, 2300 Holmes Street, Kansas City, MO 64108.

This is a subtest of the biVABA, which is distributed by VisAbilities Rehab Inc, Hoover, Ala (http://www.visabilities. com).

Table 3-4

NSUCO Oculomotor Test Scoring Criteria for Direct Observation of Pursuits

Ability

Points	Observation
1	Cannot complete half rotation in either clockwise or counterclockwise direction
2	Completes half rotation in either direction
3	Completes one rotation in either direction but not two rotations
4	Completes two rotations in one direction but less than two rotations in the other direction
5	Completes two rotations in each direction

Accuracy
(Can the client accurately and consistently fixate so that no noticeable refixation is needed when doing pursuits?)

Points	Observation
1	No attempt to follow the target or requires greater than 10 refixations
2	Refixes 5 to 10 times
3	Refixes 3 to 4 times
4	Refixes 2 times or less
5	No refixations

Head and Body Movement
(Can the client accomplish the pursuit without moving his or her head?)

Points	Observation
1	Large movement of the head or body at any time
2	Moderate movement of the head or body at any time
3	Slight movement of the head or body (>50% of time)
4	Slight movement of the head or body (<50% of time)

Reprinted with permission from the Optometric Extension Program, reference 61: Maples WC, Atchley J, Ficklin T. Northeastern State University college of optometry's oculomotor norms. J Behav Optometrist. 1992;3:143-150.

Table 3-5

NSUCO Pursuit Test Referral Criteria by Age and Sex

Sex	Ability	Accuracy	Head Movement
Boys	Less than 5	5 to 6 years: less than 2 7 to 9 years: less than 3 10 years and older: less than 4	5 to 6 years: less than 2 7 to 9 years: less than 3 10 years and older: less than 4
Girls	Less than 5	5 to 8 years: less than 3	5 to 9 years: less than 3 9 years and older: less than 5 All other ages: less than 4

Reprinted with permission from the Optometric Extension Program, reference 61: Maples WC, Atchley J, Ficklin T. Northeastern State University college of optometry's oculomotor norms. J Behav Optometrist. 1992;3:143-150.

Purpose

The client is able to employ an organized and symmetrical strategy in scanning for visual information while the client is stationary. Research with the test has shown that normal adults will employ an organized sequential scanning pattern to identify the numbers on the board using one of three patterns: clockwise, counterclockwise, or rectilinear. Most individuals will start in the upper left hand corner and scan left to right and top to bottom.

Test Materials

Scanboard and easel

Instructions

1. The client should be seated in a posturally secure position with good midline orientation (straddling a low bench is best). The board should be at eye level in the client's midline and within arm's reach so the client can touch each number on the board.

2. Instructions to the client: "There are 10 numbers on this board. Point the numbers out to me as you see them. Do not go in any particular order—just point them out as you see them. Point slowly because I will be writing down the numbers you see. Begin."

3. On the score sheet, indicate on the line under each number the order in which it was identified.

4. Do not cue the client during the test—let him indicate to you when he is finished.

5. On completion, analyze the scanning pattern for organization.

Test 2 – Scan Course[2]

Purpose

This is an informal test to observe the client's skill combining visual search with ambulation. The client is asked to walk down a hallway in which the therapist has placed 10 cards on each wall. The client is asked to point to and read each card during ambulation.

Test 3 – Warren Visual Search Subtests[2]

Purpose

Warren has developed seven visual search subtests of the biVABA: Single Letter Crowded, Search-Simple, Single Letter Search Structured, Complex Circles Search, Random Plain Circles-Simple, Random Plain Circles-Crowded, and Random Complex Circles Search. For some of these tests, the client is asked to search through an organized structured array of stimuli, and for other tests, the array is random.

Scoring

The number of correct responses is converted into a percentage score.

Validity/Reliability

There are no established reliability measures for these tests; however, Warren states in a letter to potential users of the biVABA[62]:

> *These tests are modifications of other visual search tests whose validity and reliability have been established by extensive use in research studies addressing visual search*

changes associated with inattention. The results I obtained on the field testing with brain injury and normal subjects were very consistent with what has been observed in other research studies on visual search performance.

Test 4 – Dynamic Object Search Test[27]

Description

This test is a dynamic assessment of visual search or scanning which emphasizes examining the client's ability to learn and apply a strategy within a series of search tasks. It consists of 12 pages (or trails) of 24 line-drawn objects, with the size and background distraction varying across four task conditions.

Scoring

A baseline score of independent performance is taken as well as a score with cuing provided. A learning curve or learning profile can be generated that indicates whether the client can internalize and apply targeted strategies and feedback across similar types of tasks.

Validity

After dynamic assessment procedures were given to 20 clients with right CVA and unilateral neglect, functional visual scanning tasks were initiated. Results indicated that these clients demonstrated significant changes in unilateral neglect across similar and somewhat similar tasks as compared to the control group that did not receive dynamic assessment procedures. In addition, significant differences between the two groups were observed in initiation of search on the left side and use of strategies.

TREATMENT FOR DEFICITS IN ORGANIZED SCANNING

Utilizing a Restorative Approach

1. Develop strategies with the client on how to take in visual information in an organized manner. Train the client to attend to spatial details.

2. Have the client perform functional activities for which effective scanning is required to complete the activity but is not the focus of the activity. The choice of activities should reflect input from the client regarding his or her priority functional goals.[63]

   The following are examples of functionally oriented tasks which address visual scanning (as well as saccades and fixation):

   a) Sorting silverware from the dishwasher to a bin in the drawer[8]

   b) Sorting coins from a coin holder[8]

   c) Sorting laundry by color[8]

   d) Have the client scan his or her room or clinic for specified items

   e) Take the client to a community setting, such as a grocery, department, drug, or hardware store. In a particular section of the store, have the client locate and retrieve a set of items listed by the therapist.

   f) Locate names, items, and prices, as specified by the therapist in the classified ads of the newspaper.

   g) Locate names, numbers, or addresses in a local telephone directory

3. Have the client perform tasks such as the following:

a) Cross out target letters (eg, all A's) in the paragraph of a magazine, newspaper article, or scanning worksheet designed by the therapist. Utilize the retraining principles of anchoring, pacing, density, and feedback (see number 1 below).

b) Complete paper mazes, puzzles, or other activities that require scanning ability.

4. If there is a deficit on monocular testing, train extraocular movements monocularly prior to training binocularly so that equal abilities are mastered with each eye before adding fusional demands to the task.[12]

Utilizing an Adaptive Approach

1. Provide the client with the following adaptations and cuing[63-65]:

a) Anchoring or cuing the client as to where to begin the visual search. For example, red tape or marker can be placed to the left at the beginning of all lines to be read or scanned.

b) Pacing or cuing the client about the speed of his or her response. This will help control impulsive or erratic scanning and establish an appropriate scanning rate. Slowing the client down can be accomplished simply by having him or her call out each number or letter as it appears or by placing a sticker under each one that is called out.[65]

c) Controlling the density or spacing of visual stimuli. In other words, change the distance between adjacent stimuli.

d) Providing consistent feedback to the client about his or her performance of visual scanning tasks. The client is progressed by gradually decreasing any of the cues.

2. For activities such as dressing, utilize an audiotape with instructions and stack clothes in a consistent order.[66]

3. Educate the client and his or her family about the scanning deficit and how it will affect function. Highlight areas where safety will be an issue.

4. Teach the client to self-monitor the quality of his or her pursuits (ie, make them aware of jerkiness or saccadic intrusions so they can try to correct them). For the ABI client, who may not be able to feel the eye jumps due to decreased proprioception from the extraocular muscles, cue the client every time his or her eye jumps until the client can begin to feel it on their own.[12]

Convergence and Accommodation

The vergence system aligns the eyes to maintain binocular fixation and binocular vision. The vergence system works together with the pupil and lens controlling systems for the accommodation reflex.[53] Accommodation is the process by which the refractive power of the eye changes to ensure for a clear retinal image.[45] The change in the relative position of the visual axes is termed vergence. When the angle formed by the visual axes increases, it is called convergence. When the angle decreases, it is termed divergence.[45] Divergence is associated reflexively with the relaxation of accommodation.[8] The nearest point on which the eyes can converge is termed the near point of convergence (NPC). It is visually much closer to the eye than the near point of accommodation and generally does not change with age.

Blurring of the retinal image is the primary stimulus for accommodation. There are two types of accommodation: 1) dynamic, which occurs when a target changes its distance or when we shift our attention between targets of different distances, and 2) static, which takes place after the completion of dynamic accommodation.[5] The static, or steady state, response occurs to maintain the newly acquired target in focus.[5] During accommodation, the process of convergence, or "...the simultaneous and synchronous adduction movement of the eyes...,"[67] maintains an image of an object aligned on precise corresponding points on both retinas.[2] This, in turn, ensures that a single image is seen as the object comes closer.[2] Warren summarizes the process of accommodation as follows[3]:

> *As an object approaches the eye, its point of focus on the retina is pushed further back, eventually causing the image to go out of focus. The CNS adjusts for this situation through a three step process of accommodation. As the object comes closer 1) the eyes converge (turn inward) to ensure that the light rays entering the eye stay parallel and in focus, 2) the crystalline lens of the eye thickens to refract the light rays more strongly and shorten the focal distance, and 3) the pupil constricts to reduce scattering of the light rays.*

Accommodative and convergence deficits are common as a result of ABI.[68] The most common type of deficit following trauma is accommodation insufficiency.[30] A brainstem injury can affect any or all of the components of accommodation previously described. The client will have difficulty with reading and other near tasks. The client may complain of a headache during near work, and many clients appear to have decreased concentration or comprehension.[3,68] Normally, accommodation and convergence are automatic, but with ABI, the client requires a large degree of conscious effort to clear blurred images.[68]

Decreased accommodation or convergence will lead to symptoms and stress for the client. The client may complain of fatigue with reading, writing, or any other activities requiring close focal distance. Accommodative dysfunction can "...prevent the client from returning to work, severely limit his ability to read or use a computer, and limit the progress of other rehabilitative services involving near visual tasks."[68] As Aloisio states, vergence ability is basic to all activities.[8]

EVALUATION OF ACCOMMODATION

Test 1 – Scheiman: Amplitude of Accommodation*[21]

Set-Up and Testing Strategy

It is important to position the client so that he or she is able to maximally attend and concentrate. Vertical positioning of the head is not as important with accommodation as it is with binocular vision testing. If the client normally reads with glasses, they must be used for this task.

Equipment Needed

Isolated letters, numbers, or symbols; an eye patch

You will need to make this target. To do so, simply photocopy the near visual acuity chart for both nonverbal and verbal clients. Cut out the 20/30 targets, and tape them on a tongue depressor. Place one on both sides of the tongue depressor so that you actually have two test targets.

---

*Reprinted with permission from SLACK Incorporated, Scheiman M. Understanding and Managing Vision Deficits. *Thorofare, NJ: SLACK Incorporated; 1997.*

Procedure

1. Patch the left eye.

2. It is important that the client does not know the letter or symbol on the tongue depressor before the test begins.

3. Hold the tongue depressor with the 20/30 target about 1 inch in front of the right eye. The client will be unable to identify the stimulus on the tongue depressor at this distance.

4. Slowly move the target away from the client's eye, and ask the client to report as soon as he or she can identify the target.

5. Using a ruler, measure the distance from the eye to the tongue depressor at which the client was able to identify the stimulus. Record this measurement.

6. Divide 40 by the measurement found in step 5 to determine the amplitude of accommodation. For example, say the client is able to identify the target at 8 inches. To find the amplitude, divide 40 by 8, which equals 5 D.

7. Compare the client's amplitude of accommodation to the expected amplitude for the client's age. You can determine the expected amplitude of accommodation using the following formula: The expected amplitude equals 18 minus one-third of the client's age.

Example 1—If you are working with a 9-year-old child, the expected amplitude would be:

Expected amplitude = 18 − [1/3 (9)]

Expected amplitude = 18 − 3 = 15

Example 2—If you are working with a 45-year-old, the expected amplitude would be:

Expected amplitude = 18 − [1/3 (45)]

Expected amplitude = 18 − 15 = 3

Expected Findings and Possible Responses

The amplitude of accommodation should be within 2 D of the expected finding to pass this screening test.

EVALUATION OF CONVERGENCE

Test 1 – Padula et al[13]

Procedure

A 0.5 cm silver steel ball supported by a black rod is moved in toward the client's nose. Convergence ability is recorded at the point of reported diplopia or loss of ocular alignment. Recovery is the point at which the client reports single vision or when ocular alignment is noted.

Scoring

Absent—No convergence

Impaired—Inability to converge on the target within 12 cm working distance

Intact—Convergence less than 12 cm working distance

*Test 2 – Near Point of Convergence (NPC)*7*

Purpose

To screen for adequate convergence (aiming) skills

Reprinted with permission from Lynn Hellerstein OD, Homestead Park Vision Clinic, PC 6967 S. Holly Circle, Suite 105, Englewood, CO 80112

Vision Problems Detected

Convergence insufficiency

Control

Habitual glasses, if worn by the client. Be sure client is looking through near prescription (you might need to lift glasses higher to utilize bifocal and prevent the client from tipping his head back).

Procedure

Start with the fixation target at 20 inches from the client's face. Instruct the client to stare at the target as you move it slowly toward the client's nose and to report if the target breaks into two (doubles). As you move the target toward the client's nose, watch both eyes. If one eye stops converging, the client might report seeing two targets, and you will see one eye wander outward. Where the tester sees the client's eyes no longer converge together is called the break point (may be different than where the client reports double vision). Now slowly bring the target back out. Instruct the client to report when the target jumps back into one, and observe when the eyes regain fixation. This is called the recovery point. Repeat the test several times to note whether the client fatigues over time.

Recording

Write the break point/recovery point (eg, 4/6 inch). If the client can converge to the nose, record TN (to nose).

Retest/Referral

Client should be able to converge within 6 inches from the bridge of his nose and recover within 6 inches of the bridge of his nose. Outside this range is a referral.

Test 3 – biVABA*2

Test Materials

Oculomotor Function Assessment form and penlight

Environment

Well lighted room with ambient light source; ensure that the light source is not shining directly into the client's eyes. If the client is having difficulty tracking the penlight, room illumination can be reduced to increase the contrast of the penlight.

Procedure

1. The client is seated comfortably with eyeglasses on, if worn.

2. Hold the penlight vertically so that the lighted tip can be viewed. Instruct the client to focus on the tip of the penlight.

3. Beginning at a distance of approximately 30 inches, move the penlight slowly toward the bridge of the client's nose.

4. As the penlight is moved toward the nose, observe the convergent eye movements. Both eyes should maintain fixation on the penlight and move inward, to follow the penlight as it nears the bridge of the nose (Note: observation can be aided by viewing the corneal reflections).

*Reprinted with permission from VisAbilities Rehab Services, Inc (http://www.visabilities.com), reference 2: Warren M. Brain Injury Visual Assessment Battery For Adults: Test Manual. Birmingham, Ala: VisAbilities Rehab Services Inc; 1998.

5. Record the distance from the bridge of nose at which the client breaks fixation in one or both eyes. Observe for pupillary constriction as the eyes move inward and observe the amount of effort used and the ability to maintain fixation. Fixation is broken when one or both eyes move outward or when the client reports double vision.

6. The near point of convergence in an adult is approximately 3 inches from the bridge of the nose and should be achieved without a break in fixation and with minimum effort (Note: older adults will have a farther near point than younger adults and children).

Instructions to the Client

"I am going to see how long you can stay focused on this penlight as I move it towards your nose. As I move the penlight in towards your nose, your eyes will begin to cross, and pretty soon you will find that the light appears to double or gets blurry. Please let me know as soon as this happens."

Scoring/Interpretation of Results

The primary observation is that of an inability to converge the eyes as the target moves inward. Because convergence is part of the accommodation process, inability to converge the eyes disrupts clear focusing of images at near distances. For adults, most objects (including printed materials) are held at a distance of 13 to 16 inches from the face when viewed. This distance provides the best and most comfortable focus and allows a sustained period of viewing. Although the near point of convergence is 2 to 3 inches from the bridge of the nose, few adults ever view objects that closely. Therefore, limitations in convergence are generally not functionally significant unless the client is unable to converge the eyes and easily maintain convergence to a distance of 5 inches from the bridge of the nose. An inability to converge the eyes to this distance and maintain convergence for several seconds while focusing on an object may cause the client to have difficulty performing tasks in near vision, especially those that require a sustained focus such as reading. Observation of convergence insufficiency on testing should be correlated with complaints made by the client regarding such tasks as reading, writing, quilting, or sewing.

Treatment of Accommodative and Convergence Deficits

If the client failed to pass a screening test for accommodation or convergence such as the ones described in this chapter, then a referral should be made to an optometrist or ophthalmologist. These professionals will evaluate whether vision therapy or surgery is indicated. When making the referral, the therapist should be specific about what he or she observed during the screening process as well as how the accommodative and/or convergence insufficiency is manifest during functional activities. When the client has been seen by the optometrist, he or she may be given new lenses, or prisms, which are to be worn during functional activities. The occupational therapist should maintain close communication with the optometrist relating to the effectiveness of the lenses or prisms and the client's comfort level or acceptance of their use.

As was described in the section covering organized screening, although the focus of occupational therapy intervention is not restorative, quick "warming up" activities performed at the beginning of the treatment session followed by functional near tasks can be beneficial. For example, the therapist places a spoon in the client's mouth with a bean, marble, raisin, etc. The therapist can ask the client questions about the size, color, or shape of the object that he or she will have to answer when the spoon is removed. This activity will stimulate convergence on the end of the spoon.[69]

Diplopia

Binocular vision is dependent on sensory fusion or "…the unification of corresponding retinal images into a single visual construct."[46] Diplopia, or double vision, occurs "…when the object at which the individual is looking stimulates the fovea of one eye and a nonfoveal part of the retina of the other eye."[21] In other words, there are noncorresponding retinal images. Paralytic strabismus, common to TBI clients, will result in diplopia.[18,26,30] Diplopia can cause difficulty in spatial judgment, disorientation, impaired eye hand coordination, impaired mobility, postural control, and reading.[12] To compensate for diplopia, the client may maintain an abnormal head position. This may be mistaken for poor head or postural control rather than a deliberate compensation technique by the client. He or she may squint or close one eye. The client may have near distance diplopia, which is within 20 inches of his or her face, or far distance diplopia, which is greater than 20 inches.[2] Near distance diplopia will affect activities such as reading, pouring, or writing, and far distance diplopia will affect activities such as mobility.[2]

EVALUATION OF DIPLOPIA

Test 1 – biVABA[2]

Description

The cover/uncover test is used if the therapist suspects a "tropia" (or eye deviation) is causing the diplopia. The client is instructed to fixate on a target held at eye level while the therapist quickly occludes the eye that seems to be functioning normally. The uncovered eye is observed to see if the it fixates on the target. This procedure is repeated with the other eye.

Scoring

The direction in which the uncovered eye moved is recorded.

> *Esophoria*—Eye turns in
>
> *Exophoria*—Eye turns out
>
> *Hypophoria*—Eye turns down
>
> *Hyperphoria*—Eye turns up

If both eyes are aligned equally and fixating on the target, no movement of either eye will be observed when one is covered; if the eyes are not aligned, the deviating eye will move to take up fixation when the nonaffected eye is covered.

Test 2 – biVABA[2]

Description

Alternate cover test used to detect a phoria (eye deviation held in check by fusion and, therefore, not noticeable on object fixation). Procedure as in Test 1 except the therapist occludes the eyes back and forth between the eyes every 2 seconds.

Scoring

The direction of any movement is recorded

TREATMENT OF DIPLOPIA

If the client complains of double vision and the screening indicates a problem, the therapist should refer the client to an optometrist or ophthalmologist. The therapist should communicate how the double vision is affecting functional activities.

The vision specialist may prescribe prisms, partial or full occlusion, visual training, or surgery.[1,19] The therapist should communicate to the vision specialist how the client is responding to the aid and what affect it is having (positive or negative) on client performance. For example, full occlusion may be affecting the client's balance and orientation to space, as it eliminates peripheral vision.[3] If this is the case, the therapist may explore other treatment options for the double vision with the vision specialist.

Visual Inattention

Visual inattention can be defined as a condition most often the result of right brain damage, in which there is a decreased awareness of the body and spatial environment on the side contralateral to the cerebral lesion despite the absence of a specific sensory deficit.[12,49,70-72] It can be manifest in many forms that can include impairments such as the "…dysfunction of mechanisms responsible for allocating attention to spatially coded targets; distortion of contralateral representational space; difficulty in executing motor plans aimed at the contralateral space and difficulty in allocating an appropriate motivational valance to contralateral stimuli."[73] Neglect can be associated with decreased tactile, proprioceptive, and stereognostic perception, impaired spacial orienting, impaired motor exploration, extinction (for any or all modalities), and/or hemianopia.[8,12,72] The client with the most severe form of neglect will behave as if the contralesional side of the world does not exist.[72]

Visual neglect or inattention can be apparent in many forms or degrees of severity, but all forms of neglect have the common problem of not responding to information that is contralateral to the side of the lesion.[74] Visual inattention is most common and more severe following a right hemisphere lesion, and it may occur in all three dimensions of space: horizontal (right, left), vertical (up, down), and radial (near, far).[75] It can occur with or without the presence of visual field deficits and may be seen in conjunction with body neglect.[76-78] Body-centered neglect is associated with frontal lesions, while environment-centered neglect is associated with parietal lesions.[79] Although unilateral neglect can be mistaken for hemianopia, the mechanisms underlying neglect are different than hemianopia. Neglect is "…a perceptual deficit where the neural substrates necessary for sight are intact, but the visual substrates or pathways to attend or perceive the sensory input are not."[12]

The theoretical basis of visual spatial inattention remains somewhat controversial. Some believe it is due to the interaction between a sensory deficit and mental deterioration.[76,80,81] Others attribute the deficit to an impairment of the internal representation of space.[82] Most now believe visual spatial inattention is at least in part due to disordered attention and/or orienting systems.[3,76,81,83-85]

Butter builds on the concept of an attention related deficit and divides attention into two categories: reflex and voluntary.[83] Reflex attention is triggered by stimuli with certain physical characteristics. The speed and frequency with which the stimulus has occurred also determine the degree to which it captures our attention of stimuli.[83]

Voluntary attention, on the other hand, "involves the central activation of stored representations of stimuli."[83] It is assumed that voluntary attention is related to neural structures that are located at higher cortical levels and are superimposed on the mechanisms of reflex attention.[83,86] Theoretically, reflex attention involves bottom-up processing of visual stimuli, whereas voluntary attention utilizes both top-down and bottom-up processing.

Riddoch and Humphreys support the concept of two types of attention, which they term preattentive and attentive processing.[87] Their research indicated that preattentive processing appeared relatively intact in a portion of their clients, and therefore, they believed that neglect results from an inability to "translate the information pre-attentively into a form which will support action."[87] It is a breakdown in the processes whereby visual stimuli "capture visual attention."

Some clinicians have noted a lack of systematic exploration within the extrapersonal space. Bouska et al observe that eye movement, both scanning and saccades, during activities occurs on only one side of midline within the attended space.[49] This phenomenon occurs in the absence of apraxia for eye movements and with no decrease in extraocular movements.

Rafal observes that the client with neglect in addition to not perceiving items on the left also may have a motor bias against moving his or her hand towards the left.[72] In other words, in some clients, neglect may be perceptual and, in others, more motor. He describes the following symptoms of neglect which may be manifest[72]:

...Hyperreflexive orienting toward the ipsilateral side or to local elements in the visual scene; impaired ability to disengage attention; a deranged internal representation of space that is not only shifted but contralesionally impaired; voluntary orienting toward the contralesional field; a motor bias toward the ipsilateral side that causes defective contralesional exploratory behavior; deficient ability to generate contralesional voluntary saccades; failure of contralesional stimuli to produce arousal.

Although it is accepted that neglect is a deficit associated with problems with the attentional system, it is only recently that the role of sustained attention in neglect has been examined. In his research of clients with neglect, Robertson found that sustained attention was an important modulation variable that influenced the pattern of neglect.[88] He goes on to hypothesize that impaired sustained attention may be an underlying cause of persistent neglect and that acute neglect clients who recover spontaneously may not show sustained attention deficits. Robertson believes "...the implications of this strong relationship between sustained attention and lateralized attention are considerable both for understanding normal human cognitive functioning as well as in understanding the phenomenon of unilateral neglect."[88]

Another important concept related to neglect is extinction. Visual extinction is demonstrated when the client has an inability or severe limitation in perceiving two objects briefly displayed at once while they are able to process a single visual stimuli.[85,89] The client may ignore one of two objects held in intact visual fields on either side of the midline when presented simultaneously. This may occur not only for midline opposite stimuli but for contralateral upper and lower quadrants as well. For example, a lower left quadrant stimulus can cause a simultaneous stimulus in the upper right quadrant to be neglected.

There are many theories as to why extinction occurs. The main hypotheses are that there exists 1) impaired attentional orienting to contralesional targets, 2) a problem disengaging attention from ipsilateral stimuli, or 3) an abnormal attraction of attention towards the spared side of space.[85] Recent research in the field supports the hypothesis that extinction is the result of a weaker competitive weight that is assigned to contralesional items than to ipsilateral ones.[85] The results of research conducted by Mattingley et al not only supported this hypothesis but took it one step further when they observed that a variance in competitive weight occurred from stimuli from different modalities or senses.[89] When the client was given tactile and visual stimuli at the same time, the client still extinguished the stimulus contralateral to the lesion, whether that stimulus was visual or tactile. These researchers found that extinction could be manifest within any of the primary senses and could occur within several senses in a given client.[89]

One of the main discoveries of recent research related to neglect is that of a "midline shift" of the client's world. When an individual searches for an object, he or she does so in both hemispaces.[90] Research of clients with neglect, however, has demonstrated that information to the right of the client's body midline is well attended and to the left of midline is poorly attended.[91,92] Padula et al describes the mechanism underlying the "midline shift" as follows[92]:

With an interference of information from one side of the body compared to the other, the ambient visual process attempts to create balance by expanding its concept of space on one side of the body compared to the other. In so doing, a perceived amplification of space occurs internally on one side, and a perceived compression of space occurs on the other side. This phenomena causes a shift away from the neurologically affected side.

The client with a midline shift will often describe that they feel like they are walking on a tilted floor. They will have major difficulties with balance and spatial orientation when in crowded moving environments.[92]

The client with neglect also shows a significant difference between where he or she has the initial fixation to start a visual search as compared to the normal as well as a hemianopic client.[93] Research indicated that neglect clients consistently start their search to the right of midline. Behrmann et al found clients with neglect made fewer ipsilesional than contralesional saccades, were slower to initiate leftward saccades, and adapt a rightward (rather than leftward) position for starting their visual exploration.[93] This pattern was observed for tracking single and double stimuli, viewing a scene and a face, and in reading.[93] Karnath and Perenin found similar results in their study of six neglect clients and six normal clients. They found their neglect subjects had a deviated ocular exploration, with the center shifted –15 degrees to the right of the body's midline.[90] Another interesting discovery of their research was that this midline shift was also present for tactile exploration. These and other recent studies have demonstrated that clients with neglect subjectively perceive their bodies as being oriented to the ipsilesional right side, suggesting that the egocentric midline of the body or trunk is deviated rightwards.[93] Many techniques of vision therapy, such as the use of prisms, work to readjust the client's midline perception to normalize the sensory input and gradually reduce the need for the prism as the client's perception of midline and scanning patterns improve.

To summarize, visual inattention or neglect can occur in isolation but often occurs in conjunction with associated deficits. It can occur for near (or personal) space or far (or extrapersonal) space.[90,94] It can be perceptual and/or motor in nature; it can be a spatial-based neglect or an object-based neglect. The mechanisms for neglect are now believed to be attentional-based rather than sensory-based, and the modulating affect of sustained attention appears to have an important role in neglect. Extinction can occur in any sensory modality or quadrant of vision, and finally, neglect appears to cause a "midline shift" of the client's body orientation.

Functional implications for the client with visual spatial inattention are varied and often severe. Clients will have difficulty with reading, writing, drawing, and basically any or all areas of ADL and IADLs, depending on the severity of deficit.[75,95] Neglect will generally cause the client to be more prone to accidents than hemianopic clients because they are most often not aware of the deficit.[12] Neglect is associated with lower scores not only for ADLs but with sensory-motor and cognitive measures as well.[47] The most impacted areas will be "...those areas that require inspection and integration of significant amounts of visual detail and those completed in dynamic environments."[3] These can include driving, shopping, and, in general, all community mobility.

EVALUATION OF VISUAL INATTENTION

General Guidelines for Evaluation

Clinical Observations

Applying the information previously described regarding the nature and concepts related to visual inattention, the therapist should ask the following:

1. What is the client's posture and head position? Is there any head turning/tilt?
2. What is the level of the client's sustained attention?
3. Where does the client start his visual search (ie, initial point of fixation)?

Table 3-6

Comparison of Search Patterns:
Persons With Visual Field Deficit Versus Persons With Hemi-Inattention

Visual Field Deficit	Hemi-Inattention
• Search pattern is abbreviated toward blind field	• Search pattern is asymmetrical: initiated/confined to the right side
• Client attempts to direct search toward blind side	• Client makes no attempt to direct search toward left side
• Search pattern is organized and generally efficient	• Search pattern is random and generally inefficient
• Client rescans to check accuracy of performance	• Client does not rescan to check accuracy of performance
• Time spent on task is appropriate to level of difficulty	• Client completes task quickly; level of effort applied is not consistent with difficulty of task

Reprinted with permission from reference 2: Warren M. Brain Injury Visual Assessment Battery For Adults: Test Manual. Birmingham, Ala: VisAbilities Rehab Services Inc; 1998:4-43.

4. Does he or she perform visual search in an organized manner within his or her intact visual fields? Refer to Table 3-6 for a description of search patterns of the hemianopic client versus the client with visual inattention. Is the speed of the search decreased?

5. Does the client's performance improve if the visual array is set up in an organized structured manner?

6. Does neglect become apparent primarily for intrapersonal activities or activities involving extrapersonal space?

7. Does it appear to be on object-based neglect or spatial neglect?

8. Does increasing the complexity of the visual array decrease performance?

9. Does verbal cuing help performance, especially preattentive cuing? Does tactile, auditory, proprioceptive, or kinesthetic cuing help?

10. What specific functional activities appear to be affected by the inattention? Does neglect mostly appear during activities such as eating, reading, or hygiene? Or is it more prevalent during mobility (ie, decreased awareness of doorways, turning wheelchair only in one direction)?[8] How does altering the task and/or the environment affect performance?

Test 1 – Behavioral Inattention Test[96]

Description

The Behavioral Inattention Test (BIT) is an objective behavioral test of everyday skills relevant to visual neglect. It has nine behavioral subtests and six conventional pencil and paper subtests.* Conventional subtests include line crossing, letter cancellation, star cancellation, figure and shape copying, line bisection, and representational drawing. The behavioral subtests are picture

*Results of a study of 54 right hemisphere CVA subjects indicated that the therapist may only need to administer the conventional subtests to identify neglect.

scanning, telephone dialing, menu reading, article reading, telling and setting the time, coin sorting, address and sentence copying, map navigation, and card sorting.

Scoring

In each subtest, the number of omissions is recorded. In addition, errors of commission and/or other types of errors are noted but not incorporated into the score. The total score from the conventional subtests determines the presence of unilateral visual neglect. Behavioral subtests can then be used to identify how the neglect is causing everyday problems and as a guide in treatment strategy. Detailed information on scoring is contained in the test manual.

Validity

1. A comparison of scores on the behavioral battery to those on the conventional tests was made. The correlation was 0.92 (p < 0.001).

2. Behavioral scores were compared with a short questionnaire completed by the therapist at the time of assessment. The correlation was 0.67 (p < 0.001).

3. Forty Israeli subjects (CVA) were evaluated with the BIT, performance tasks, and a checklist of ADLs. Results supported the construct and predictive validity of most of the BIT subtest as functional measures of unilateral neglect.

Reliability

1. Inter-rater reliability was established at 0.99 (p < 0.001).

2. Parallel form reliability was established between two test versions at 0.91 (p < 0.001).

3. Test-retest reliability was established at 0.99 (p < 0.001).

Procedure

The instructions for two of the conventional subtests and two of the behavioral subtests are presented as examples.

Conventional Subtests

Line Crossing[97]

Description

Subjects are presented with a page containing 40 1-inch (25 mm) lines. The page is placed directly in front of them. The lines appear to be randomly spaced about the page but are in fact grouped into three columns containing six lines on either side of the midline.

Instructions

"On this page, we have many lines pointing in different directions. Follow my pen as I indicate these lines." (Move pen right to left, top to bottom over all the lines on the page.) "Now with this pen, I want you to cross out all the lines that you can see on the page, like this." (Illustrate by crossing out two of the four central lines.)

Some clients may initially cross out only those lines that appear to correspond to the orientation of the example. In such cases, the client should be instructed to cross out all the lines, irrespective of orientation.

Scoring

The total number of lines crossed is noted. The maximum is 36 (18 left, 18 right). The four lines of the central column are not scored.

Reprinted with permission from Thames Valley Test Co, reference 97: Wilson B, Cockburn J, Halligan P. Behavioural Inattention Test. *Bury St. Edmunds, England: Thames Valley Test Co; 1987.*

Star Cancellation*[97]

Description

Subjects are presented with a page containing 52 large stars, 13 randomly positioned letters, and 10 short words, interspersed with 56 smaller stars.

Instructions

"This page contains stars of different sizes. Look at the page carefully; this is a small star. Every time you see a small star, cross it out like this." (Illustrate by crossing out the two small stars immediately above the centralizing arrow on the stimulus sheet.) "I would like you to go through this page and cross out all the small stars without missing any of them."

Scoring

The total number of small stars canceled is noted. The response sheet can be further divided into six sections by the scoring template for further analysis of omissions. Total number of stars is 54 (27 left, 27 right).

Behavioral Subtests

Article Reading*[97]

Description

The subject is presented with a short, three column article and is instructed to read it. (This is obviously not appropriate for some language impaired clients.)

Instructions

"Here is a short article from a newspaper. Please read it out loud, slowly and carefully."

Scoring

This is based on the percentage of words omitted in all three columns. Word omission, incomplete words, and partial or whole substitutions of words are scored. The examiner uses a photocopy of the original article to record the relevant errors made.

Coin Sorting*[97]

Description

The subject is presented with an array of coins (six denominations in all, three of each denomination). He is asked to indicate the coins according to the denomination called out. This is arranged according to a preset order.

Instructions

"Here, we have a selection of coins, which I would like you to look at. There are three rows altogether" (indicate). "I am now going to call out various names of coins, and I'd like you to point to the coin or coins I name. Be sure to point out all the coins of each type called out."

Scoring

All coins identified are recorded on a score sheet. The score is based on the number of omissions. Location of omissions can be noted on the score sheet.

Test 2 – Alternating Simultaneous Stimuli (Extinction)**[98]

Procedure

The therapist is seated at arm's length directly facing the client. The client is instructed to focus on the therapist's nose. Using the index fingers of both hands approximately 8 inches in front of the client's face, the therapist wiggles one of two fingers two times, a total of 7 to 10 trials.

Reprinted with permission from Thames Valley Test Co, reference 97: Wilson B, Cockburn J, Halligan P. Behavioural Inattention Test. Bury St. Edmunds, England: Thames Valley Test Co; 1987.
**Reprinted with permission from Santa Clara Valley Medical Center, reference 96: Zoltan B, Jabri J, Panikoff L, Ryckman D. Perceptual Motor Evaluation for Head Injured and Other Neurologically Impaired Adults. San Jose, Calif: Santa Clara Valley Medical Center, Occupational Therapy Department; 1983.*

X = Finger moves

0 = Finger does not move

Ask the client to indicate which finger he sees moving, by either pointing or a verbal response.

Note: The rating should not overlap with the client's field cut, as you would be sketching field loss and not neglect. Test for neglect within the client's visual field and on the border of the field deficit, if present.

Directions

Say, "For this test, keep your eyes on my nose at all times. Tell me how many fingers I move—one or two. Point to what moved."

Observe whether the client is able to attend consistently to visual stimuli presented simultaneously or whether he neglects right or left stimuli.

Note: Visual confrontation on only the affected side may reveal no apparent neglect. However, subsequent simultaneous confrontation may show visual neglect of stimuli in the presence of intact peripheral vision.

Scale

1—Present, visual spatial neglect noted.

0—Absent, attends to visual stimuli correctly.

Test 3 – biVABA[2]

The scanboard, scancourse, and visual search subtests are used as an indication and measurement of the speed and organization of the client's visual search patterns. The quality and style of the client's search pattern can provide information that may help differentiate between a hemianopic client and the client with visual inattention (see Table 3-6). In addition, please refer to the references for detailed information pertaining to the administration, scoring, and interpretation of these tests.[2]

Test 4 – Dynamic Object Search Test[99]

Please refer to the description of this test in the section on Organized Scanning on page 80.

Dynamic Assessment

During dynamic assessment of visual neglect, the therapist provides cues that may help improve performance. Golisz and Toglia provide the following examples[100]:

- Do you think you got all the information on the left page?
- See if you can find any information that you may have missed.
- What did you do to make sure you were looking over to your left?
- Let's try this again, but this time, I want you to make sure to touch your left hand as you look toward the left side of the paper to make sure you are all the way over the left.

During dynamic assessment, the therapist identifies the potential underlying causes of poor performance and repeats the activity with modifications.[100] Some activity parameters will stay the same, while one activity parameter is changed. For example, if the therapist feels performance errors are due to the complexity/density of the visual array, the activity would be repeated with a less dense or complex array.

TREATMENT OF VISUAL INATTENTION

Utilizing a Restorative Approach

A restorative approach to visual inattention should only be utilized if the client can be made aware of the neglect deficit and how it is affecting his or her function. Recent research has, in fact, indicated that disability awareness training with neglect clients resulted not only in increased awareness but also in improved ability to perform various ADL tasks for which they had not been specifically trained.[21,101] The client should also have the capacity to learn new strategies for attention and visual search. Note, however, that the client generally is able to recognize a problem he or she is having with sustained attention but not his or her problems with neglect. With these clients, because they understand and accept that they have an attention problem, they are open to activities that work to improved sustained attention. Research has shown the client may be taught to compensate for his attention deficit, which will in turn help ameliorate the neglect problem.[88] It is hypothesized that this method is effective because of the functional anatomical connections between the two systems underlying the two disorders.[88]

1. Provide activities that stimulate the reorganization of the patient's scanning patterns.[3,27] Activities should be arranged to teach, first, a left to right linear pattern (for reading and scanning of small visual detail) and, second, a left to right clockwise or counter clockwise pattern (for viewing unstructured visual arrays in the extrapersonal environment [ie, grocery stores, for driving]).[2]

2. Warren outlines the following principles when working on activities to reorganize the client's scanning[3]:

   a) Treatment activities should require the client to scan as broad a visual space as possible.

   b) Treatment activities will be more effective if the client is required to interact physically with the target once it is located.

   c) Treatment activities should emphasize conscious attention to visual detail and careful inspection and comparison of targets.

   d) Practice the search strategy within the context to ensure carry over of application to ADLs.

3. Due to the close relationship of sustained attention to visual neglect, utilize activities designed to increase the client's sustained attention (refer to Chapter 8).

4. When speaking to the client, sit or stand in the neglected space to force the client to turn his or her head and scan the neglected space to find you. Add a motor component such as having the client hand something to you or, for example, have the client place a piece of a puzzle that you are holding in its appropriate spot.

5. Place items the client needs during treatment in the neglected space. For example, clothes during dressing training. Have the client wear a watch on the neglected side, and periodically ask him what time it is.

6. Provide verbal, auditory (bell, finger snapping), tactile, and kinesthetic cuing to encourage the client to look to the unattended space. For example, if the client will not reach into unattended space, the therapist should physically guide him to complete the task or tap his or her shoulder to look to the left or right instead of a verbal cue. This is more effective with the aphasic client. Preattentive cuing has been shown to increase speed and accuracy of visual attention[102,103]—for example, using auditory cuing or using an arrow to point to a stimulus, such as a video or an approaching stairwell.

7. Some researchers indicate the use of dynamic stimuli (eg, flashing lights) versus static stimuli to be effective in the reduction of visual inattention.[83,104]

8. Research has indicated that videotaping the client and having the client view his or her performance on the tape can significantly improve client performance.[105]

9. Provide computer training with software designed especially for the remediation of visual inattention.

10. For the client who exhibits a midline shift, utilize an NDT approach to help re-establish a normal body scheme. For example, facilitate normal postural control through handling and weight shifting activities. Incorporate reaching into the neglected space during NDT activities. Combine NDT activities and handling with previously described scanning activities to increase the effect of the treatment.

11. Provide constraint induced therapy as described in Chapter 1.

12. Refer the client to the optometrist for evaluation for prism use to treat the client with a midline shift and neglect. Research has shown prism therapy to be an effective way to achieve long-term success in neglect treatment.[106,107]

Utilizing an Adaptive Approach

This approach should be utilized with the client who is unable to be made aware of his or her deficit and, as a result, cannot be taught new scanning strategies.

1. Increase client and family awareness of the visual inattention and how it will affect the client functionally. Activities where safety is an issue should be highlighted. Also, emphasize the need for visual scanning during activities.

2. If possible, have the client identify his or her own compensation strategies, and provide tasks that allow the client to apply these strategies. Carry out the tasks in a variety of contexts or environments.

3. Utilizing a Dynamic Interactional frame of reference—identify how a given task can be altered to facilitate performance. For example, does simplifying the visual array of the task improve performance, or does the client perform better if he or she is asked to point to a target before reading it?

4. Emphasize visual scanning activities, and show the client how head and eye movements can compensate.[49] Progress the client as follows[49]:

    a) Movements leading the eye from attended to unattended space

    b) Eye movements into the unattended space

    c) Eye movements without the use of head movements

    d) Incorporate the client's increased awareness and scanning into more difficult visual perceptual and visual motor tasks

5. Help the client become aware of the problem by having him cue himself before starting an activity—for example, stating, "when I look at things, I tend not to see things on my left. So when I start this and I pick a place to look, I am probably not looking in the correct place, so I will look farther to the left than the first spot I pick to start looking."

6. Research has indicated the use of visual imagery can be an effective technique with neglect clients.[22] In a study of 16 clients with neglect, they were asked to imagine their eyes as horizontal sweeping beams of a lighthouse and were shown a picture of a lighthouse. They were then asked to use this image in functional and therapy training tasks. The

---

Table 3-7

Functions/Limitations of Visual, Vestibular, and Somatosensory Systems Related to Posture, Movement, Perception, and the Environment

System	Function	Limitation
Vestibular	Provides posture and balance control; this includes orientation to gravity through the otoliths; provides a way to distinguish movement in the environment from self motion. Maintain visual fixation during head and/or body movement	Unable to distinguish body tilt or body motion from head motion
Somatosensory (information from muscles and joint receptors)	Provides information on the relationship of one body segment to another and of the support surface; provides the first means of adjustment for regaining balance during disturbances	Unable to differentiate surface tilts from head tilts
Visual	Provides vertical orientation; detects optic array movements; provides depth perception of objects moving towards/away from the individual	Inadequate in distinguishing movement of the environment from movement of the body

Adapted from reference 108: Rosen A, Cohen A, Trebing S. The integration of visual and vestibular systems in balance disorders-a-clinical perspective. In: Suchoff IB, Ciuffreda KJ, Kapoor N, eds. Visual and Vestibular Consequences of Acquired Brain Injury. Santa Ana, Calif: Optometric Extension Program; 2001.

---

treatment group was matched with controls for diagnosis, race, and age. The treatment group showed significant improvement as compared to the control group with visual inattention as measured by a facility rating scale and family reports.[22]

7. Place all necessary items for functional independence within the client's field of vision. Design the client's environment to reduce the risk of injury and increase the potential for successful interaction with the environment.[75]

Visual/Vestibular Processing

The ability to maintain one's balance and posture is the outcome of the integration of the visual, vestibular, and somatosensory systems.[108] The interaction of these systems is necessary for "...adequate preceptor of motion and for distinguishing between self-motion and motion in the individual's surroundings."[109] As a result of injury to one or more of these systems, there is a lack of or conflict in sensory information that results in a complex of symptoms.[110] The functions and limitations of each of these systems as they relate to posture, movement, perception, and the environment are described in Table 3-7. In addition, functional manifestations of problems with posture, balance, and dizziness and the likely underlying cause are summarized in Table 3-8.

Many ABI clients with decreased visual acuity often complain about postural instability as well as vertigo or dizziness.[111] When evaluating the integrity of the visual processing system, symptoms associated with vestibular dysfunction may be apparent.[11] Binocular deviations such as fixation disparity, phorias, convergence insufficiency, and accommodative deficits are all often associated with symptoms of vestibular dysfunction.[108] These associated clinical visual vestibular deficits are the manifestation of the inter-related underlying neuroanatomical structures and

---

Table 3-8

Functional Manifestation of Dizziness and Balance Problems and Likely Underlying Cause

Functional Manifestation	*Likely Underlying Cause*
Symptoms occur during activities such as making a bed, walking up and down stairs, reaching or looking up, riding in a car around curves, riding elevators, and making quick stops	Directly related to vestibular stimulation
Symptoms occur during activities such as shopping in crowded stores (eg, grocery shopping) or in visually busy environments (eg, rows of trees along the road)	Visual dependency and hypersensitivity
Symptoms occur in activities such as difficulty walking in the dark, falling or losing balance when closing their eyes	Inadequate use of somatosensory cues

Adapted from reference 108: Rosen A, Cohen A, Trebing S. The integration of visual and vestibular systems in balance disorders-a-clinical perspective. In: Suchoff IB, Ciuffreda KJ, Kapoor N, eds. Visual and Vestibular Consequences of Acquired Brain Injury. Santa Ana, Calif: Optometric Extension Program; 2001.

---

systems. For example, the same vestibular neurons that respond to vestibular stimulation also respond to smooth pursuit and optokinetic stimuli.[59] Central vestibular and ocular connections are highly integrated with the visual ocular stabilizing pathways, and both systems share the final common pathways of ocular motor neurons.[59]

Vestibular inputs travel to the vestibular nucleus in the brainstem, vestibulocerebellum, and reticular formation in the brainstem, all of which also receive sensory inputs from the visual and somatosensory systems.[112] Also of note is the fact that the exact position of the semicircular canals within the skull geometrically mirrors the functional actions of the extraocular muscles as a result of their insertion on the eyeballs.[108] As a result, the CNS integrates and "recalibrates" the input from the vestibular system of the inner ears to the motor output of the extraocular muscles.[108]

Vestibular, ocular, and postural or cervical responses and reflexes maintain a steady gaze on the fovea during head and body movements.[2,60,113] A stable gaze depends on 1) vestibular controlled eye movements, 2) visually controlled eye movements (saccades, optokinetic, smooth pursuit), and 3) head movements.[112] This is accomplished by the vestibular ocular reflex (VOR), which is activated in the labyrinth (semicircular canals) during head movements,[77,114,115] and the optokinetic reflex, which is activated during sustained movement and takes over the function of the VOR.[2,53] When there is an impairment of the VOR, the client will be unable to maintain stable gaze during head movement, which will result in blurred vision.[30,60,79,113,116] In addition, the vestibular nucleus receives information from visual, somatosensory, and auditory systems and, in association with the VOR, is important to maintaining a stable visual world during head and body movements. The VOR stabilizes gaze by producing an eye movement of equal velocity and opposite direction to the head movement. The ratio of the eye velocity to head velocity is referred to as the gain. The gain tells you how active the VOR is or if there is any VOR at all.[112] The ideal gain in a normal individual is 1".[60,108]

As previously described, each semicircular canal has major connections to one ipsilateral and one contralateral extraocular muscle. These connections are the basis of the vestibularocular reflex.[108] Since the three pairs of semi-circular canals represent all rotational movement in three-dimensional space, vision can be maintained for all directions of head movement.[108] When we are able to maintain fixation when our head is rotating at high speeds, the VOR is being utilized to maintain that fixation. When we are moving our head at slow speeds, we are utilizing the pursuit

---

Table 3-9

Types of Nystagmus and Their Symptoms

Type	Symptoms
Downbeat nystagmus	Defective vertical gaze holding. The eyes tend to drift up, and a corrective downward saccade is generated; almost always present in the primary position, and causes difficulty in reading and sometimes oscillopsia
Upbeat nystagmus	May be present in primary position or only in upgaze
Gaze evoked nystagmus	Difficulty in maintaining eccentric gaze. The eyes drift back towards the center, and a corrective saccade to reposition the eyes more peripherally is required; the nystagmus is often symmetrical right to left; this type of nystagmus may occur in normals at the extremes of gaze; therefore, the stability of fixation should be assessed at roughly 40 to 50 degrees from primary position
Seesaw nystagmus	A variety of disconjugate vertical nystagmus (ie, one eye moves up as the other moves down). The upward moving eye will intort while the downward moving eye extorts; bitemporal visual field deficits are associated with this deficit
Disassociated nystagmus	Nystagmus of only the abducting eye when gaze is directed to the side opposite the lesion; the client often has diplopia because of the limited adduction of the ipsilateral eye
Jerk nystagmus	Commonly consists of a slow drift to one side followed by a corrective saccade (ie, right jerk nystagmus = slow movement to the left with fast to the right); primarily due to asymmetric vestibular input
Pendular nystagmus	Relatively symmetric (ie, not an identifiable slow and fast phase and shows relatively equal amplitude in speed in separate direction)

Adapted from reference 1: Morton RL. Visual dysfunction following brain injury. In: Ashley MJ, ed. Traumatic Brain Injury Rehabilitation and Case Management. 2nd ed. Boca Raton, Fla; CRC Press; 2004.

---

system.[15] The VOR has two components: 1) angular VOR, which is mediated through the otoliths, and 2) linear VOR, which comes into play where near targets are being viewed and the head is being moved at a relatively high frequency.[117]

Injuries as a result of TBI that can cause vestibular dysfunction can include inner ear concussion, temporal bone fractures, intracranial pressure, and/or damage to the central vestibular structure.[118] The client with damage to the central vestibular structure may exhibit ocular dysmetria, cogwheeling during smooth pursuit movement, optokinetic asymmetries, and spontaneous nystagmus.[118] Spontaneous nystagmus means that the vestibular apparatus or its connections to or from the brain may be damaged or there is damage to the CNS.[112]

Nystagmus is a repetitive oscillatory to-and-fro movement of the eyes.[119] These involuntary rhythmic oscillations of one or both eyes can be the result of any lesion or trauma that causes an imbalance to the pursuit, optokinetic, and vestibular systems, which keep fixation stable.[21] Clients with nystagmus will often also complain of problems with tinnitus, balance, and vertigo.[1] Vertigo is a unidirectional shift of the environment and is the result of large amplitude nystagmus.[119] Depending on the location and magnitude of the lesion or trauma, various types of nystagmus may be observed. These specific types of nystagmus are summarized in Table 3-9.

Clients who present with nystagmus may also complain of oscillopsia, or the sensation of the world moving.[1] Oscillopsia related to nystagmus occurs when the head is stationary and, when occurring with head movements, can be the result of weakness of an extraocular muscle[115] or caused by "...excessive slipping of visual images on the retina due to inadequate vestibular, cervical, and ocular responses during head movement."[2] Oscillopsia that is brought on or exacerbated by head movement is thought to reflect an inappropriate VOR gain or phase.[91,120] Oscillopsia can interfere with the ability to see clearly while moving or even standing still. It can cause difficulty reading signs or identifying faces while moving or reading the dashboard while driving.[116] It will affect postural stability and total body function required for ADLs and IADLs.[58] Oscillopsia tends to worsen with irregular head movements such as those that occur with ambulation.[58] Clients may complain that objects that are far away appear to be jumping or bouncing.[58]

Visual vestibular system dysfunction is common following an ABI and can have a major impact on the client's functional independence. Vestibular processing problems that cause blurred vision, nystagmus, oscillopsia, postural instability, and spatial disorientation can interfere with everything from reading or reaching for objects to driving and community mobility.[116] For this reason, most ABI clients require a therapy program that addresses both systems to assist the client in reaching his or her highest potential for independence. Research has demonstrated that a comprehensive multidisciplinary approach combining visual and vestibular therapy results in the greatest therapeutic benefit.[108]

EVALUATION OF VISUAL/VESTIBULAR PROCESSING

Test 1 – Doll's Head Reflex[1]

Description/Procedure

The client's head is rotated to one side by the examiner. The head is rapidly rotated to midline from an initial position of 30 degrees off midline. This is done with the client maintaining fixation on a target. This tests the integrity of the pathways from the vestibular nucleus to the lateral gaze center.[1]

Scoring

The response is considered positive if the eyes have to make a saccade to refixate.

Test 2 – Dynamic Visual Acuity[60,121]

Description/Procedure

This tests visual acuity during head movement and is a method of assessing the VOR. The VOR can be tested in the dark. This tests the visual-vestibular interaction to stabilize gaze.[112] The client's static visual acuity is measured first with a wall chart such as the Snellen Eye Chart. The client is then asked to read the same chart while the client's head is rotated by the examiner through a 60-degree arc at a frequency of one to two cycles per second.

Scoring

Normal—May lose one line of visual acuity

Unilateral vestibular loss—May lose two to four lines

Bilateral vestibular loss—May lose five to six lines

Also note any complaints by the client of dizziness, oscillopsia, nausea, or blurring of vision. This test will measure how much the client can still see when making rapid head movements and is a good indicator if the client should still be driving.[60,117]

Test 3 – Post Head Shake Nystagmus[121]

Procedure

Passively rotate or have the client actively rotate his or her head at a high frequency for 10 to 20 seconds and then stop abruptly.

Scoring

Clients with severe unilateral vestibular loss will have nystagmus with the initial slow phase directed toward the affected side and a subsequent reversal phase toward the unaffected side. Bilateral vestibular hypofunction and acute unilateral hypofunction do not produce any nystagmus after head shaking.

Test 4 – Optokinetic Nystagmus[121]

Procedure

The therapist moves a series of alternating black and white stripes in front of the client's visual fields. The stripes are moved first to the right and then to the left in front of the client's visual fields at 20 to 40 degrees per second.

Scoring

The following abnormalities may be noted: nystagmus is induced in one direction but not the other; optokinetic nystagmus is normal at lower speeds but abnormal when the speed is increased; no nystagmus can be elicited in either direction.

If the results of the preceding test indicate dysfunction, the client should be referred to an optometrist for evaluation as to whether techniques such as patching would help reduce symptoms.

TREATMENT OF VISUAL/VESTIBULAR PROCESSING DEFICITS

Although there is a strong indication of successful treatment of clients with deficits as a result of a peripheral vestibular injury, the efficacy of treatment with clients with a central vestibular problem appears less certain at this time. Preliminary research, however, indicates that vestibular rehabilitation with ABI clients does cause improvement but requires a longer period of treatment than the peripherally impaired clients.[117,122] Some hypothesize that the longer recovery time relates to the neural basis of CNS compensation of vestibular problems.[25] The neural basis of CNS compensation of vestibular dysfunction is not limited to one specific part of the brain but is distributed throughout the CNS. Therefore, lesions in the cerebrum, cerebellum, spinal cord, brainstem, and sensory systems can all reduce or prevent the CNS's capacity for compensation.[113] Recent research, however, is encouraging and has shown that vestibular rehabilitation in addition to other rehabilitation programs causes improvement in performance of ADLs as well as in specific symptoms such as gaze stabilization problems, dizziness, and/or vertigo and balance problems.[112,116]

The subsequent treatment sections focus on techniques primarily related to gaze stabilization. Although improvement in gaze stabilization will indirectly result in improvement in balance and symptoms of dizziness or vertigo, specific treatments for these deficits are not described. The reader is referred to the references for information related to these areas.

Utilizing a Restorative Approach

The goals of gaze stabilization treatment are to improve visual tracking, improve gaze stabilization during head movements, and improve visual modulation of the VOR.[58,90,118] The overall goal is to evaluate how gaze stabilization problems are affecting occupational performance and to incorporate this information into occupation-based activities whenever possible.

General Guidelines/Assumptions

1. Poor gaze stability, which results in impaired visual cues to postural stability, will affect postural stability, which will in turn affect balance, which in turn will affect functional performance. Exercises that improve gaze stability, therefore, will help postural stability, balance, and overall total body function.[117]

2. CNS compensation or habituation (reduction of symptoms produced by specific movements), occurs as a result of repetitive exposure to the movement or movements that bring on the symptoms.[58,60]

3. Underlying mechanisms of the recovery of gaze stability that can occur can include the recovery of the VOR itself, alterations of saccadic amplitude and direction, improved function of the cervico-ocular reflex (COR), central processing, and limiting head movement and activity.[113,117] Horak outlines, therefore, the physiological goal of gaze stabilization or eye-head coordination exercises as follows[112]:

    a) Increase the cervico-ocular reflex

    b) Better programming of eye movements in anticipation of head movements (ie, eyes move first, then the head)

    c) Enhance saccadic and smooth pursuit systems

    d) Decrease the amplitude and velocity of head movements.

4. Adaptation of the VOR is context specific; therefore, activities should stress the system in different ways (ie, different frequencies or different head positions).[60]

5. Graded exercises and activities that cause exposure to eye, head, and body movements as well as general physical activities are the core activities of the restorative approach to visual vestibular deficits.[111-113,116,119] Addressing the client's symptoms of anxiety is also an important element of treatment.

Specific Progression of Gaze Stabilization Exercises[91,113,118]

1. Saccadic and smooth pursuit tracking exercises while the head is still

2. Stabilize gaze on a still object in midline while the head is moving either horizontally or vertically. Increase the time as the client progresses. Progress from slow to faster movements and self-imposed to therapist passively moving the client's head

3. Stabilize gaze on two still objects at periphery (eye-head movements)

4. Stabilize gaze on object moving in-phase with head

5. Stabilize gaze on object moving out-of-phase with head

6. Moving targets (predictable and unpredictable)

7. Neck still on trunk

8. Head on trunk movements

Start the treatment progression in supported sitting and progress to standing and walking. Also, progress from a firm support surface to compliant and irregular surfaces.[113,118]

Sample Functionally Oriented Treatment Activities/Progressions

1. Make the activity progressively more challenging as the client improves by changing speed or amplitude of the stimulus, changing directions, postures, visual, or surface environment.[112] For example, progress from a stimulus presented on a blank wall to a checkered or patterned background.[112] Whitney and Herdman provide the following example of progressively challenging treatment activities with the ultimate goal of the client being able to handle grocery shopping[60]:

    a) First, the client walks down a hallway while moving his or her head right and left and up and down.

b) Client performs the same activity, but the therapist adds items that the client has to avoid while walking.

c) Client walks down the aisle of an uncrowded (then more crowded) drugstore.

d) Client walks in the most complex visually stimulating environment (ie, grocery store or shopping mall).

2. Tape a word (progress to sentence, paragraph) on a mirror, and have the client move his or her head back and forth and read the word (sentence, paragraph).[112]

3. Cohen et al describe the following graded, purposeful activities, which were utilized in the treatment of a client with vestibular dysfunction.[123] These activities specifically related to the task or situation that produced symptoms during the assessment.

a) Sitting and dealing cards into two piles spaced about 3 ft apart.

b) Sitting and leaning to the floor to retrieve objects.

c) Playing catch in sitting position.

4. In supine position, rolling side to side to move bean bags from one side of the treatment mat or bed to the other.

5. Standing and moving cups from a low shelf to an overhead shelf.

6. Playing catch in standing position.

7. Standing and dealing cards along a 6-ft counter.

8. Rotating and handing cards one at a time to the therapist.

9. Dribbling a ball back and forth across the room while bouncing a ball off the wall, alternating right and left.

10. Walking back and forth across the room while bouncing a ball off the wall, alternating right and left.

11. Walking back and forth across the room while reading signs on the wall, alternating right and left.

12. Walking around the room and stooping to retrieve objects on the floor.

13. Sidestepping back and forth across the room while reading signs on the wall, first to the front, then over one shoulder.

Utilizing an Adaptive Approach

1. If the client's ABI results in decreased ability to utilize proprioceptive and tactile cues to maintain balance and total body function, have the client utilize visual cues (ie, visual scanning) while walking.

2. If the client's ABI results in an inability to utilize visual cues for balance and total body function, have him or her utilize tactile or proprioceptive cues—for example, running his or her hand along the wall while walking down a hallway.

3. If the client has oscillopsia that is worsened by head movement, have the client perform the activity while the head and body are still—for example, standing still in a store aisle to read a label.[21]

4. If the client has a reduced gain of the VOR, causing difficulty with fine visual discrimination tasks when the head is not stationary, stabilize the client's head against a headrest to perform these activities.[116]

5. Rearrange the client's environment so that functional activities can be performed without having to utilize the postures or movements that elicit symptoms—for example, do not place important items in the kitchen in a lower cabinet, which requires bending, if this is a movement that causes problems.

6. Keep the client's environment as visually simple and uncluttered as possible—for example, painted walls instead of wallpaper or a solid tablecloth instead of a patterned one.

References

1. Morton RL. Visual dysfunction following traumatic brain injury. In: Ashley MJ, ed. *Traumatic Brain Injury Rehabilitative Treatment and Case Management*. Boca Raton, Fla: CRC Press; 2004.
2. Warren M. *Brain Injury Visual Assessment Battery For Adults: Test Manual*. Birmingham, Ala: VisAbilities Rehab Services Inc; 1998.
3. Warren M. Evaluation and treatment of visual deficits. In: Pedretti L, ed. *Occupational Therapy: Practice Skills For Physical Dysfunction*. St. Louis, Mo: Mosby Inc; 2001.
4. Cohen AH, Rein LD. The effect of head trauma on the visual system: the doctor of optometry as a member of the rehabilitation team. *J Am Optom Assoc*. 1992;63(8):530-536.
5. Cuiffreda KJ, et al. Normal vision function. In: Gonzales EG, Myers S, Edelstein J, Lieberman J, Downey J, eds. *Downey and Darling's Physiological Basis of Rehabilitation Medicine*. Boston, Mass: Butterworth Heimann; 2001.
6. Warren M. Visuospatial skills: assessment and intervention strategies. *AOTA Self Study Series: Cognitive Rehabilitation*. Bethesda, Md: The American Occupational Therapy Association, Inc; 1994.
7. Hellerstein L, Freed S. Rehabilitative optometric management of a traumatic brain injury patient. *J Behav Optometry*. 1994;5(6):143-147.
8. Aloisio L. Visual dysfunction. In: Gillen G, Burkhardt A, eds. *Stroke Rehabilitation: A Function-Based Approach*. St. Louis, Mo: Mosby Inc; 2004.
9. Falk NS, Askionoff EB. The primary care optometric evaluation of the traumatic brain injury patient. *J Am Optometr Assoc*. 1992;63(8):547-553.
10. Gianutsos R, Ramsey G, Perlin RR. Rehabilitative optometric services for survivors of acquired brain injury. *Arch Phys Med Rehabil*. 1988;69(8):573-579.
11. Bryan VL. Management of residual physical deficits, In: Ashley MJ, Krych DK, eds. *Traumatic Brain Injury Rehabilitative Treatment and Case Management*. Boca Raton, Fla: CRC Press; 2004:319-366.
12. Suter PS. Rehabilitation and management of visual dysfunction following traumatic brain injury. In: Ashley MJ, ed. *Traumatic Brain Injury Rehabilitative Treatment and Case Management*. Boca Raton, Fla: CRC Press; 2004.
13. Padula WV, Argyris S, Ray J. Visual evoked potentials: evaluating treatment for post-trauma vision syndrome in patients with traumatic brain injuries. *Brain Inj*. 1994;8(2):125-133.
14. Atria M. Neurology: a summary of brain anatomy and function for the vision therapist. In: *Vision Therapist: Working With the Brain Injured, 35(1)*. Santa Ana, Calif: Optometric Extension Program; 1993.
15. Suchoff IB, Ciuffreda KJ, Kapoor N. An overview of acquired brain injury and optometric implications. In: Suchoff IB, Cuiffreda KJ, Kapoor N, eds. *Visual and Vestibular Consequences of Acquired Brain Injury*. Santa Ana, Calif: Optometric Extension Program, Inc; 2001.
16. Cormican D. Seeing the whole picture. *OT Practice*. 2004;9(7):14-17.
17. Braun J. Divided attention: narrowing the gap between brain and behavior. In: Jochen B, ed. *Visual Attention and Cortical Circuits*. Cambridge, Mass: MIT Press; 2001.
18. Warren M. A hierarchical model for evaluation and treatment of visual perceptual dysfunction in adult acquired brain injury, part 2. *Am J Occup Ther*. 1993;47(1):55-65.
19. O'Dell MW, Bell KR, Sandel ME. Medical rehabilitation of brain injury: AAPMR study guide in brain injury rehabilitation. *Arch Phys Med Rehabil*. 1998;79:S10-S15.
20. Bailey C, Gouras P. The retina and phototransduction. In: Kandel ER, Schwartz JH, eds. *Principles of Neural Science*. 2nd ed. New York, NY: Elsevier Science; 1985.
21. Scheiman M. *Understanding and Managing Vision Deficits*. Thorofare, NJ: SLACK Incorporated; 1997.

22. Niemeier JP. The lighthouse strategy: use of a visual imagery technique to treat visual inattention in stroke patients. *Brain Inj.* 1998;12(5):399-406.

23. Richman J, Garzia P. *Developmental eye movement test.* Test booklet. South Bend, Ind: Bernell Corporation; 1987.)

24. Post RB. Leibowitz HW. Two modes of processing visual information: implications for assessing visual impairment. *Am J Optom Physiol Opt.* 1986;63(2):94-96.

25. Vision Associates, 4209 US Highway 90 W #312 Lake City, FL 32055.

26. Warren M. A hierarchical model for evaluation and treatment of visual perceptual dysfunction in adult acquired brain injury, Part 1. *Am J Occup Ther.* 1993;47(1):42-54.

27. Toglia J. A dynamic interactional approach to cognitive rehabilitation. In: Katz N, ed. *Cognition and Occupation Across The Life Span.* Bethesda, Md: The American Occupational Therapy Association, Inc; 2005.

28. Gianutsos R, Perlin R, Mazerolle KA, et al. Rehabilitation optometric services for persons emerging from coma. *J Head Trauma Rehabil.* 1989;4(2):17-25.

29. Warren M. Providing low vision rehabilitations services with occupational therapy and ophthalmology: a program description. *Am J Occup Ther.* 1995;49(9):877-883.

30. Hellerstein L. Visual problems associated with brain injury. In: Scheiman M, ed. *Understanding and Managing Vision Deficits.* Thorofare, NJ: SLACK Incorporated; 1997.

31. Zasler N. Medical aspects. In: Raskin SA, Mateer CA, eds. *Neuropsychological Management of Mild Traumatic Brain Injury.* New York, NY: Oxford University Press; 2000.

32. Brazier J, Smith SE. Disorders of the pupil. In: Easty DL, Sparrow JM, eds. *Oxford Textbook of Ophthalmology.* New York, NY: Oxford University Press; 1999.

33. Baily C. Neuro-ophthalmic history and examination. In: Easty DL, Sparrow JM, eds. *Oxford Textbook of Ophthalmology.* Vol 2. New York, NY: Oxford University Press; 1999.

34. Ciuffreda KJ, Han Y, Kapoor N, et al. Oculomotor consequences of acquired brain injury. In: Suchoff IB, Ciuffreda KJ, Kapoor N, eds. *Visual and Vestibular Consequences of Acquired Brain Injury.* Santa Ana, Calif: Optometric Extension Program, Inc; 2001.

35. Bronstein AM, Hood D. The cervico-ocular reflex in normal subjects and patients with absent vestibular function. *Brain Res.* 1986;373:399-408.

36. Watson GR, Whittaker S, Steciw M. *Pepper Visual Skills for Reading Test.* 2nd ed. Lilburn, Ga: Bear Consultants, Inc; 1995.

37. Engelhardt N, et al. *Sight Unseen. Advance for Directors in Rehabilitation.* 2003:69-74.

38. Vezzetti D. Capacity, content, control: a model for analyzing the cognitive demands of activity. *Occup Ther Pract.* 1989;1(1):9-17.

39. Whitney SL, Wrisley DM, Marchetti GF, Furman JM. The effect of age on vestibular rehabilitation outcomes. *Laryngoscope.* 2002;112(10):1785-1790.

40. Freeman P. Low vision: overview and review of low vision evaluation and treatment. In: Scheiman M, ed. *Understanding and Managing Vision Deficits.* Thorofare, NJ: SLACK Incorporated; 2002.

41. Waddell PA, Gronwall DMA. Sensitivity to light and sound following minor head injury. *Acta Neurol Scand.* 1984;69:270-276.

42. Beaver KA, Mann WC. Overview of technology for low vision. *Am J Occup Ther.* 1995;49(9):913-921.

43. Lampert J, Lapolice DJ. Functional considerations in evaluation and treatment of the client with low vision. *Am J Occup Ther.* 1995;49(9):885-890.

44. Raskin S. Cognitive remediation of mild traumatic brain injury in an older age group. In: Raskin S, Mateer C, eds. *Neuropsychological Management of Mild Traumatic Brain Injury.* New York, NY: Oxford University Press; 2000.

45. Von Noordon GK. *Binocular Vision and Ocular Motility.* 3rd ed. St. Louis, Mo: CV Mosby Co; 1985.

46. Neger RE. The evaluation of diplopia in head trauma. *J Head Trauma Rehabil.* 1989;4(2):27-34.

47. Kelly JP. Anatomy of the central visual pathways. In: Kandel ER, Schwartz JH, eds. *Principles of Neural Science.* 2nd ed. New York, NY: Elsevier Science; 1985.

48. Gianutsos R, Suchoff I. Visual fields after brain injury: management issues for the occupational therapist. In: Scheiman M, ed. *Understanding and Managing Vision Deficits.* Thorofare, NJ: SLACK Incorporated; 1997.

49. Bouska MJ, Kauffman NA, Marcus SE. Disorders of the visual perceptual system. In: Umphred DA, ed. *Neurological Rehabilitation.* 2nd ed. St. Louis, Mo: CV Mosby; 1990.

50. Kennard C. Disorders of visual perception. In: Easty DL, Sparrow JM, eds. *Oxford Textbook of Ophthalmology.* Vol 2. New York, NY: Oxford University Press; 1999.

51. Kandel ER. Processing of form and movement in the visual system. In: Kandel ER, Schwartz JH, eds. *Principles of Neural Science.* 2nd ed. New York, NY: Elsevier Science; 1985.

52. Frohman E, Zee D. Supranuclear eye movement abnormalities. In: Easty DL, Sparrow JM, eds. *Oxford Textbook of Ophthalmology.* Vol 2. New York, NY: Oxford University Press; 1999.

53. Gouras P. Oculomotor system. In: Kandel ER, Schwartz JH, eds. *Principles of Neural Science.* 2nd ed. New York, NY: Elsevier Science; 1985.

54. Abrams RA. Planning and producing saccadic eye movements. In: Rayner K, ed. *Eye Movements and Visual Cognition.* New York, NY: Springer Verlag; 1992.

55. Vogel MS. An overview of head trauma for the primary care practitioner: part II-Ocular damage associated with head trauma. *J Am Optometric Assoc.* 1992;63:542-546.

56. Heide W, Kompf D. Specific parietal lobe contribution to spatial constancy across saccades. In: Tier P, Karnath HO, eds. *Parietal Lobe Contributions to Orientation in 3D Space.* New York, NY: Springer Herlag; 1997.

57. Fischer, Burkhart. Saccadic reaction time: implications for reading, dyslexia, and visual cognition. In: Rayner K, ed. *Eye Movements and Visual Cognition.* New York, NY: Springer Verlag; 1992.

58. Herdman SJ, Clendaniel RA. Assessment and treatment of complete vestibular loss. In: Herdman SJ, ed. *Vestibular Rehabilitation.* Philadelphia, Pa: FA Davis; 2000.

59. Honrubia V. Quantitative vestibular function tests and clinical examination. In: Herdman SJ, ed. *Vestibular Rehabilitation.* Philadelphia, Pa: FA Davis; 2000.

60. Whitney SL, Herdman SJ. Physical therapy assessment of vestibular hypofunction. In: Herdman SJ, ed. *Vestibular Rehabilitation.* Philadelphia, Pa: FA Davis; 2000.

61. Maples WC, Atchley J, Ficklin T. Northeastern State University college of optometry's oculomotor norms. J Behav Optometrist. 1992;3:143-150.

62. Warren M. Letter to potential users of the biVABA. VisAbilities Rehab Services. 1634-A Montgomery Hwy #194, Hoover, AL 35216-4902.

63. Gordon WA, Hibbard MR, Egelko S, et al. Perceptual remediation in patients with right brain damage: a comprehensive program. *Arch Phys Med Rehabil.* 1985;66(6):353-359.

64. Diller L, Gordon W. Interventions for cognitive deficits in brain-injured adults. *J Consult Clin Psychol.* 1981;49(6):822-834.

65. Piasetsky E, Ben-Yishay Y, Weinberg J. The systematic remediation of specific disorders: selected application of methods derived in a clinical research setting. In: Trexler LE, ed. *Cognitive Rehabilitation Conceptualization and Intervention.* New York, NY: Plenum Press; 1982.

66. Cook EA, Luschem L, Sikes S. Dressing training for an elderly woman with cognitive and perceptual impairments. *Am J Occup Ther.* 1991;45(7):652-654.

67. Cohen M, GrossWasser Z, Banchadske R, Appel A. Convergence insufficiency in brain-injured patients. *Brain Inj.* 1980;3(2):187-191.

68. Leslie S. Accommodation in acquired brain injury. In: Suchoff IB, Cuiffreda KJ, Kapoor N, eds. *Visual and Vestibular Consequences of Acquired Brain Injury.* Santa Ana, Calif: Optometric Extension Program Inc; 2001.

69. Valenti C. Brain injured patients in vision therapy: perspective. *Vision Therapy: Working With The Brain Injured.* 35(1). Santa Ana, Calif: Optometric Extension Program; 1999.

70. Anton HA, Hershler C, Lloyd P, Murray D. Visual neglect and extinction: a new test. *Arch Phys Med Rehabil.* 1988;69:1013-1016.

71. Butter CM, Kirsch N. Combined and separate effects of eye patching and visual stimulation on unilateral neglect following stroke. *Arch Phys Med Rehabil.* 1990;73(12):1133-1138.

72. Rafal RD. Neglect. In: Parasuraman R, ed. *The Attentive Brain.* Cambridge, Mass: The MIT Press; 1998.

73. Katz N. Functional disability and rehabilitation outcome in right hemisphere damaged patients with and without neglect. *Arch Phys Med Rehabil.* 1999;80:379-384.

74. Robertson L. Visualspatial attention and parietal function: their role in object perception. In: Parasuraman R, ed. *The Attentive Brain.* Cambridge, Mass: MIT Press; 1998.

75. Heilman KM, Valenstein E, Watson RT. Neglect and related disorders. *Semin Neurol.* 2000;20(4):463-470.

76. Caplan B. Assessment of unilateral neglect: a new reading test. *J Clin Exp Neurophysiol.* 1986;9(4):359-364.

77. Caplan B. Stimulus affects in unilateral neglect? *Cortex.* 1985;21:69-89.

78. Finkel LJ, Sajda P. Constructing visual perception. *Am Scientist.* 1994;82(3):224-237.

79. Cohen AH. The role of optometry in the management of vestibular disorders. *Brain Inj.* 2005;3(3):7-10.

80. Parker RS. *Traumatic Brain Injury and Neuropsychological Impairment.* New York, NY: Springer-Verlag; 1990.

81. Zoltan B. Visual, visual perceptual and perceptual-motor deficits in brain injured adults: evaluation, treatment and functional implications. In: Kraft GH, Berrol S, eds. *Physical Medicine and Rehabilitation Clinics of North America.* Philadelphia, Pa: WB Saunders Co; 1992.

82. Baynes K, Holtzman JD, Volpe BT. Components of visual attention: alterations in response pattern to visual stimuli following parietal lobe infarction. *Brain.* 1986;109(Pt 1):99-114.

83. Butter CM, Kirsch NL, Reeves G. The effect of lateralized dynamic stimuli on unilateral spatial neglect following right hemisphere lesions. *Neurol Neurosci.* 1990;2:39-46.

84. Calvanio, Petrone PN, Levine D. Left visual spatial neglect is both environment-centered and body-centered. *Neurology.* 1987;37(7):1179-1183.
85. Di Pellegrino G, Basso G, Frassinetti F. Spatial extinction on double asynchronous stimulation. *Neuropsychologia.* 1997;35(9):1215-1223.
86. Cabay M, King LJ. Sensory integration and perception: the foundation for concept formation. *Occup Ther Pract.* 1989;1(1):18-27.
87. Riddoch MJ, Humphreys GW. Perceptual and action systems in unilateral visual neglect. In: Jeannerod M, ed. *Neurophysiological and Neuropsychological Aspects of Spatial Neglect.* New York, NY: North-Holland; 1987.
88. Robertson IH, Tegner R, Tham K, Lo A, Nimmo-Smith I. Sustained attention training for unilateral neglect: theoretical and rehabilitation implications. *J Clin Exp Neuropsychol.* 1995;17(3):416-430.
89. Mattingley JB, Driver J, Beschin N, Robertson IH. Attention competition between modalities: extinction between touch and vision after right hemisphere damage. *Neuropsychologia.* 1997;35(6):867-880.
90. Karnath HO, Perenin MT. Tactile exploration of peripersonal space in patients with neglect. *NeuroReport.* 1998;9:2273-2277.
91. Kasten E, Poggel DA, Sabel BA. Computer-based training of stimulus detection improves color and simple pattern recognition in the defective field of hemianopic subjects. *J Cognitive Neuroscience.* 2000;12(6):1001-1012.
92. Padula WV, Argyris S. Post trauma vision syndrome and visual midline shift syndrome. *NeuroRehabilitation.* 1996;6:165-171.
93. Behrmann S, Watt S, Black SE, Barton JJ. Impaired visual search in patients with unilateral neglect: an oculographic analysis. *Neuropsychologia.* 1997;35(11):1445-1458.
94. Walker R, Findlay M. Eye movement control in spatial and object-based neglect. In: Tier P, Karnath HO, eds. *Parietal Lobe Contributions to Orientation in 3D Space.* New York, NY: Springer Verlag; 1997.
95. Chen Sea MJ, Henderson A, Cermak S. Patterns of visual spatial inattention and their functional significance in stroke patients. *Arch Phys Med Rehabil.* 1993;74(4):355-360.
96. Wilson B, Cockburn J, Halligan P. Development of a behavioral test of visuospatial neglect. *Arch Phys Med Rehabil.* 1987;68(2):98-102.
97. Wilson B, Cockburn J, Halligan P. *Behavioural Inattention Test.* Bury St. Edmunds, England: Thames Valley Test Co; 1987.
98. Zoltan B, Jabri J, Panikoff L, Ryckman D. *Perceptual Motor Evaluation for Head Injured and Other Neurologically Impaired Adults.* San Jose, Calif: Santa Clara Valley Medical Center, Occupational Therapy Department; 1983.
99. Toglia J. Multicontext treatment approach. In: Crepeau E, Cohn ES, Schell BAB, eds. *Willard and Spackman's Occupational Therapy.* Philadelphia, Pa: Lippincott, Williams and Wilkins; 2003.
100. Golisz K, Toglia J. Perception and cognition. In: Crepeau EB, Cohn ES, Schell BAB, eds. *Willard and Spackman's Occupational Therapy.* Philadelphia, Pa: Lippicott, Williams and Wilkins; 2003.
101. Chen Sea MJ, Henderson A, Cermak SA. Patterns of visual spatial inattention and their functional significance in stroke patients. *Arch Phys Med Rehabil.* 1993;74(4):355-360.
102. Eimer M. An ERP study on visual spatial priming with peripheral onsets. *Psychophysiology.* 1994;31:154-163.
103. Robertson IH, Mattingley JB, Rorden C, Driver J. Phasic alerting of neglect patients overcomes their spatial deficit in visual awareness. *Nature.* 1998;395(6698):169-172.
104. Dick RJ, Wood RG, Bradshaw JL, Bradshaw JA. Programmable visual display for diagnosing, assessing and rehabilitating unilateral neglect. *Med Biol Eng Comput.* 1987;25:109-111.
105. Tham K, Ginsburg E, Fisher AG, Tegner R. Training to improve awareness of disabilities in clients with unilateral neglect. *Am J Occup Ther.* 2001;55(1):46-53.
106. Frassinetti F, Angeli V, Meneghello F, Avanzi S, Làdavas E. Long-lasting amelioration of visuospatial neglect by prism adaptation. *Brain.* 2002;125(3):608-623.
107. Pierce SR, Buxbaum LJ. Treatments of unilateral neglect: a review. *Arch Phys Med Rehabil.* 2002;83:256-265.
108. Rosen A, Cohen A, Trebing S. The integration of visual and vestibular systems in balance disorders-a clinical perspective. In: Suchoff IB, Ciuffreda KJ, Kapoor N, eds. *Visual and Vestibular Consequences of Acquired Brain Injury.* Santa Ana, Calif: Optometric Extension Program; 2001.
109. Dieterich M, Brandt T. Brain activation studies on visual-vestibular and ocular motor interaction. *Curr Opin Neurol.* 2000;13:3-18.
110. Hellerstein L, Winkler P. Vestibular dysfunction associated with traumatic brain injury: collaborative optometry and physical therapy treatment. In: Suchoff IB, Ciuffreda KJ, Kapoor N, eds. *Visual and Vestibular Consequences of Acquired Brain Injury.* Santa Ana, Calif: Optometric Extension Program Foundation; 2001.

111. Gurr B, Moffat N. Psychological consequences of vertigo and the effectiveness of vestibular rehabilitation for brain injury patients. *Brain Inj.* 2001;15(5):387-400.
112. Horak F. Vestibular rehabilitation for dizziness and balance disorders. Workshop presented by North American Seminars Inc. Escondido, Calif: April 23-24, 2005.
113. Shumway-Cook A, Horak F. Rehabilitation strategies for patients with vestibular deficits. *Neurol Clinics N Am.* 1990;8:441-457.
114. Farber S, Zoltan B. Visual vestibular systems interaction: treatment implications. *J Head Trauma Rehabil.* 1989;4(2):9-15.
115. Leigh JR. Pharmacological and optical methods of treating vestibular disorders and nystagmus. In: Herdman SJ, ed. *Vestibular Rehabilitation.* Philadelphia, Pa: FA Davis; 2000.
116. Cohen HS. Disability in vestibular disorders. In: Herdman SJ, ed. *Vestibular Rehabilitation.* Philadelphia, Pa: FA Davis; 2000.
117. Herdman SJ. Advances in the treatment of vestibular disorders. *Phys Ther.* 1997;77(6):602-615.
118. Shumway-Cook A. Vestibular rehabilitation of the patient with traumatic brain injury. In: Herdman SJ, ed. *Vestibular Rehabilitation.* Philadelphia, Pa: FA Davis; 2000.
119. Lyons C. Nystagmus. In: Easty DL, Sparrow JM, eds. *Oxford Textbook of Ophthalmology.* Vol 2. New York, NY: Oxford University Press; 1999.
120. Lieberman S, Cohen AH, Rubin J. NYSOA K-D test. *J Am Optom Assoc.* 1983;54(7):631-637.
121. Roland PS, Otto E. Rehabilitation for posttraumatic vestibular dysfunction. In: Ashley MJ, ed. *Traumatic Brain Injury Rehabilitative Treatment and Case Management.* Boca Raton, Fla: CRC Press; 2004.
122. Shepard NT, Telian SA. Programmatic vestibular rehabilitation. *Otolarygol Head Neck Surg.* 1995;112(1):173-182.
123. Cohen H, Miller LV, Kane-Wineland M, Hatfield CL. Vestibular rehabilitation with graded occupations. *Am J Occup Ther.* 1995;49(4):362-367.

Resources

Baillet R, Blood K, Bach-y-Rita P. Visual field rehabilitation in the cortically blind. *J Neurol Neurosurg Psychiatry.* 1985;48(11):1113-1124.

Chronister K. The missing link in fall-prevention programs. OT Practice. 2004;9:11-14.

Cohen H. Vestibular rehabilitation improves daily life function. *Am J Occup Ther.* 1994;48(10):919-925.

Corbetta M. Functional anatomy of visual attention in the human brain: studies with positron emission tomography. In: Parasuraman R, ed. *The Attentive Brain.* Cambridge, Mass: The MIT Press; 2000.

Eimer M. Spatial cuing, sensory gating and selective response preparation: an ERP study on visuo-spatial orienting. *Electroencephal Clin Neurophysiol.* 1993;88(5):408-420.

Ferro JM, Kertesz A, Black SE. Subcortical neglect. *Neurology.* 1987;37:1487-1492.

Findlay, John M. Programming of stimulus elicited saccadic eye movements. In: Rayner K, ed. *Eye Movements and Visual Cognition.* New York, NY: Springer Verlag; 1992.

Gianutsos R, Matheson P. The rehabilitation of visual perceptual disorders attributable to brain injury. In: Meir MJ, Benton AL, Diller L, eds. *Neuropsychological Rehabilitation.* New York, NY: Guilford University Press; 1987.

Hain TC, Ramaswamy TS, Hillman MA. Anatomy and physiology of the normal vestibular system. In: Herdman SJ, ed. *Vestibular Rehabilitation.* Philadelphia, Pa: FA Davis; 2000.

Hartman-Maeir A, Katz N. Validity of the behavioral inattention test (BIT): relationships with functional tasks. *Am J Occup Ther.* 1985;49(6):507-516.

Hayhoe MH, Lachter J, Moeller P. Spatial memory and integration across saccadic eye movements. In: Rayner K, ed. *Eye Movements and Visual Cognition.* New York, NY: Springer Verlag; 1992.

Heilman K, Barret A, Adair J. Possible mechanisms of anosognosia: a defect in self-awareness. *Phil Trans R Soc Lond B Biol Sci.* 1998;353(1377):1903-1909.

Hibbard MR, Gordon WA, Kenner B. The neuropsychological evaluation: a pathway to understanding the sequelae of brain injury. In: Suchoff IB, Ciuffreda KJ, Kapoor N, eds. *Visual and Vestibular Consequences of Acquired Brain Injury.* Santa Ana, Calif: Optometric Extension Program Inc; 2001.

Lepore FE. Disorders of ocular motility following head trauma. *Arch Neurol.* 1995;52:924-926.

Macdonald J. An investigation of body scheme in adults with cerebral vascular accident. *Am J Occup Ther.* 1960;14:72-79.

Malec J. Training the brain-injured client in behavioral self-management skills. In: Edelstein BA, Couture ET, eds. *Behavioral Assessment and Rehabilitation of the Traumatically Brain Damaged.* New York, NY: Plenum Press; 1984.

Nakayama K, Joseph JS. Attention, pattern recognition and pop out in visual search. In: Parasuraman R, ed. *The Attentive Brain.* Cambridge, Mass: The MIT Press; 2000.

Niebur E, Koch C. Computational architectures for attention. In: Parasuraman R, ed. *The Attentive Brain.* Cambridge, Mass: The MIT Press; 2000.

Padula WV, Shapiro J. Post-traumatic vision syndrome caused by head injury. In: Padula WV, ed. *A Behavioral Vision Approach for Persons with Physical Disabilities.* Santa Ana, Calif: Optometric Extension Program Foundation Inc; 1988.

Parasuraman R, ed. *The Attentive Brain.* Cambridge, Mass: The MIT Press; 2000.

Paulus WM, Straube A, Brandt T. Visual stabilization of posture: physiological stimulus characteristics and clinical aspects. *Brain.* 1984;107(Pt 4):1143-1163.

Perenin MT. Optic ataxia and unilateral neglect: clinical evidence for dissociable spatial functions in posterior parietal cortex. In: Thier P, Karnath HO, eds. *Parietal Lobe Contributions to Orientation in 3D.* New York, NY: Springer Verlag; 1997.

Petit L, Orssaud C, Tzourio N, Mazoyer B, Berthoz A. Superior parietal lobule involvement in the representation of visual space: a PET review. In: Thier P, Karnath HO, eds. *Parietal Lobe Contributions to Orientation in 3D Space.* New York, NY: Springer Verlag; 1997.

Poggel DA, Kasten E, Sabel BA. Attentional cuing improves vision restoration therapy in patients with visual field defects. *Neurology.* 2004;63:2069-2076.

Rayner K. Eye movements and visual cognition: introduction. In: Rayner K, ed. *Eye Movements and Visual Cognition.* New York, NY: Springer Verlag; 1992.

Rossi PW, Kheyfets S, Reding MJ. Fresnel prisms improve visual perception in stroke patients with homonymous hemianopia or unilateral visual neglect. *Neurology.* 1990;40(10):1597-1599.

Tham K, Borell L, Gustavsson A. The discovery of disability: a phenomenological study of unilateral neglect. *Am J Occup Ther.* 2000;54(4):398-405.

Uomoto JM. The contribution of the neuropsychological evaluation to traumatic brain injury rehabilitation. In: Ashley MJ, ed. *Traumatic Brain Injury Rehabilitative Treatment and Case Management.* Boca Raton, Fla: CRC Press; 2004.

Warren M. Including occupational therapy in low vision rehabilitation. *Am J Occup Ther.* 1995;49(9):857-859.

Whitney SL, Rossi MM. Efficacy of vestibular rehabilitation. *Otolaryngol Clin N Am.* 2000;33(3):659-672.

Yuen HK, Benzing P. Treatment methodology. Guiding of behavior through redirection in brain injury rehabilitation. *Brain Inj.* 1996;10(3):229-238.

Zihl J. Cerebral disturbances of elementary visual functions. In: Brown JW, ed. *Neuropsychology of Visual Perception.* Hillsdale, NJ: Lawrence Erlbaum Assoc; 1989.

Zoltan B. Remediation of visual-perceptual and perceptual-motor deficits. In: Rosenthal M, Griffith ER, Bond MR, Miller JD, eds. *Rehabilitation of the Adult and Child with Traumatic Brain Injury.* Philadelphia, Pa: FA Davis; 1990.

CHAPTER 4

APRAXIA

Acquired brain injury (ABI) can affect the client's ability for skilled action performance, which in turn will impair his or her ability to carry out everyday activities without error.[1] The ABI client can have difficulty with naturalistic action, or the behavior an individual uses to accomplish everyday, simple tasks, such as hair combing, and more complex or extended activities, such as grooming or dressing, and which require one to use objects and sequence multiple steps to achieve goals.[2] This impaired ability to perform naturalistic actions is termed *apraxia* and is defined as the inability to perform certain skilled purposeful movements in the absence of motor power, sensation, or coordination. It is a cognitive motor disorder that involves the loss or impaired ability to program motor systems to perform purposeful skilled movements.[3] Although there may be some degree of spontaneous recovery from apraxia, generally some degree of impairment persists and causes a deficit that interferes with activities of daily living (ADLs).[3] Praxis is a performance skill and forms the foundation for the development of performance patterns and occupations.[4]

Although the conceptualization of apraxia as a motor programming disorder has been universally accepted, the exact nature of the programming deficit has remained controversial.[5-9] Heilman and Rothi envision a model of motor planning in which there are visuokinesthetic motor engrams stored in the left parietal lobe.[7] Information from this area then activates the premotor cortex in the left and then the right hemispheres through the corpus callosum. Building on these concepts, some studies have provided evidence that apraxia may result "from lesions disconnecting the areas where stimuli instigating the movement are processed from the center, where the plan of action must be evoked and programmed, in order to activate the motor cortex neurons."[10] Others support this notion of stored engrams, or schemas related to motor planning.[11,12]

Humphreys and Forde describe a concept called "contention scheduling" to explain how an individual executes routine tasks.[11] The individual stores schemas for routine tasks, and when a triggering stimulus activates the schema above its threshold, that schema would remain active until the goal is reached or the schema is inhibited by competing schemas.[11] Norman and Shallice expand on this and describe a second system called the supervisory attention system (SAS), which they hypothesize is involved in higher order cognitive control or willed actions, which are required when dealing with novel situations.[12] Anderson et al also describe a class of areas or system that relates to attention, intention, and decisions.[13] They describe it as an intermediate stage between sensory and motor structures that contains abstract representation of space and the mental operations important for planning movements.[13] The concept of a "schema" as the fundamental unit of organized behavior is embedded in their theory of the performance of everyday actions. They describe "intermediate level actions" as everyday actions. These activities, making a cup of coffee for example, require both object knowledge and action sequences. Their model of action addresses this level of activity or action and contains the following assumptions[13]:

1. *The fundamental unit of organized behavior within the intermediate domain is the schema. Schemas are goal directed. Schemas are effective methods for achieving goals.*

   Cooper and Shallice provide the following example to illustrate this assumption[14]:

   Thus, a goal might be that a particular mug of coffee is sweet. A schema for achieving this goal might comprise: picking up a spoon, dipping the spoon into some sugar contained within a sugar-bowl, filling the spoon with sugar, transporting it, and then tipping it into the mug. The same goal might be achieved by any number of other schemas, such as one involving sugar cubes. The schema that is most appropriate in any particular situation will depend on a variety of factors, including the objects available in the environment and individual preferences.

2. *Schemas consist of a partially ordered set of subgoals. The schema network is task dependent in that different tasks will require networks made up of different schemas and goals.*

3. *Schemas have an associated activation value. This value is a real number that varies over time. Schema activation may be affected by the presence (or absence) of appropriate triggering situations in the environment. Thus, the presence of small portable objects in the environment may excite the schema for picking up such objects. Schemas may also be excited by "top-down" influences from higher level schemas. Thus, a schema for add sugar from sugar bowl to coffee mug may excite a lower-level schema for pick up teaspoon.*

4. *Schema activations are influenced by five factors: top-down influence, environmental influence, self-influence, lateral influence, and random noise.*

5. *In the absence of any influence, schema activations tend to persist (ie, if a schema is highly active and all influences are removed from it, its activation will slowly decay to its resting value).*

6. *Schemas have associated "triggering conditions." The environmental influence on a schema is dependent on the extent to which its triggering conditions are satisfied by the (system's representation of the) current condition. For example, "...the schema for 'pick-up' is triggered by situations in which there is a free hand and a small portable object within reach of that hand." Higher-level schemas are activated solely by the presence of the objects involved in their component subschemas (so, the schema for prepare instant coffee is activated by all coffee-related objects).*

7. *Schemas have a state; they may be either selected or unselected. If a schema is selected, it may pass excitation to its component schema, as illustrated in the example provided in assumption number 4.*

8. *When a basic-level schema is selected, it triggers execution of its corresponding action.*

9. *When a schema's activation exceeds the selection threshold, its state changes to selected.*

Table 4-1

Component Skills of Motor Planning

Cognitive Formulation of Movement Intention
  Selecting a Goal
  Planning the Movement
  Anticipating the Result

Knowledge of The Functional Properties of Objects
  Actions and Action Sequences
  Attentional Processes
  Integration of Tactile-Kinesthetic Information
  (such as where the body is in space, how the parts of the body
  relate to each other during movement, and how the body and
  limbs are positioned)

Adapted from reference 15: Golisz K, Toglia J. Perception and cognition. In: Crepeau E, Cohn ES, Schell BAB, eds. Willard and Spackman's Occupational Therapy. *Philadelphia, Pa: Lippincott Williams and Wilkins; 2003.*

10. *When a selected schema's activation falls below that of one of its competitors or when the state of a selected schema's source schema changes, the selected schema is deselected.*

Golisz and Toglia describe many skills associated with motor planning.[15] These component skills are summarized in Table 4-1. These skills require cognitive, language, tactile, visual, kinesthetic, and vestibular processing. For example, vestibular input provides a sense of body position, or language can help the client translate verbal commands into action.[15]

Many theorize that apraxia is a disturbance to a complex functional system involving two basic functional processes (ie, planning and execution).[16,17] Roy and Square elaborate on this assumption in their belief that there are two systems that allow us to act in the world: conceptual and production.[8] The conceptual system incorporates three types of knowledge relative to motor planning. These categories of knowledge include knowledge of objects and tools in terms of the action and function they serve, knowledge of actions independent of tools or objects but into which tools or objects may be incorporated, and knowledge relevant to the seriation of single actions into a sequence. In addition to this internal knowledge, perceptual and contextual information provide the individual with an "externalization" of knowledge about the function of the conceptualization of action. The first component is focused on the object or tool to be used for a particular function. The next component focuses on the actions performed in carrying out these functions. Perceptual abilities come into play next in selecting an object to perform an action. For example, if the appropriate object is not nearby, the individual may use an object or tool that shares the same characteristics or attributes with the appropriate one.

The second, or production system of motor action, is hypothesized to consist of a number of parallel systems that may operate somewhat independently.[8] Control may shift from one level to another with performance of action involved with a delicate balance between higher- and lower-level processes. Higher level processes demand attention and keep the action sequence directed toward the intended goal. The lower-level system is more autonomous and involves action programs that require minimal attention demands and "…which adaptations to environmental constraints are made through existing neural networks."[8]

Apraxia can be a problem in the production system through a temporal-spatial disorder or a disruption to fine motor control. Errors in motor sequencing can occur as a result of damage to either hemisphere.[9,18] Depending on the location of damage, the type of motor planning deficit that can occur will change. Deficits associated with right brain damage, for example, include difficulties with visual synthesis and analysis for interpreting imitation, commands, spatial organization and spatial thinking for movement production, and unilateral inattention for the interpretation of imitation and production of movements.[9,19,20] Clients with frontal apraxia will often show object substitutions and object misuse, as for example, pouring coffee grinds into orange juice or putting butter in coffee.[1,16,17]

Apraxia has also been seen in damaged areas such as the thalamus.[21] Recent fMRI studies of normals indicate the left intraparietal sulcus is a critical area involved in the development of apraxia for tool use.[22]

Apraxia is commonly seen with aphasia, but aphasia does occur without apraxia. Some hypothesize that praxis and language use two different but partly overlapping networks. At times, aphasic disorders may be confused with apraxic disorders. For example, clients who do not understand verbal commands may be labeled apraxic when they do not move to a verbal command.[7] The opposite may also happen (ie, clients with apraxia are occasionally mistakenly thought to have a comprehension deficit when their failure to follow a verbal command is actually the result of an inability to produce the correct movements).[7]

Apraxia, or motor planning problems, may be subtle or extremely obvious. The client may be unaware of the problem but, more likely, become very frustrated by it. Many times, there is an abnormal clumsiness of the nonparetic hand.[23]

When evaluating the client with apraxia, it must be determined which part or parts of the processing system are impaired. Research has shown "… the functional systems and the neural systems of praxis for various parts of the body are sufficiently different that composite measures of praxis probably have no meaning."[24] A comprehensive evaluation, therefore, requires the inclusion of items testing motor planning with specific body parts. Recent research also indicates a performance difference in clients between less representational acts and more representational acts as well as improvement of performance on imitation. Apraxia evaluation has also recently expanded and is no longer limited to gesture production. It now includes the evaluation of the client's ability to recognize and discriminate gestures.[9] The therapist must differentiate between the client's ability to perform transitive movements (those directed at object manipulation) and intransitive movements (those meant to express ideas of feelings).[10]

In summary, apraxia may take several different forms, with a breakdown occurring in the conceptual and/or production systems. The deficit may be associated with spatiotemporal or temporal problems. The major types of apraxia that may be manifest in the client with ABI include ideomotor, ideational, oral, constructional, and dressing apraxia. The definition, evaluation, and treatment of these categories of deficits are described in the following sections.

Ideomotor Apraxia

Ideomotor apraxia, one of the most common and widely studied forms of apraxia, is the inability to imitate gestures or perform a purposeful motor task on command even though the client fully understands the idea or concept of the task.[25-27] The client knows what to do but cannot perform the action successfully.[28] These clients, although unable to perform on command, retain kinesthetic memory patterns and the ability to carry out many old habitual motor tasks automatically.[29] Often associated with left hemisphere damage, ideomotor apraxia is hypothesized by some to take two forms.[7,30] The first form is the result of lesions or trauma where visuokinesthetic motor engrams are stored. The second form is related to damage to the areas where the engrams are connected to the motor area of the frontal lobes. Clinically, damage to either area will result in the client having trouble performing movements on command. Clients with "disconnection" lesions where the engrams remain intact, however, should be able to discriminate between poor and correct task performance.[3]

Ideomotor apraxia is a multi-dimensional disorder involving different sensory motor connections.[31] It involves the modality of elicitation, different motor programs that relate to the body part utilized, different conceptual representations or levels of meaningfulness, and "different anatomies for the various interactions of body part and modality."[31] All these dimensions must be included in any comprehensive evaluation of ideomotor apraxia.

Performance should be assessed at the command, imitation, and real object level. The client's ability to motor plan utilizing different body parts, such as buccofacial, limb, and total body movements, is also important information.

It has also been found that intransitive movements, or those movements which convey ideas or feelings, are good measures of ideomotor apraxia.[10] These movements relate to a repertoire of motor acts that are well practiced. In addition, they can be designated with a verbal label and have a definite conformation. This allows for easy comparison against the established standard.

One final consideration in the evaluation of ideomotor apraxia is the need for a qualitative analysis of the client's performance. The client with ideomotor apraxia will exhibit common errors in motor performance. These errors are outlined as follows[7,15,28,32]:

1. Body parts as objects
2. Altered proximity
3. Altered plane
4. Fragmentary responses
5. Poor distal differentiation
6. Gestural enhancement
7. Vocal overflow
8. Perseveration
9. Manipulation of body part
10. Timing errors
11. Spatial errors
12. Sequencing errors

Functionally, ideomotor apraxia is considered to be less severe than the related deficit of ideational apraxia.[27] The client with ideomotor apraxia is unable to perform skilled movements on command but improves with imitation and further improves with the use of the actual object.[10,26,31] Research has also indicated that these clients improve in certain aspects of their movements when visual and somesthetic cues are provided.[5]

Ideational Apraxia

The concept of ideational apraxia as a separate entity from ideomotor apraxia has been somewhat controversial.[10] Ideational apraxia is probably the least recognized type of apraxia because approximately 90% of these clients also have aphasia or dementia.[26] The majority of theorists, researchers, and clinicians believe, however, the two can be differentiated. Ideational apraxia has traditionally been described as a disability in carrying out complex sequential motor acts, which is caused by a disruption of the conception, rather than the execution, of the motor act.[25,32,33] It is an inability to carry out a series of acts or an "ideational plan."[7] The deficits the client with ideational apraxia display are characterized by a loss of knowledge of tool function as well as by a conceptual

---

Table 4-2

Conceptual Apraxia

Type of Deficit	Observed Behavior
Content error-tool-object-action knowledge	Inability to select the actions associated with the use of a specific tool. For example, when asked to use a screwdriver, they use it like a hammer.*
Tool-object association knowledge	Unable to recall which tool is associated with which object. For example, will use a screwdriver instead of a hammer when shown a piece of wood with a partially hammered nail.
Mechanical knowledge	Does not understand the mechanical advantage of certain tools. For example, when presented with a partially driven nail without an available hammer, they will not choose an alternative tool that is hard, rigid, and heavy (ie, wrench) but may choose something flexible and light weight.

Note: The client with object agnosia can also use a tool as if it were another tool. If the client can name the tool he or she is using, then the client is not considered agnostic.
Adapted from reference 3: Heilman KM, Rothi LJG, Valenstein E. Two forms of ideomotor apraxia. Neurology. 1982;32:342-346.

---

disturbance related to the sequential organization of actions involving objects.[20] The errors of the client with ideational apraxia generally occur not from the utilization of single objects in isolation, but in planning more complex events.[32]

For the client with ideational apraxia, the mental process for conceptual sequencing that allows one to relate the symbolism of object names and visual imagery to a related motor performance is lost.[34] Frequently, complex acts cannot be performed, whereas simple isolated acts or parts of acts remain. In responding to a command, the more hypothetical the request, the more difficulty the client has.[34]

In recent years, many have used the term "conceptual apraxia" for those clients who are unable to select and use tools and utensils despite normal sensation, motor power, and coordination.[3,22,35] These theorists differentiate clients who cannot sequence acts (ideational apraxia) from those whose deficits are the result of a conceptual problem (conceptual apraxia). Conceptual apraxia is hypothesized to occur in two domains: 1) associative knowledge (tool-action association such as hammer/pound; tool-object association such as hammer/nail) and 2) mechanical knowledge (such as knowing what is the advantage of using a particular tool).[35] A description of observed client behavior, depending on what type of conceptual apraxia the client has, is contained in Table 4-2.[3]

The client with ideational apraxia will perform poorly with activities that require a series of movements.[28] These clients are also at a loss when attempting activities such as using a screwdriver, unlocking a padlock, or cutting bread with a knife.[22] As Moll et al describe, "...at times, they look so bewildered when faced by such everyday tasks that they may be erroneously diagnosed as demented."[22] This client cannot pretend to perform an act or describe the function of an object. For example, if given a cigarette and a match and told to light the cigarette, the client may put the match in his mouth or put the unlighted match to the cigarette. He or she also cannot describe the match's function.

Ideational apraxia always affects performance bilaterally.[32] There should be no significant difference between right and left hand performance beyond that expected from natural hand preference. As with the client with ideomotor apraxia, there should be a qualitative assessment of the client's motor performance. Common errors that characterize performance include the following:

1. Elements occur in the wrong order. The client might pour milk in the bowl before putting in cereal.

2. Sections of the sequence are omitted. The kettle is put on the stove with no water inside.

3. Two or more elements may be blended together. The client lifts sugar toward the cup while at the same time making a stirring motion.

4. The action remains incomplete. When cutting their meat, such clients take one slice at it and try to eat it even though it has not been completely cut.

5. The action overshoots what is necessary. When asked to take off his coat, the client proceeds to take off all his clothes. Instead of a drop of milk in the cup for the tea, he will fill the whole cup.

6. Objects are used inappropriately, either for the context or overall. Instead of spooning sugar into the cup of tea, the client eats the sugar from the spoon. A pencil might be used as a comb. The candle is struck instead of the match.

7. Movements may be made in the wrong plane or wrong direction. The client might "stir" his tea by lifting the spoon up and down. He might make a pulling-away motion when trying to push in a plug.

8. Many of these errors can be interpreted as perseveratory. After pouring the tea from the pot into the cup, the client might then perform a similar act with the sugar bowl instead of spooning it in.

9. Many clients, in their endeavors to testify what they realize is wrong, make several abortive runs at a task before succeeding or becoming frustrated and giving up.

Infrequently, the ideational or conceptual objective of a motor performance is lost while the motor remains intact, because the motor sequence belongs to the intact hemisphere whereas the ideational sequence is found in the damaged hemisphere. Denny-Brown refers to this syndrome as adextrous apraxia.[36] For example, a left-handed man has learned to write with his right hand. After a right-sided brain lesion, he is unable to conceptualize and form an intelligible word; however, he retains the skill to form written letters with his right hand.[36]

EVALUATION OF IDEOMOTOR AND IDEATIONAL APRAXIA

As previously described, these apraxias are very similar and difficult to differentiate. The test is the same for both of them; only the quality of the response varies slightly. When asked to do a task, a client with motor or ideomotor apraxia would not be able to do it on command but could do it automatically at the appropriate time. A client with ideational apraxia could not do it even automatically although he or she has the motor capacity to do it.

General Guidelines for Evaluation

1. Prior to praxis testing, perform a detailed assessment of the client's sensory and physical functioning. In addition, evaluate the client's language status, and consult with the speech pathologist as needed.

2. Evaluate visual agnosia prior to praxis testing to rule out difficulties with object recognition as a cause of poor performance.[28]

3. Evaluate motor planning skills of both hands whenever possible.

4. In addition to observing the client's performance, observe whether the client is bothered by his or her errors or can recognize that he or she has made errors.[3]

5. Golisz and Toglia recommend the following guidelines[15]:

   * Identify under what conditions limb or total body apraxia occurs.

   * What is the client's response to cuing (any modality)?

   * What is the client's awareness of his or her performance?

   * Have the client predict his or her performance before performing the movement tasks.

Test 1 – Praxis Subtest of the LOTCA[37]

Description

The praxis subtest of the LOTCA contains three parts: motor imitation, utilization of objects, and symbolic actions.

Scoring

1 point—Client is unable to produce any task
2 points—Client is only able to imitate movements
3 points—Client is able to imitate movements and to manipulate with objects
4 points—Client performs all tasks

Reliability

Inter-rater reliability with Spearman's rank correlation coefficient between raters ranged from 0.82 to 0.97 for the various subtests.

Validity

Wilcoxin's two-sample test was used to compare each client group with the control group. Tests differentiated at the 0.001 level of significance between the control group and each of the client groups.

DYNAMIC ASSESSMENT

Test 1 – Toglia[38]

Description

Table 4-3 illustrates a sample functional dynamic assessment.[38] Tasks range from simple to complex and are presented with 3 to 4 unnecessary items.

Scoring

The ability to perform each substep is recorded using codes described in Table 4-3, and the number and type of cues are recorded. This information is then analyzed in terms of what conditions facilitate client performance during treatment.

OCCUPATION-BASED EVALUATIONS

Test 1 – Multi-Level Action Test[19,39]

Description

The Multi-Level Action Test (MLAT) is composed of three primary tasks: making a slice of toast with butter and jam, wrapping a present, and packing a lunchbox. These tasks are performed

Table 4-3

Sample Dynamic Assessment of Clients With Aphasia and Apraxia

Task Directions	Objects on Table	Task Steps	Results	Number of Cues	Type of Cues
Peel the banana	Banana, orange, apple	Selects banana Orients banana Peels all sides	E	0	
Butter the bread, and cut it in half	Knife, spoon, fork, plate, butter, bread, cream cheese, sugar	Selects knife Holds knife properly Opens butter Puts butter on knife Spreads butter on bread Repeats spreading Cuts bread	E • C O • O C	 2 3	 P/G P/A/G
Pour the soda into the glass, and drink it with the straw	Soda can, glass, straw, fork, can opener, coffee mug	Selects can Opens can Pours into glass Opens straw Places straw in glass Drinks	E • O C O C	 1 3	 G P/T/G
Fit the letter into the envelope, put a stamp on it	Letter (8.5 x 11), envelope, stamp, letter opener, scissors, pen	Selects paper Folds paper Selects envelope Puts paper in envelope Takes stamp off packet Places stamp properly	E C E C C E	 2 3 2	 G/P P/T/G T/G
Make yourself a bowl of cereal	Cereal, milk, bowl, spoon, fork, knife, can of soda box of pancake mix, orange juice, can opener, scissors	Selects cereal Opens cereal box Pours into bowl Selects milk Opens milk Pours milk Selects spoon Holds spoon properly Eats cereal	E E C C C* C C O C	 1 2 1 2 1 1	 G A/T G G P G

Note: O = Client performs step without cues; • = Client performs step in an awkward and clumsy manner without cues; C = Client performs step with cues; E = Examiner performs this step. Even with cues, client is unable to perform this step; * = Step occurred out of sequence.

Cues may include but are not limited to the following: V = Verbal cues: Repeating, rephrasing, simplifying directions, stating name of key object; SR = Stimuli reduction: Removing the unnecessary items; P = Visually focusing attention by pointing; A = Auditorily focusing attention by tapping; G = Visual gesturing action without object; G/O = Visual gesturing action with object; T = Tactile cues to initiate movement; TS = Task segmentation: Removing all items; Presenting one item at a time in the order in which it is used. If examiner places object in client's hand, then an E is used for item selection because the examiner performed this step.

Adapted from Treatment of Individuals With Limb Apraxia, by J Toglia, December 1993, presented at AOTA Neuroscience Institute: Treating Adults With Apraxia, Denver, CO. Reprinted with permission from Republication Licensing Service (RLS) Copyright Clearance Center, Inc.

Table 4-4

MLAT Error Taxonomy

Step Omission

For example, fail to use stamp on letter; fail to use cream in coffee

Sequence

Anticipation/omission (eg, seal thermos before filling; close lunch box before packed)
Reversal (eg, stir mug of water, then add grinds)
Perseveration (eg, make two sandwiches)

Semantic Substitution

For example, stir coffee with fork (instead of spoon); place bread on hot-plate (instead of toaster)

Action Addition

Action not interpretable as step in task; includes "utilization behavior" and anomalous actions (eg, cut gift box, pack extraneous items into schoolbag)

Gesture (Manner)

Correct object used with incorrect gesture (eg, spoon [rather than pour] cream into cup)

Grasp/Spatial Misorientation

Misorientation of the object relative to the hand or to another (reference) object (eg, grasp wrong end of scissors [misoriented relative to hand]; place stamp on envelope sideways [misoriented relative to reference object])

Spatial Misestimation

Spatial relationship between two or more objects incorrect; act otherwise well executed (eg, cut paper much too small for gift)

Tool Omission

For example, spread jelly with finger (instead of knife)

Quality

Inappropriate or inexact quantity (spatial or volume) (eg, fill thermos with juice to point of overflow)

Reprinted with permission from Psychology Press (http://www.psypress.co.uk/journals.asp), reference 19: Buxbaum LJ, Schwartz MF, Crew TG. The role of semantic memory in objective use. Cogn Neuropsychol. 1997;14(2):233.

under four conditions: 1) Solo-Basic (all and only the materials needed are present), 2) Solo-Distractors (functionally related and often visually similar distractor items are also presented [eg, hot dogs are a distractor of lunchmeat, masking tape for scotch tape]), 3) Dual-Basic (client performs one primary task, and an additional task, in any order [eg, preparing a slice of toast and a cup of instant coffee]), and 4) Dual-Search (some materials needed to perform the two tasks are in a closed drawer, along with other irrelevant items). All conditions are untimed.

Scoring

Error scores are generated. Refer to Table 4-4 for a summary of MLAT Error Taxonomy and Table 4-5 for MLAT Scoring Guidelines.

*Test 2 – Naturalistic Action Test**

Description

The Naturalistic Action Test (NAT) is a shortened version of the MLAT with more simplified scoring procedures. The three core tasks are still making toast and coffee, wrapping a gift, and

*The Naturalistic Action Test can be purchased through Harcourt Assessment Inc, 19500 Bulverde Road, San Antonio, TX 78259, 1-800-211-8378.

Table 4-5
MLAT Accomplishment Score Guidelines

Toast (3 points maximum)

3: Toasts bread, then applies butter and jelly (any order)
2: Toasts bread, applies just jelly or just butter
1: Does not toast bread, applies butter and jelly; or toasts bread, does not apply either
0: Does not toast bread, applies butter or jelly

Letter (3 points)

3: Folds and inserts letter, seals filled envelope, and applies stamp
2: Folds and inserts letter, seals envelope, but does not apply stamp
1: Folds and inserts letter only; or applies stamp to empty envelope
0: Folds letter only; or seals empty envelope

Coffee (3 points)

3: Adds grinds, cream, and sugar (any order)
2: Adds grinds and cream; or grinds and sugar
1: Adds grinds alone
0: Adds sugar and/or cream without grinds

Present (4 points)

4: Boxes the present, wraps the packed box, adds bow
3: Wraps present directly, adds bow; or wraps packed box without bow
2: Boxes the present, adds bow to unwrapped box; or wraps present directly, no bow
1: Boxes the present only; or wraps the empty box, no bow
0: Cuts paper, adds bow to empty box; inserts present without closing box

Schoolbag (2 points)

2: Puts paper in binder or binder pocket, pens and pencils into case, necessary items into schoolbag (necessary items are: binder/paper, pencil case, magic markers, pens/pencils)
1: Puts paper into binder or pocket, packs into schoolbag; or puts pencils/pens into case and packs into school-bag
0: Packs paper and binder without assembling; or packs pencils/pens directly; or packs empty pencil case

Lunch Box (6 points)

Assign 1 point for each of following steps:
• Takes cookies from container and wraps them
• Makes sandwich
• Fills thermos
• Seals filled thermos with at least bottom lid
• Packs cookies, wrapped sandwich, and filled/sealed thermos into lunch box

packing a lunchbox. The maximum time to complete each task is 30 minutes. Physical assistance is given when needed after the client has clearly indicated his or her intention to perform an action. Acceptable initiation cues, generic cues, and time-based cues are described in the test manual.

Scoring

The client is scored for accomplishment of steps performed as well as on selected errors. These two scores are combined for a single NAT score ranging from 0 to 6 with a maximum score of 18.

Norms

Demographic and clinical data were collected on a sample of 45 right cerebral vascular accidents (RCVAs), 30 left cerebral vascular accidents (LCVAs), 25 traumatic brain injuries (TBIs), and 28 controls. The mean total NAT score for subjects was 10.9 (SD 5.5) and for controls 17.3 (SD 1.2) (U = 355, p < 0.001).

Reliability

Inter-rater across the three tasks of the NAT, median weighted Kappa for accomplishment score was 0.98 (range 0.95 to 1.0).

Internal Consistency

Cronbach's coefficient alpha = 0.79 for the entire sample and 0.75 for the client sample.

Concurrent Criterion Validity

Correlated (around 0.5) with both the physical and cognitive subscales of the Functional Independence Measure (FIM).

Construct Validity

Correlated with measurements of processing speed/arousal (r = 0.68), visual spatial attention (r = 0.61), and working memory (p < 0.001)

Predictive Validity

The NAT was assessed against the instrumental activities of daily living (IADL) scale, and a significant correlation was found between discharge NAT and follow up IADL in bivariate analysis (r = 0.58) and in multiple regression analysis. A correlation between the NAT administered at the same time as the IADL measure was also strong (r = 0.64).

TREATMENT FOR IDEOMOTOR AND IDEATIONAL APRAXIA

Utilizing a Restorative Approach

1. Provide proprioceptive, tactile, and kinesthetic input prior to and during a task. For example, take the client's leg through the required motion to propel his wheelchair.*

2. Combine tactile and kinesthetic input with visual and verbal mediation. Cue the client to look at what he or she is doing, and demonstrate the movements for the client to get a visual model.[28] Use these techniques with the client verbalizing what he or she wants to do—for example, "I want to reach for my shirt" or "I am closing my fingers around a cup."[28]

3. Place your hand over the hand of the client, and guide him or her through the required task. For example, during hygiene activities, if the client used his toothbrush on his hair, do not verbally cue him that he has made a mistake. Guide his hand with the toothbrush, without verbalizations, away from his hair and into his mouth or down to the faucet in an appropriate sequence (Bonifils, personal communication). Frequently, this will elicit recognition on the client's part, and he may be able to take over the normal sequence of movement. "Guiding can be a way of respectfully communicating by stopping one engram and replacing it with another without words" (Bonifils, personal communication).

Utilizing an Adaptive Approach

1. Keep verbal commands to a minimum, and place activity on a subcortical level. For example, instead of the verbal command, "Lock your brakes," say to the client, "There's something on your brakes."

Note: Single case study research results indicated that the addition of sensory stimulation (tactile and proprioceptive) to verbal and visual cues enhanced motor performance and that this was maintained long term even when sensory input was removed.[28,40]

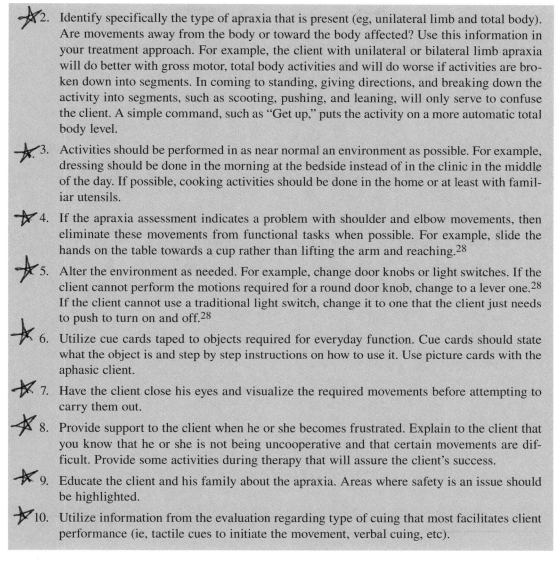

2. Identify specifically the type of apraxia that is present (eg, unilateral limb and total body). Are movements away from the body or toward the body affected? Use this information in your treatment approach. For example, the client with unilateral or bilateral limb apraxia will do better with gross motor, total body activities and will do worse if activities are broken down into segments. In coming to standing, giving directions, and breaking down the activity into segments, such as scooting, pushing, and leaning, will only serve to confuse the client. A simple command, such as "Get up," puts the activity on a more automatic total body level.

3. Activities should be performed in as near normal an environment as possible. For example, dressing should be done in the morning at the bedside instead of in the clinic in the middle of the day. If possible, cooking activities should be done in the home or at least with familiar utensils.

4. If the apraxia assessment indicates a problem with shoulder and elbow movements, then eliminate these movements from functional tasks when possible. For example, slide the hands on the table towards a cup rather than lifting the arm and reaching.[28]

5. Alter the environment as needed. For example, change door knobs or light switches. If the client cannot perform the motions required for a round door knob, change to a lever one.[28] If the client cannot use a traditional light switch, change it to one that the client just needs to push to turn on and off.[28]

6. Utilize cue cards taped to objects required for everyday function. Cue cards should state what the object is and step by step instructions on how to use it. Use picture cards with the aphasic client.

7. Have the client close his eyes and visualize the required movements before attempting to carry them out.

8. Provide support to the client when he or she becomes frustrated. Explain to the client that you know that he or she is not being uncooperative and that certain movements are difficult. Provide some activities during therapy that will assure the client's success.

9. Educate the client and his family about the apraxia. Areas where safety is an issue should be highlighted.

10. Utilize information from the evaluation regarding type of cuing that most facilitates client performance (ie, tactile cues to initiate the movement, verbal cuing, etc).

Limb-Kinetic Apraxia

The client with limb-kinetic apraxia has difficulty or is incapable of making fine, precise movements with the limb contralateral to a central nervous system (CNS) lesion.[3] Spatial accuracy, timing, and joint coordination can all be affected.[41] The client is unable to translate motor programs into the muscle contractions necessary to achieve the action required.[26] These clients have a loss of fine and precise movements, independent finger movements and difficulty coordinating simultaneous movements.[42] The deficit is especially evident when the client performs rapid movements such as tapping but is also seen when he or she pantomimes, imitates, or uses objects.[3] All types of movements can be affected. The client with limb-kinetic apraxia understands the action required, and engages in appropriate motor programs; however, actions are performed in a clumsy manner because the muscle activity is incorrectly specified.[26] The neuroanatomic correlates of limb-kinetic apraxia remain unclear.[3]

EVALUATION OF LIMB-KINETIC APRAXIA

Test items from previously described apraxia tests that require unilateral limb movement and fine motor coordination will reveal limb-kinetic apraxia. In addition, the therapist should observe the client during ADLs for unusual clumsiness.

TREATMENT OF LIMB-KINETIC APRAXIA

Utilizing a Restorative Approach

1. Provide proprioceptive, tactile, and kinesthetic input prior to and during a task. For example, to improve writing skills, have the client write utilizing a clayboard and pencil shaped dowel for increased proprioceptive input.

2. Provide activities that try to tap into the client's previous memory for performing a given task. For example, if the client has difficulty grasping a cup, provide cups of different materials and weight (ie, paper, plastic, ceramic) to cue the client as to how much pressure to apply.

Utilizing an Adaptive Approach

1. Identify which occupational performance activities are affected and alter as needed. For example, if the client is unable to hold and manage a straight edge razor, have him use an electric razor instead. If the client is unable to manage the fine motor skills required to use a manual can opener, have him or her use an electric can opener.

2. Alter the environment as needed to facilitate improved performance in occupational performance (ie, change door knobs, light switches, slip on versus tie shoes, Velcro adaptations to clothes, etc).

Oral Apraxia

Oral apraxia is the difficulty in forming and organizing intelligible words, though the musculature required to do so remains intact. This differs from dysarthria, in which the muscles are affected and the speech is slurred. These clients may be able to use the tongue for automatic acts such as chewing and swallowing but may not be able to stick it out when asked. Some believe oral apraxia is a disorder of the linguistic-conceptual system.[43-45] The wrong movement is selected for execution at the highest level of programming the motoric act. Others believe it is a problem with the productions system. Roy and Square believe both systems are involved and state, oral apraxia "involves both top-down and bottom-up influences, which operate in parallel."[8]

EVALUATION AND TREATMENT FOR ORAL APRAXIA

Evaluation and treatment for oral apraxia are usually done by the speech pathologist. If there is no speech pathologist available, however, a simple screening test can be used. First, ask the client to lick his or her lips. If he or she cannot do so on command, put some honey or peanut butter on the client's lips and observe whether he or she automatically licks it off. If the client can lick his or her lips automatically but not on command, he or she is probably apraxic. If the client cannot lick them at all, he or she is probably dysarthric. Some of the evaluations previously described in the ideomotor/ideational section also contain items that test for oral apraxia.

Constructional Apraxia

Constructional apraxia is the impairment in producing designs in two or three dimensions (copying, drawing, or constructing) whether upon command or spontaneously.[46,47] This failure cannot be attributed to perceptual impairments, ideomotor apraxia, organizational impairments, or primary motor or sensory impairments.[15] The performance of constructional tasks, in fact, presupposes normal visual acuity—the ability to perceive several elements of the model as well as their spatial relationship and sufficient motor ability.[48] These clients have lost the ability to assemble and organize an object from disarticulated pieces.[49] This constructional ability or visuomotor organization combines perceptual activity with motor response.[50]

Constructional apraxia results from lesions in either cerebral hemisphere and limits the client's ability to perform purposeful acts while using objects in his or her environment.[51] The planning of constructive processes might be impaired after dominant hemisphere damage, and the "…inability to make use of movement to relevant spatial and configurative (visual) information might underlie constructional apraxia after damage of the nondominant hemisphere."[40]

Controversy exists about the occurrence of constructional apraxia among clients with right- and left-sided brain damage. It is widely believed that clients with right-sided damage show a greater incidence of the deficit.[52] However, others hypothesize an equal distribution of the symptoms of both right and left groups.[53] The authors, hypothesizing an equal distribution of symptoms in both groups, insist that aphasic clients often have the deficit but are not included in test groups for clients with left-sided brain damage since they are frequently either confused or unable to understand directions.

Although clients with both right and left hemiplegia display this deficit, a distinct difference between the two groups, supported more by observation of quality of response than by objective perceptual testing, has been widely described in the literature.[54] It seems clients with apraxia with right-sided lesions, with or without visual field deficits, are characterized by a visual-spatial disability, such that they lack perspective, the exact location of a figure in space, and the ability to analyze parts in relation to each other.[30,55-57] Clients with apraxia with left-sided lesions have spatial problems only if a visual field deficit exists simultaneously but, overall, exhibit an executive or planning problem.[55,57-59] Thus, these clients, regardless of whether they are able to see things in correct perspective, have trouble initiating a planned sequence of movements when trying to construct an object.

Clients with right-sided cerebral damage tend to be less hesitant in their drawings and use a piecemeal approach rather than an orderly one.[58] They frequently draw on the diagonal, neglect the left side of the drawing, and have no particular way for using the space on the page.[56] Their designs are often very complex, often unrecognizable, but do include many pieces of the drawing scattered with proper spatial relationships to one another.[18,24,60,61] Frequently, lines in the drawing are overscored in an attempt to correct or finish the task.[58] Their drawings show that they have a great deal of difficulty with perspective, and constructing anything with three dimensions, such as blocks or bricks, is extremely difficult.[47] These clients are usually not helped by the presence of a model, and when given some landmarks (eg, part of the drawing filled in), their work is unaffected or they become more confused.[56,60] Short-term visual memory is hypothesized to be poor, and the client seems unable to keep the model in mind. After several trials at a particular task, no learning appears to take place.[60,62]

On the other hand, clients with left-sided damage tend to be very hesitant in their task and produce designs of great simplicity.[63] They often cannot draw angles, their designs are poor in outline, and they have apparent difficulty in execution.[58] These clients seem to have more general intellectual impairment, and it is thought that their ability to establish the program task is lost or diminished. Their performance is often facilitated by the presence of a model, and often they tend to move closer and closer to it (called the closing-in effect by Mayer-Gross)[64] until finally their copy is superimposed on the model.[56] Landmarks, such as part of the picture filled in, appear helpful.[60] After several trials, these clients seem to learn the task and can repeat it more easily.[43] Memories for visual and auditory images are thought to be short; thus, drawing on command or from memory is affected more than copying a model.

Functionally, constructional apraxia has been related to body scheme problems, dressing apraxia, and meal preparation.[65-69] In a study of 54 head injured clients, Neistadt found a significant correlation between constructional praxis and meal preparation. Neistadt concludes that constructional abilities may contribute to meal preparation performance and believes it is "...functionally relevant for rehabilitation specialists to use block design type tests to evaluate the constructional skills of the clients who have brain injury."[70] In a study of 101 cerebral vascular accident (CVA) clients, Warren found that disorders of body scheme and constructional apraxia jointly contributed to the presence of dressing apraxia.[68]

Lorenze and Cancro,[71] using the WAIS block design and object assembly subtests, found that clients who did poorly on these tests did not acquire dressing and grooming skills even after practice in dressing. In clients with right-sided lesions, the presence of severe constructional apraxia with perceptual problems has been found to relate to the same lack of independence in daily living skills.[72]

Historically, occupational therapists have used primarily a restorative approach to treat constructional apraxia.[70] The effectiveness of this approach, however, has come into question. In a study of 45 adult male TBI clients, both a restorative and adaptive treatment approach were given. The subject group that received the restorative approach received training in parquetry block designs. The group receiving the adaptive approach received training in food preparation. The results of the study indicated that they had task specific learning. In other words, the parquetry group did better on post-test on parquetry tasks, and the functional group performed better on the specific functional task on post-test. There was no transfer of learning to other functional or constructional tasks or activities. This important study suggests two possible directions in treatment decision making. First, for transfer of learning to occur, training must occur in a variety of environments using targeted strategies for task completion.[73] Second, since learning appears to be task specific, an adaptive functional approach would have more impact than a restorative approach.

EVALUATION FOR CONSTRUCTIONAL APRAXIA

Test 1 – Copying Designs, Two-Dimensional

Description

The therapist hands the client paper and pencil and asks him to copy the design on the stimulus card. A separate sheet of paper is used to copy each stimulus card. There are several variations of this test, and none of them are standardized. Following are examples:

- Copy a previously drawn line drawing of a house (Figure 4-1), a flower, and a clock face.[74]
- Copy geometric designs (Figure 4-2).

Scoring

Nonstandardized
Each drawing is scored on a scale of 1 to 3.

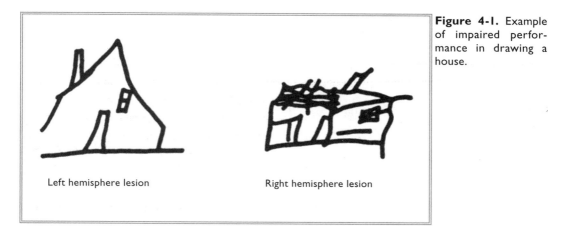

Figure 4-1. Example of impaired performance in drawing a house.

Left hemisphere lesion

Right hemisphere lesion

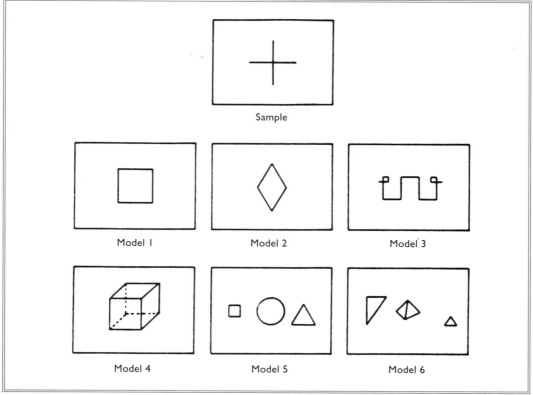

Sample

Model 1

Model 2

Model 3

Model 4

Model 5

Model 6

Figure 4-2. Copy geometric designs test.[71] (Adapted from Lorenze EJ, Cancro R. Dysfunction in visual perception with hemiplegia: its relation to activities of daily living. *Arch Phys Med.* 1962;43:514-517.)

Score 1—If the drawing is essentially correct, no lines are omitted or added, and spatial arrangement is correct.

Score 2—If the drawing is partially defective owing to omissions of some lines, rotations, or disproportions between single parts, but not to such an extent as to prevent identification of the figure.

Score 3—If the drawing is unrecognizable.

Intact—Scores of drawings mostly 1

Impaired—Scores of drawings mostly 2

Severe—Scores of drawings mostly 3

Validity

To improve validity, rule out incoordination, especially if the client is using his nondominant hand and unilateral neglect. Right and left hemiplegics have qualitative differences in their drawings (see description of deficit on page 125).

Test 2 – Graphic Designs, Santa Clara Valley Medical Center[75]

Description

The client is asked to copy from prepared cards each of the following: horizontal line, vertical line, cross, circle, square, triangle, diamond, cube, house, and clock.

Scoring

Severely impaired—Design is almost totally unrecognizable

Impaired—Design lacks perspective, is rotated, or is partially unrecognizable

Intact—Design is copied accurately

Validity

To improve validity, rule out incoordination, unilateral neglect, visual field cuts, and other visual problems.

Reliability

Inter-rater reliability ($r = 0.98$) was established for this test in a study of adult clients who sustained head trauma.[76] In the same study, frequency data indicated no variance in performance for copying horizontal and vertical lines, a cross, a square, and a triangle. All other items appeared to be good discriminators of dysfunction.

Test 3 – Block Design, Santa Clara Valley Medical Center[75]

Description

The client is asked to duplicate block designs from prepared models.

Scoring

Severely impaired—Design is almost completely unrecognizable

Intact—Design is copied accurately

Validity

To improve validity, rule out motor apraxias.

Reliability

Inter-rater reliability (r = 0.96) was established for this test in a study of adult head trauma clients.[76] In addition, item analysis indicated a high degree of test reliability (alpha = 0.87) for this test given in conjunction with the Santa Clara Valley Medical Center graphic design test.[76]

Other Tests

Almost any constructional task can be utilized as a constructional praxis evaluation. Some of them have been described elsewhere in this chapter, and only some of the more common ones are listed here: copying pegboard designs, puzzles, copying block designs similar to design on the Wechsler Adult Intelligence Scale, Draw-A-Man Test, and Frostig's Spatial Relations Test.

VALIDITY OF CONSTRUCTIONAL PRAXIS TESTS

Benton believes that the various "constructional apraxia" tests are not necessarily testing the same skill.[77] He found that his Visual Retention Test (a test of copying geometric figures) correlated only weakly with his Three-Dimensional Constructional Praxis Test. Pehoski also found only a weak correlation between her copy drawing test and Benton's Three-Dimensional Constructional Praxis Test.[78]

The tests vary in complexity, in the type of movement and dexterity required to do the task, in the demands of higher intellectual function, and in the involvement of two or three spatial dimensions. For example, the task of copying geometric designs requires more precise graphic movements and a higher degree of sensorimotor integration than block building.[77]

TREATMENT FOR CONSTRUCTIONAL APRAXIA

Utilizing a Restorative Approach*

1. Have the client practice various two- and three-dimensional table top activities. The activities should be occupation-based whenever possible (ie, if the client was a telephone repairman prior to the ABI, have him put together a telephone, or if the client was an architect, have him or her work on generating blue print-type drawings). Utilize techniques such as backward chaining.[66]

2. Provide tactile and kinesthetic cues to the client by having the client explore a three-dimensional model with his hands before constructing his model.

3. Provide tactile kinesthetic guiding to the client during constructional tasks. For example, if the client is working on a work-related nuts and bolts assembly task, place your hand over the client's hand and guide him or her through the necessary sequence. Reduce or remove guiding as the client takes over the task.

4. Along with constructional tasks retraining, simultaneously work on visual analysis tasks (ie, analysis of similarities and differences), on understanding of the relationship of parts to one another, and reasoning about the nature of the stimuli.[66] This is recommended because visual analysis and visuoconstructive skills are often used this way in everyday task performance.[66]

Utilizing an Adaptive Approach

1. Identify performance components that are impaired as the result of constructional apraxia (ie, meal preparation and vocational tasks). Provide assistive techniques such as backward

---

Note: There is some question as to whether the restorative approach is effective in treating constructional apraxia. The therapist should constantly evaluate client progress and use occupation-based constructional activities whenever possible when utilizing a restorative approach.

chaining during the task.[66] Present a partially completed task, and ask the client to complete it—for example, placing the knife and glass in a partially completed place setting.[66]

 2. Apply concepts from the Dynamic Interactional Approach: identify what task characteristics can be altered to improve performance—for example, the client may be able to perform assembly tasks if the pieces are laid out in a specific order or marked with sequential numbers for assembly.

 3. Educate the client and his or her family about the constructional deficits and how they will affect function. Areas where safety is an issue should be highlighted.

Dressing Apraxia

Dressing apraxia is the inability to dress oneself because of a disorder in body scheme and/or spatial relations. This apraxia is related more to body scheme and spatial deficits than to a difficulty in the motor performance of dressing.[36] The client makes mistakes of orientation in putting clothes on backwards, upside-down, or inside-out.[49] Often, clients with right-sided lesions will neglect to dress the left side of the body or put both legs in the same pant leg.

Some believe this type deficit is more a manifestation of hemispatial neglect and that a more generalized dressing deficit relates to a client's inability to align the axis of the garment with the body axis.[79] As Devinsky and D'Esposito have observed, clients usually do not have a primary disorder of praxis, but the impaired dressing skills, rather, can result from the following[49]:

> ...impaired body image and defective visuospatial constructional ability. Clients' awareness of the left side may be diminished (sensory neglect), or they may fail to activate motor programs (motor neglect). In the former instance, they omit dressing or insufficiently dress that side; in the latter, they do not make the hand, arm, and truncal adjustments needed to place the left arm through a shirt or jacket sleeve.

Pehoski provides the following example of the client with dressing apraxia.[78]

1. The subject was unable to find the correct sleeve. He looked at the shirt in a puzzled manner and finally put his involved arm into a sleeve, but it was the wrong sleeve.

2. He then had some difficulty getting the sleeve up the involved extremity, but he finally managed to slide it past the elbow and onto the involved shoulder.

3. He then reached around his back as a normal response to find the other sleeve. Since the correct sleeve had not been used at the beginning, the second arm hole was not in back as it should have been, but remained in front. He then came back to the material in front of him, found the second arm hole, and put in his uninvolved extremity. The shirt was then on as if it were to be buttoned down the back. He looked puzzled for a moment and then put the material that was in front over his head to the back. Now he had the bulk of the material behind his neck with the two shirt tails hanging over his shoulder in front. Feeling at the back of his neck, he asked, "Where is the collar?" After several seconds of fumbling for the collar and trying to pull the shirt down, he said, "I've fouled up somewhere along the line. The collar is nowhere." (Total time: 3 minutes, 34 seconds.)

Dressing apraxia has been associated with posterior parietal lesions, especially those involving the right hemisphere.[49,79] The level of awareness and concern the client demonstrates over his or her inability to dress is an important factor in the severity of the dressing apraxia.[80]

EVALUATION FOR DRESSING APRAXIA

The test for this is strictly a functional one (ie, observe the client during dressing). Does he or she have trouble in deciding where to begin or where to find the right armhole? Does he or she neglect to dress the left half of his or her body (indication of unilateral neglect)? Does he or she put the shirt on inside out or backwards? Does he or she button it so the buttons are not aligned correctly? All these are signs of dressing apraxia and not just the inability to dress because of motor paralysis. Because there is usually a high degree of correlation between dressing and constructional apraxia, some people have used tests for constructional apraxia to assist in diagnosing or predicting dressing apraxia.[71,76]

TREATMENT FOR DRESSING APRAXIA

Utilizing a Restorative Approach

1. The client is encouraged to start dressing on his or her own with visual or verbal cues. If the client does not start dressing, try a verbal cue: "Get dressed please." Then, wait to see if the client is able to recognize the language combined with the visual cue.[81] Provide non-verbal tactile-kinesthetic client guiding at the beginning and during dressing. As needed, reduce or remove guiding as the client takes over the activity. If there is a breakdown in the sequence or the client is having difficulty, provide guiding again.

2. Apply concepts from the Neurodevelopmental Approach. Provide weight bearing, weight shifting, and handling techniques prior to and during dressing as needed.

Utilizing an Adaptive Approach

1. Apply concepts from the Dynamic Interactional Approach. Identify how changing the surface characteristics of dressing can alter performance. For example, does laying one garment at a time versus all clothes at once improve performance? Try dressing training in a variety of ways (ie, sitting on edge of the bed, in wheelchair, etc).

2. Apply concepts from a Functional Adaptive Approach by providing the following to help the client compensate.

   a) Use labels to distinguish back from front and right from wrong side.

   b) If garment does not have distinguishing labels, the therapist can color code the garment for right-left, back-front, and wrong side-right side.

   c) If the client has trouble matching buttons to the right buttonhole, tell him or her to start at the bottom of the shirt, find the last button, and match it to the last buttonhole. Continue matching upward from there. The therapist can also color code the bottom button and buttonhole.

   d) Have the client circle the button with his other finger to feel that he or she has it all the way through the buttonhole.

3. If the client cannot manage a button down shirt, have him or her use a pullover whenever possible. If he or she cannot manage zippers, utilize pull on pants or skirts, and try Velcro fastening. If the client cannot manage tying shoes, try slip-ons or Velcro fastenings.

4. Educate the client and his or her family regarding his or her dressing problems and why he or she is having difficulty. Emphasize that this problem is not related to poor motivation. Train the client and the family on compensation techniques.

References

1. Schwartz MF. Analysis of a disorder of everyday action. *Cogn Neuropsychol.* 1995;12(8):863-892.
2. Giovannetti T, Libon DJ, Buxbaum LJ, Schwartz MF. Naturalistic action impairments in dementia. *Neuropsychologia,* 2002;40(8):1220-1232.
3. Heilman KM, Rothi LJG, Valenstein E. Two forms of ideomotor apraxia. *Neurology.* 1982;32:342-346.
4. May-Benson T. Praxis is more than just motor planning: clinical reasoning for understanding intervention for praxis. *OT Practice.* 2004;9:CE1-CE8.
5. Clark MA, Merians AS, Kithari A, et al. Spatial planning deficits in limb apraxia. *Brain.* 1994;117:1093-1106.
6. Harrington DL, Haaland KY. Motor sequencing with left hemisphere damage: are some cognitive deficits specific to limb apraxia? *Brain.* 1992;115:857-874.
7. Heilman M, Rothi LJG. Apraxia. In: Heilman KM, Valenstein E, eds. *Clinical Neuropsychology.* 4th ed. New York, NY: Oxford University Press; 2003.
8. Roy EA, Square PA. Common considerations in the study of limb, verbal and oral apraxia. In: Roy EA, ed. *Neuropsychological Studies of Apraxia and Related Disorders.* New York, NY: North-Holland; 1985.
9. York CD, Cermak SA. Visual perception and praxis in adults after stroke. *Am J Occup Ther.* 1995;49(6):543-550.
10. DeRenzi E. Methods of limb apraxia evaluation and their bearing on the interpretation of the disorder. In: Roy EA, ed. *Neuropsychological Studies of Apraxia and Related Disorders.* New York, NY: North-Holland; 1985.
11. Humphreys GW, Forde EME. Disordered action schema and action disorganization syndrome. *Cogn Neuropsychol.* 1998;15(6/7/8):771-811.
12. Norman DA, Shallice T. Attention to action: willed and automatic control of behavior. In: Davidson RJ, Schwartz GE, Shapiro D, eds. *Consciousness and Self Regulation.* New York, NY: Plenum Press; 1996.
13. Andersen RA, Snyder LH, Bradley DC, Xing J. Multimodal representation of space in the posterior parietal cortex and its use in planning movements. *Annu Rev Neurosci.* 1997;20:303-330.
14. Cooper R, Shallice T. Contention scheduling and the control of routine activities. *Cogn Neuropsychol.* 2000;17(4):297-338.
15. Golisz K, Toglia J. Perception and cognition. In: Crepeau E, Cohn ES, Schell BAB, eds. *Willard and Spackman's Occupational Therapy.* Philadelphia, Pa: Lippincott Williams and Wilkins; 2003.
16. Goodgold-Edwards SA, Cermak S. Integrating motor control and motor learning concepts with neuropsychological perspectives on apraxia and developmental dyspraxia. *Am J Occup Ther.* 1990;44(5):431-439.
17. Hodges JR, Bozeat S, Lambon Ralph MA, et al. The role of conceptual knowledge in object use evidence from semantic dementia. *Brain.* 2000;123(pt 9):1913-1925.
18. Arnadottir G. *The Brain and Behavior: Assessing Cortical Dysfunction Through Activities of Daily Living.* St. Louis, Mo: CV Mosby; 1990.
19. Buxbaum LJ, Schwartz MF, Carew TG. The role of semantic memory in object use. *Cogn Neuropsychol.* 1997;14(2):219-254.
20. Rumiati R, Zanini S, Vorano L, Shallice T. A form of ideational apraxia as a selective deficit of contention scheduling. *Cogn Neuropsychol.* 2001;18(7):617-642.
21. Pramstaller PP, Marsden CD. The basal ganglia and apraxia. *Brain.* 1996;119(Pt 1):319-340.
22. Moll J, De Oliveira-Souza R, De Souza-Lima F, Andreiuolo PA. Activation of intraparietal sulcus using a fMRI conceptual praxis paradigm. *Arq Neuropsiquiatr.* 1998;56(4):808-811.
23. Sunderland A. Recovery of ipsilateral dexterity after stroke. *Stroke.* 2000;31(2):430-433.
24. Barron A, Mattila WR. Response slowing of older adults: effects of time-limit contingencies on single- and dual-task performances. *Psychol Aging.* 1989;4(1):66-72.
25. Hopkins HL. Occupational therapy management of cerebrovascular accident and hemiplegia. In: Willard H, Spackman C, eds. *Occupational Therapy.* 4th ed. Philadelphia, PA: JB Lippincott Co; 1971.
26. Marsden CD. The apraxias are higher order defects of sensorimotor integration. In: *Novartis Foundation Symposium 218.* New York, NY: John Wiley and Sons; 1998.
27. Square-Storer P. *Acquired Apraxia of Speech.* New York, NY: Taylor and Francis; 1989.
28. Butler JA. Evaluation and intervention with apraxia. In: Unsworth C, ed. *Cognitive and Perceptual Dysfunction: A Clinical Reasoning Approach to Evaluation and Treatment.* Philadelphia, Pa: FA Davis; 1999.
29. Balliet R, Blood K, Bach-y-Rita P. Visual field rehabilitation in the cortically blind? *J Neurol Neurosurg Psychiatry.* 1985;48(11):1113-1124.
30. Gulyas B, Heywood CA, Popplewell DA, Roland PE, Cowey A. Visual form discrimination from color or motion cues: functional anatomy by positron emission tomography. *Proc Natl Acad Sci.* 1994;91:9965-9969.
31. Baker-Nobles L, Bink MP. Sensory integration in the rehabilitation of blind adults. *Am J Occup Ther.* 1979;33(9):559-564.
32. Miller N. *Dyspraxia and Its Management.* Gaithersburg, Md: Aspen Publications; 1986.

33. Ochipa C, Rothi LJG, Heilman KM. Ideational apraxia: a deficit in tool selection and use. *Ann Neurol.* 1989;25:190-193.
34. Crovitz HF, Harvey MT, Horn RW. Problems in the acquisition of imagery mnemonics: three brain-damaged cases. *Cortex.* 1979:225-234.
35. Heilman M, Maher LM, Greenwald ML, Rothi LJ. Conceptual apraxia from lateralized lesions. *Neurology.* 1997;49(2):457-464.
36. Denny-Brown D. The nature of apraxia. *J Nerv Ment Dis.* 1958;126:9-32.
37. Jongbloed L, Stacey S, Brighten C. Stroke rehabilitation: sensorimotor integrative versus functional treatment. *Am J Occup Ther.* 1989;43(6):391-397.
38. Toglia J. A dynamic interactional approach to cognitive rehabilitation. In: Katz N, ed. *Cognition and Occupation Across the Life Span.* 2nd ed. Bethesda, Md: American Occupational Therapy Association Press; 2005.
39. Buxbaum LJ, Schwartz MF, Montgomery MW. Ideational apraxia and naturalistic action. *Cogn Neuropsychol.* 1998;15(6/7/8):617-643.
40. Platz T, Mauritz KH. Human motor planning and use of new task-relevant information with different apraxic syndromes. *Eur J Neurosci.* 1995;7:1536-1547.
41. Rapcsak SZ, Ochipa C, Anderson KC, Poizner H. Progressive ideomotor apraxia: evidence for a selective impairment of the action production system. *Brain Cogn.* 1995;27(2):213-236.
42. Heilman M, Meador KJ, Loring DW. Hemispheric asymmetries of limb-kinetic apraxia: a loss of deftness. *Neurology.* 2000;55(4):523-526.
43. Berrol S. Issues in cognitive rehabilitation. *Arch Neurol.* 1990;47:219-220.
44. Duchek J. Cognitive dimensions of performance. In: Christiansen C, Baum C, eds. *Occupational Therapy: Overcoming Human Performance Deficit.* Thorofare, NJ: SLACK Incorporated; 1991.
45. Stoer P. Chromaticity and achromaticity: evidence for a functional differentiation in visual field defects. *Brain.* 1987;110:869-886.
46. Cohen RF, Mapou RL. Neuropsychological assessment for treatment planning: a hypothesis-testing approach. *J Head Trauma Rehabil.* 1988;3(1):12-23.
47. Hecaen H, Penfield W, Bertrand C, Malmo R. The syndrome of apractognosia due to lesions of the minor cerebral hemisphere. *Arch Neurol Psychiat.* 1956;75(4):400-434.
48. Damasio A, Tranel D, Rizzo M. Disorder of complex visual processing. In: Mesulam, ed. *Principles of Behavioral and Cognitive Neurology.* 2nd ed. New York, NY: Oxford University Press; 2000.
49. Devinsky O, D'Esposito M. The right hemisphere, interhemispheric communication, and consciousness. In: *Neurology of Cognitive and Behavioral Disorders.* New York, NY: Oxford University Press; 2004.
50. Averbach S, Katz N. Cognitive rehabilitation: a retraining model for clients with neurological disabilities. In: Katz N, ed. *Cognition and Occupation Across the Life Span.* 2nd ed. Bethesda, Md: American Occupational Therapy Association Press; 2005.
51. Fahle M. Figure-ground discrimination from temporal information. *Proc R Soc Lond B Biol Sci.* 1993;254(1341):199-203.
52. Fisher B. Effect of trunk control and alignment on limb function. *J Head Trauma Rehabil.* 1987;2(2):72-79.
53. Finlayson MA, Garner SH. *Brain Injury Rehabilitation: Clinical Considerations.* Philadelphia, Pa: Lippincott, Williams and Wilkins; 1994.
54. Crook T. Psychometric assessment in the elderly. In: Raskin A, Javick L, eds. *Psychiatric Symptoms and Cognitive Loss in the Elderly.* New York, NY: Hemisphere Publishing Co; 1979.
55. DeRenzi E, Faglioni P. The relationship between visuo-spatial impairment and construction. *Cortex.* 1967;3:327-342.
56. Piercy M, Hecaen H, De Ajuriaguerra J. Constructional apraxia associated with unilateral cerebral lesion: left and right sided cases compared. *Brain.* 1960;83:225-242.
57. Podolsky S, Schachar R. Clinical manifestations of diabetic retinopathy and other diseases of the eye in the elderly. In: Ordy JM, Bizzee KR, eds. *Aging. Vol 10. Sensory Systems and Communication in the Elderly.* New York, NY: Raven Press; 1979.
58. Gainotti G, Tiacci C. Patterns of drawing disability in right and left hemispheric patients. *Neuropsychologia.* 1970;8:379-384.
59. Bumpa-Tel, Inc. *Instructo-Clinic: A Psychophysical Testing Apparatus.* Cape Gir, Mo: Bumpa-Tel, Inc; 1973.
60. Hecaen H, Assal G. A comparison of constructive deficits following right and left hemispheric lesions. *Neuropsychologia.* 1970;8:289-303.
61. Kahan HJ, Whitaker HA. Acalculia: an historical review of localization. *Brain Cogn.* 1991;17:102-1151.
62. Neistadt ME. Occupational therapy treatment for constructional deficits. *Am J Occup Ther.* 1991;46(2):141-148.
63. McFie J, Zangwill OL. Visual-constructive disabilities associated with lesions of the left cerebral hemisphere. *Brain.* 1960;83:243-259.
64. Mayer-Gross W. Some observations of apraxia. *Proc Roy Soc Med.* 1934-1935;28:1203-1212.

65. Baum B, Hall K. Relationship between constructional praxis and dressing in the head injured adult. *Am J Occup Ther.* 1981;35(7):438-442.
66. Bouska MJ, Kauffman NA, Marcus SE. Disorders of the visual perceptual system. In: Umphred DA, ed. *Neurological Rehabilitation.* 2nd ed. St. Louis, Mo: CV Mosby; 1990.
67. Neistadt ME. The relationship between constructional and meal preparation skills. *Arch Phys Med Rehabil.* 1993;74:144-148.
68. Warren M. Relationship of constructional apraxia and body scheme disorders to dressing performance in adult CVA. *Am J Occup Ther.* 1981;35(7):431-437.
69. Williams N. Correlations between copying ability and dressing activities in hemiplegia. *Am J Phys Med.* 1967;46:1132-1340.
70. Neistadt ME. A critical analysis of occupational therapy approach for perceptual deficits in adults with brain injury. *Am J Occup Ther.* 1990;44:299-304.
71. Lorenze EJ, Cancro R. Dysfunction in visual perception with hemiplegia: its relation to activities of daily living. *Arch Phys Med.* 1962;43:514-517.
72. Gregory ME, Aitkin JA. Assessment of parietal lobe function in hemiplegia. *Occup Ther.* 1971;34:9-17.
73. Toglia JP. Generalization of treatment: a multicontextual approach to cognitive perceptual impairment in the brain injured adult. *Am J Occup Ther.* 1991;45(6):505-516.
74. Deitz JC, Tovar VS, Thor DW, Beeman C. The test of orientation for rehabilitation patients: inter-rater reliability. *Am J Occup Ther.* 1990;44(9):784-790.
75. Zoltan B, Jabri J, Panikoff L, Ryckman D. *Perceptual Motor Evaluation for Head Injured and Other Neurologically Impaired Adults.* San Jose, Calif: Santa Clara Valley Medical Center, Occupational Therapy Department; 1983.
76. Baum B. The establishment of reliability and validity of a perceptual evaluation on a sample of adult head trauma patients. Thesis. University of Southern California, December 1981.
77. Benton AL, Fogel ML. Three-dimensional constructional praxis, a clinical test. *Arch Neurol.* 1962;7:347-354.
78. Pehoski C. Analysis of perceptual dysfunction and dressing in adult hemiplegics. Thesis. Sargent College, Boston University; 1970.
79. Weintraub S. Neuropsychological assessment of mental state. In: Mesulam, M-Marsel, ed. *Principles of Behavioral and Cognitive Neurology.* 2nd ed. New York, NY: Oxford University Press; 2000.
80. Takayama Y, Sugishita M, Hirose S, Akiguchi I. Anosodiaphoria for dressing apraxia: contributory factor to dressing apraxia. *Clin Neurol Neurosurg.* 1994;96:254-256.
81. Bonfils K. Affolter approach. In: Pedretti L, ed. *Practice Skills for Physical Dysfunction.* St. Louis, Mo: CV Mosby; 1995.

Resources

Anderson SW, Tranel D. Awareness of disease states following cerebral infarction, dementia, and head trauma: standardized assessment. *Clin Neuropsychol.* 1989;3(4):327-339.
Doehring DG, Reitan RM, Klove H. Changes in patterns of intelligence test performance associated with homonymous visual field defects. *J Nerv Ment Dis.* 1967;132:227-233.
Fetherlin JM, Kurland L. Self-instruction: a compensatory strategy to increase functional independence with brain-injured adults. *Occup Ther Pract.* 1989;1(1):75-78.
Fraser C, Turton A. The development of the Cambridge apraxia battery. *Brit J Occup Ther.* 1986;49:348-252.
Glisky E, Schacter D. Remediation of organic memory disorders: current status and future prospects. *J Head Trauma Rehabil.* 1986;1(3):54-63.
Madden DJ. Adult age differences in the time course of visual attention. *J Gerontol.* 1990;45:9-16.
Papagno C, Della Sala S, Basso A. Ideomotor apraxia without aphasia and aphasia without apraxia: the anatomical support for a double dissociation. *J Neurol Neurosurg Psychiatry.* 1993;56(3):286-289.
Pascal GK, Suttell B. *The Bender-Gestalt Test—Its Quantification and Validity for Adults.* New York, NY: Grune & Stratton; 1951.
Schwartz M, Segal ME, Veramonti T, et al. *The Naturalistic Action Test.* Bury St. Edmunds, England: Thames Valley Test Company, Ltd; 2002.
Shiffman LM. Cerebrovascular accident. In: Early MB, ed. *Physical Dysfunction Practice Skills for the Occupational Therapy Assistant.* St. Louis, Mo: Mosby Year-Book Inc; 1998.
Solet JM. Solet test for apraxia. Thesis. Boston University; 1974.

CHAPTER 5

Body Scheme Disorders

Body Scheme

An individual's body scheme is a representation of the spatial relations among the parts of the body and is different from the psychodynamic sense of identity.[1-6] <u>Body scheme has been viewed as an unconscious automated system that is required for environmental exploration through move-</u><u>ments and static posture.</u>[7] Neonatal imitation of movement points towards an implicit knowledge of the body structure that precedes the adult body scheme.[8] As Hari et al describe, an individual's bodily awareness relies on a stable body scheme, which may in part be genetically determined and may change after a brain lesion.[9]

<u>Through the integration of proprioceptive, tactile, and pressure input, the body scheme becomes</u> <u>the neural foundation for perception of body position and the relationship of the body and its</u> <u>parts.</u>[10] Prior and current sensory input (including muscle, proprioceptive, cutaneous, vestibular, tactile, visual, and auditory) form an awareness of our body and the spatial relations of its parts.[2,8,11] Attention, memory, and language also contribute to an individual's body scheme.[11]

An intact body scheme allows for the spatial indexing of sensory input and is involved in the triggering and guidance of movement.[12] It is the foundation for future skills in environmental perception.[37,56,60,61] An intact body scheme allows the individual to know and understand the body's orientation in space, which is crucial for interacting with the environment.

Many professionals believe there are multiple distinct yet interacting representations that contribute to an individual's body awareness or knowledge.[14] Sirigu et al hypothesize that there are at least four kinds of representations that contribute to body knowledge processing.[15] These representations are described as follows[15]:

1. The first contains semantic and lexical information about body parts, such as names; the functional relations that exist between body parts, such as the wrist and the ankle (eg, articulations); the functional purpose of the mouth or the ear, etc. These representations are in large part prepositional and are likely to be more strongly linked to the verbal systems.

2. The second contains the category-specific visuospatial representations of an individual's own body but also of bodies in general. These representations define a structural description of the body and specify in a detailed manner the position of individual parts on the body surface (eg, the nose is in the middle of the face), the proximity relationships that exist among body parts (eg, the nose is next to the eyes, the leg is between the ankle and the knee etc), and most importantly, the boundaries that define each body part. These representations are necessary for "part/whole" analysis. They are likely to be more strongly linked to the nonverbal, visual, and somatosensory systems.

3. The third level is the emergent body-reference system and is conceptualized as a dynamic, actual body image. It gives information about the position and the changes in position of an individual's own body parts relative to each other and in relation to external space.

4. Motor representations also contribute to the construction of a spatial representation of the body. It is further hypothesized that these components of the body representation system are relatively independent but can also interact with each other. The degree of interaction depends on the particular task demands.

The parietal cortex (especially the right) and the cerebellum have been linked with body scheme disorders.[2,16] Since the body scheme has multiple representations, impairment can occur at different levels of body knowledge processing.[1,15,17]

Clinically, the client may exhibit different types of problems. For example, the client may be able to localize body parts on himself but not on others or be able to name body parts spatially but not functionally. In addition, the client's body alignment and positioning may influence the degree of body knowledge.[18] Disturbances in body scheme can include autotopagnosia, anosognosia, unilateral body neglect, impaired right-left discrimination, and finger agnosia. The definition, evaluation, and treatment of these disorders are subsequently described. It is important to note that one study indicated that clients who were unable to perform on some of the subsequent tests in real life did not exhibit body neglect or an inability to reach various parts of their body.[7] Other studies, however, indicated that no matter what level or component of body scheme is impaired, associated problems with various self-care activities will be evident.[10] If a client appears to have difficulty (not due to a motor, planning, or primary sensory impairment) with activities such as dressing, then a detailed evaluation of body scheme through the appropriate subsequent tests is recommended.

Autotopagnosia

Autotopagnosia, a disturbance in the previously described body scheme, is the lack of awareness of body structure and the failure to recognize one's body parts and their relationship to each other. Clients can recognize body parts individually, indicating the problem is not with knowledge of the parts themselves.[4] In addition, they can move a body part when the examiner points to it, which indicates that the problem is not linguistic.[4] A client who has such a deficit also has difficulties in his or her reference point to the outside world. A client with this difficulty may have trouble using his or her contralateral limbs, may confuse the sides of the body, and may not differentiate properly his or her own body parts and those of the examiner.[6,13,15,16]

Many clients, upon evaluation, will grope uncertainly along his or her body.[7] They may point to a body part near the target or point to one that has a similar function.[2,7] Denes et al notes that body parts that are perceptually well defined, such as the nose, are more easily localized than those without specific boundaries, such as the cheek.[7]

Semenza provides the following classification of errors that can provide important qualitative information[19]:

Contiguity (spatial) errors—Same limb as stimulus; this group includes errors that reflect misreaching.

Conceptual errors—Different types of errors are included under this label: joint for joint, eye-ear-nose substitutions, and *contiguity errors* where alternative response choices are presented as cut-out parts in a multiple choice display. This last type of error is not classified as spatial because it cannot possibly result from a spatially vague indication. It is indeed likely to derive from a disorder in the conceptual representation or in its output.

Random errors—Include all the remaining.

Macro- and microsomatognosia are disorders in body scheme that distort a person's perception of his or her own body. A client may see his or her whole body or part of it as abnormally small (micro) or exceptionally large (macro).

In clients who have autotopagnosia without an accompanying problem in spatial relations, the prospects for successfully attaining skills of daily living are high.

EVALUATION OF AUTOTOPAGNOSIA

The therapist should rule out aphasia, attentional deficits, visual or tactile agnosia, apraxia, or primary motor problems as causes of poor performance on the subsequent tests.[19,20]

Test 1 – Point to Body Parts on Command[21-24]

Description

Therapist asks the client to point or indicate in some way the body part named on him- or herself, on the examiner, and on a human figure puzzle, or doll. There is no standardized form for this test. The therapist can make up the commands. Following are some examples excluding "left" and "right" from the command:

1. Show me your knees.
2. Show me your mouth.
3. Show me your stomach.
4. Show me your nose.
5. Show me you feet.
6. Show me your shoulders.
7. Show me your elbows.
8. Show me your hair.
9. Show me your back.

Scoring

Nonstandardized

Intact—Client correctly indicates all parts named in a reasonable length of time.

Validity

Sauguet, MacDonald, and Boone use variations of this to measure body scheme.[21,23,25] It is used mainly to test a client's verbal understanding. Sauguet separated his sample into people with left hemiplegia, people with right hemiplegia without receptive aphasia, and people with right hemiplegia with receptive aphasia. Only the clients with receptive aphasia made errors on this test. Boone found that if the words "right" and "left" were excluded from the command, most of the errors were eliminated.

To improve validity, rule out aphasia as a cause of poor performance.

Reliability

Research conducted with adult TBI clients on a variation of this test established inter-rater reliability (r = 0.94).[26] Item analysis of this subtest given with four additional subtests (ie, Draw-A-Person, Right/Left Discrimination, Body Puzzle, and Face Puzzle) indicated good internal consistency (coefficient alpha = 0.60).[26]*

Test 2 – Point to Body Parts, Imitation[1,25]

Description

The client is told to imitate movements of the examiner, who touches different parts of his or her own body. Mirror image responses are acceptable. There is no standardized form of this test. Therapists can make up their own commands. Touching 6 to 10 body parts is sufficient. Examples follow:

1. Touch your left hand.
2. Touch your right cheek.
3. Touch your left leg.
4. Touch your left elbow.
5. Touch your right palm.
6. Touch your right knee.
7. Touch your left shoulder.
8. Touch your right ear.
9. Touch your right forearm.
10. Touch your left wrist.

Scoring

Nonstandardized

Intact—Client correctly indicates all parts named within a reasonable length of time.

Validity

This test eliminates most of the verbal problems of the last test. Indeed, in Sauguet's study, 90% of the right hemiplegics with aphasia had a normal performance, as compared with 100% of the right hemiplegics without aphasia and left hemiplegics.[25]

To improve validity, rule out apraxia as a cause of poor performance.

Test 3A – Body Visualization and Space Concepts

(Norm descriptive statistics available in adaptation by Taylor)[27]**

A coefficient alpha measure of 0.50 was considered acceptable for the establishment of reliability.
**Developed by AJ Ayres, ADI Auxiliary Publication Project, Document 8179, Library of Congress, Washington, DC*

Table 5-1

Normative Descriptive Statistics

Age	Number of Subjects	Mean Score	Standard Division
50 to 64	90	27.5	1.3
65 to 74	60	26.9	1.2

Adapted from reference 28: Taylor MM. Analysis of dysfunction in the left hemiplegia following stroke. Am J Occup Ther. 1968;22:512-520.

Description

The examiner reads questions to the client. Instruct the client to "Think of yourself sitting as you are now when answering the following questions."

1. Ordinarily, are a person's teeth inside or outside his mouth?
2. Are your legs below your stomach?
3. Which is farther from your nose, your feet or your stomach?
4. Is your mouth above your eyes?
5. Which is closer to your mouth, your neck or your shoulder?
6. Is your shoulder between your neck and your elbow?
7. Are your fingers between your elbow and your hand?
8. Which is farther from your toes, your heel or elbow?
9. Which is nearer to your head, your arms or your legs?
10. Which is on top of your head, your hair or your eyes?
11. Is your back behind you or in front of you?
12. Is your stomach behind you or in front of you?
13. Is your elbow above or below your shoulder?
14. Is your nose above or below your neck?

Scoring

Although this test has not been standardized for adults, Taylor[28] provides some normative data presented in Table 5-1. However, until a more extensive normative study can be done, interpretation of scores is nonstandardized.

Intact—Client correctly answers all questions within a reasonable length of time.

Validity

To improve validity, rule out aphasia as a cause of poor performance.

Test 3B – Body Revisualization

MacDonald has devised a shorter version of this test in which the client only has to answer "true" or "false."[23] An expressive aphasia client can indicate "true" or "false" by pointing to one of two cards marked "true" and "false."

Description

Ask the client whether these statements are true or false:

1. Your mouth is below your chin.

2. Your eyes are above your forehead.

3. Your knees are below your hips.

4. Your hands are at the end or your arms.

5. Your have one chin, one nose, and one mouth.

Scoring

Nonstandardized

Intact—Client correctly answers all within a reasonable length of time.

Validity

To improve validity, rule out receptive aphasia.

Test 4 – Draw-A-Man[23,24,30]

Description

Client is given a blank piece of paper and a pencil and is asked to draw a man.

Scoring

Nonstandardized

The following scoring is taken from MacDonald.[23] The Goodenough-Harris Drawing Test[31] and the Denver Developmental Screening Test[32] both have standardized scoring systems for children. The first is more complicated than MacDonald's; the second is less complicated. The second scoring system included in this section is from Zoltan et al.[24]

Scoring System No 1

1. Total of four points for presence of all body parts

   Point distribution:

   1 point—Head

   1 point—Trunk

   2 points—Two arms if full figure, one arm if profile

   2 points—Two legs if full figure, one leg if profile

2. Total of three points for correct proportion of body parts to trunk

   Point distribution:

   1 point—Area of head not more than one-half or less than one-half the length of the trunk

   1 point—At least one arm not longer than twice the length of the trunk or less than one-half the length of the trunk

   1 point—At least one leg not longer than twice the length of the trunk or less than the length of the trunk.

3. Total of one point for correct postural alignment (ie, figure in normal standing or sitting position)

4. Total of two points for correct juxtaposition of extremities with trunk

   Point distribution:

   1 point—Arms emerge from upper one-half of trunk

   1 point—Legs emerge from lower one-half of trunk

   Intact—Total score of 10 points

Scoring System No 2

Total of 10 body parts:

Head	Right hand
Trunk	Left hand
Right arm	Right foot
Left arm	Left foot
Right leg	Left leg

Intact—Scores 10

Minimally impaired—Scores 6 to 9

Severely impaired—Scores 5 or below

Validity

This test is also used as a means of identifying or diagnosing unilateral neglect and anosognosia. It is a constructional task and, therefore, overlaps into disorders of spatial judgment and apraxia, which should be ruled out. The validity of this test as a test of body scheme is controversial. Maloney and Payne[30] treated a group of developmentally delayed teenagers with sensory-motor training based on the work of Kephart, and pre- and post-tested them with three tests of body image, including the Draw-A-Man Test. On the post-testing, the group made significant gains on the two other tests of body image but not on the Draw-A-Man Test. They concluded that the test does not reflect changes in body image occurring as a result of sensory-motor training. The Draw-A-Man Test is also used as a personality projective test, ie, to determine how one feels about one's body. Gregory and Aitken[29] found that depressed clients often drew a miserable looking man whose size was very small on the page. This test is also used as a test of intelligence.[31]

Reliability

Research conducted on a sample of clients with TBI utilizing this scoring system established inter-rater reliability (r = 0.86)[26] As noted with the pointing to body parts test, the Draw-A-Man Test, when given to adult clients with head trauma with four other subtests, had an overall reliability of coefficient alpha = 0.60.[26]

TREATMENT FOR AUTOTOPAGNOSIA

Utilizing a Restorative Approach

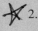 1. Provide tactile input/stimulation—For example, have the client rub his arm with a rough cloth while naming the body part or before placing arm in sleeve.

2. Practice particular tasks that reinforce body knowledge—For example, the client identifies body parts as they are touched by the therapist as he or she dresses.

3. Apply concepts from the neurodevelopmental frame of reference as follows:

   a) Incorporate into treatment bilateral activities that facilitate normal movement and improved body scheme.

   b) Provide appropriate handling techniques to educate the client about what it feels like to move normally. Provide treatment in a variety of ways and positions to facilitate retention of motor learning.

4. Utilize techniques described in Chapter 1 for constraint-induced therapy.

Utilizing an Adaptive Approach

1. Identify where in the body knowledge representation the breakdown occurs. Educate the client and his family regarding the client's body scheme deficits and how they affect function. Train the family in how to assist the client in affected self-care tasks in order to compensate.

2. If the client has a functional awareness of body parts but not a spatial awareness, or vice versa, utilize this in your approach and client cuing to maximize function—for example, "Move the part of the body that you use to hold things," instead of "Move your hand."

3. If the client is able to localize a body part near the correct one (ie, pointing to shoulder when asked to point to arm), utilize this in your approach and client cuing. For example, if you ask the client to move his arm and he moves his shoulder, say, "Move the part of your body just below the one you just moved."

Unilateral Body Neglect

Unilateral body neglect is the inability to integrate and use perceptions from one (usually left) side of the body.[33] This deficit may occur independently of visual field cuts or visual inattention or be compounded by these deficits. The client with unilateral body neglect will ignore one half of his body. For example, a male client may forget to shave one side of his face or forget to dress one side of his body.

EVALUATION FOR UNILATERAL BODY NEGLECT

Test 1 – Draw-A-Man

Description

Client is given separate sheets of blank paper and told to draw a man.

Scoring

Subjective

> *Intact*—Drawing includes all parts in proper place.
>
> *Impaired*—Some parts are missing from the left side, body parts are thinner on left side, or parts are skewed to the right.

Validity

To improve validity, rule out constructional and motor apraxias.

Test 2 – Functional

Description

Probably the best test of unilateral body neglect is observation during functional activities. Does the client ignore one half of his or her body while performing self-care activities such as brushing teeth, shaving, or dressing?

Scoring

Subjective

> *Intact*—Client shows no signs of unilateral body neglect during self-care activities.
>
> *Impaired*—Client shows signs of unilateral body neglect in some but not all self-care activities.
>
> *Severely Impaired*—Client shows signs of unilateral body neglect in all self-care activities.

TREATMENT FOR UNILATERAL BODY NEGLECT

Utilizing a Restorative Approach

1. Provide tactile or proprioceptive stimulation to the neglected side prior to self-care tasks. Examples follow:

   a) Therapist rubs affected arm of client while client watches, using either his or her own hand, a rough cloth, or vibrator.

   b) Client rubs himself with his nonaffected hand while he watches it.

   c) While watching himself, client self-ranges the affected arm and hand to assist if he has little muscle power.

2. Apply concepts from a neurodevelopmental frame of reference. Have the client participate in bilateral tasks to facilitate increased total body awareness. Specific handling techniques and proprioceptive facilitation through weight bearing activities will also help.

3. Set up activities that will "force the use" of the neglected extremities. Please refer to the section in Chapter 1 for specific guidelines for constraint-induced therapy.

4. Provide tactile kinesthetic guiding during self-care tasks.

Utilizing an Adaptive Approach

1. Educate the client and his or her family about the client's unilateral body neglect and how it will affect function. Train the family in how to assist the client in affected self-care tasks in order to compensate. Highlight activities where safety is an issue.

2. Provide visual cues or reminders to the client—for example, a sign on the client's mirror reading, "Have I shaved both sides of my face?" or "Have I washed both arms?"

3. Provide verbal cuing to the client during self-care tasks, as needed, to compensate for body neglect.

4. Train the client to self-monitor his performance. For example, after he feels he has completed a task, such as putting on a shirt, he asks himself, "Have I put each arm through a sleeve?," or after shaving, the client asks, "Have I shaved both sides of my face?" The client should then check himself if he has completed the task correctly before moving on

to the next task. If necessary, the client could utilize a daily activity checklist to monitor his performance after task completion.

Anosognosia

Anosognosia is a relatively transient, severe form of neglect to the extent that the client fails to recognize the presence or severity of his or her paralysis.[34-36] The course of anosognosia may differ among clients, with those who have sustained static injuries such as ischemia or trauma showing improved insight over time.[34-36] Research has shown that anosognosia will affect the rehabilitation process and outcome.[37] Anosognosia may be simply unconcern for the paralysis (anosodiaphoria) or, at the other extreme, may be a complete denial of paralysis. When asked whether anything is wrong, the client denies his illness.[38] If confronted by the fact that the side is paralyzed and will not move in response to his or her efforts, the client may reply that the limb has "a will and purpose of its own," that "it is tired," or that "it always was a lazy arm."[29] The client may make excuses for left-sided weakness by stating it is because he or she is right handed.[1] When asked to move the weak extremity, the client will perform the task with the intact one and, despite contrary evidence, insist he or she followed the therapist's directions.[34]

The client with anosognosia is unable to form a consistent and accurate picture of the reality of his or her paralysis.[39] The deficit is often associated with mental confusion or intellectual impairments; however, the deficit may occur independently.[35] The lack of awareness may be evident in the client's verbal or nonverbal behavior. Many anosognostic clients also have visual neglect.[39] Denial may take the form of confabulation, and the client will persist in his or her belief despite repeated demonstration of disability.[36] As the denial decreases, the client may become agitated, frustrated, and/or depressed. This is different from psychological denial, which would be associated with avoidance behaviors.[40]

It has been recently theorized that anosognosia requires both cognitive impairment and sensory, especially proprioceptive, loss.[34,39] Others believe that insight or discovery into weakness is dependent on attempted action, and anosognosia occurs due to learned non-use.[41] Others believe it results from diffuse cognitive impairment.[34,39,42] The awareness of a sensorimotor deficit, for example, is hypothesized not as an immediate sensory phenomenon, but rather as a result of discovery or the product of observation and inference. The anosognosic client cannot make any inference of why he or she cannot perform a task. The client's reasoning skills are impaired. Levine hypothesizes that cognitive deficits impairing the ability to infer will distinguish those individuals with sensory loss and paralysis who are anosognosic from those who discover and become aware of their paralysis.[39]

Ullman has attempted to interpret anosognosia as a way in which the client experiences his body.[42] Even transient cerebral vascular accident (CVA) clients have described a limb as feeling like it is "not there" or not belonging to the body. For the client with brain damage, abstract thinking may be diminished so that he or she is tied to subjective experience. Thus, if the arm does not feel a part of him or does not hurt, he cannot make reasonable judgments about it. Another variable is the client's premorbid personality; that is, the client may have always been one to go through life verbally denying that anything was wrong no matter what the crisis or disturbing event. With these two factors working together, the client does not have to deal with an illness he cannot perceive and can separate himself from a stressful situation. In his way, the client is preserving his own intactness. The following example illustrates these concepts[42]:

A client lying in bed noticed his arm protruding from a blanket. He remarked spontaneously, *"When I was put in bed, this arm was sticking out. I told the nurses and doctors.*

They think it's my arm, but it's not. That's been sticking out like this ever since I was put in here."
"Whose hand is it?"
"I wouldn't know. It was here when they put me in bed. I always had an idea I was laying on top of a corpse because this hand was laying out there motionless."

EVALUATION FOR ANOSOGNOSIA

There are no standardized assessments specific to anosognosia. Please refer to the evaluation section in Chapter 10 on decreased awareness for assessments, which includes a portion devoted to decreased sensory motor awareness. Generally, the therapist should record relevant spontaneous behavior as well as behavior as a result of his or her inquiries.[35]

Evaluation, clinical observation, and informal interviewing during occupation-based activities are recommended.

TREATMENT FOR ANOSOGNOSIA

Please refer to treatment suggestions in Chapter 10 for decreased awareness. Please also refer to information on specific guidelines for constraint-induced therapy. Research suggests that this is likely an effective treatment strategy for anosognosia.

Right-Left Discrimination

Right-left discrimination is a skill that develops relatively late.[12] In most people, it is not mastered until seven years of age or later.[43] Successful right-left orientation requires many cognitive abilities including mental rotation.[20] In addition to a spatial ability, it requires a somewhat high level of conceptualization.[44]

The client who has sustained an ABI may exhibit difficulty with right-left discrimination. This difficulty is generally characterized by a selective incapacity to apply the right-left distinction to symmetrical parts of the body.[45] It is a specific disorder of spatial orientation confined to the sagittal plane of the client's body or that of the confronting therapist.[45] Clients are spared other spatial concepts such as up-down or front-back.[20]

Generally associated with parietal lobe dysfunction, right-left disorientation is considered by some to be a rare but striking disorder.[12,20] It is usually evaluated by assessing the client's ability to point to the side of the body indicated by the therapist on verbal command or imitation.[10] The skills required for this assessment are verbal, sensory, and conceptual.[45] The client must understand the term and retain it in short-term memory for the time necessary to execute the command. The client must also be able to discriminate sensory input from the opposite one. Finally, for tasks that involve right-left discrimination on others, the client must be able to manipulate his or her personal orientation, which requires a high degree of conceptual skill.

Deficits such as aphasia, decreased short-term memory, and sensory impairment must be ruled out as causes of impaired performance on the subsequently described tests.

EVALUATION OF RIGHT-LEFT DISCRIMINATION

Test 1 – Ayres' Right-Left Discrimination Test
(Subtest of the Southern California Sensory Integration Tests)[46]

Description
Therapist sits facing the client and gives the client a series of commands:

1. Show me your right hand.

2. Touch your left ear.

3. Take this pencil with your right hand. (Hold pencil in both hands, hands resting on knees.)

4. Now put it in my right hand. (Hold hands palm up on knees.)

5. Is this pencil on your right or left side? (Hold pencil in left hand, one foot in front of client's right shoulder.)

6. Touch your right eye.

7. Show me your left foot.

8. Is this pencil on your right or left side? (Hold pencil in right hand in front of client's left shoulder.)

9. Take this pencil with your left hand. (Hold pencil in both hands, hands resting on knees.)

10. Now, put it in my left hand. (Hold hands palm up on knees.)

Scoring

Score two points if correct within 3 seconds and one point if correct within 4 to 10 seconds. If the client first makes a wrong response, and then corrects himself, the score is based on the time of correct response. If the command is repeated, the score can be no more than one. This test has been standardized only for children. In testing its reliability for children aged 4.0 to 8.11 years, the test-retest correlations ranged from r = 0.15 to 0.54. Scoring for adults is nonstandardized.

> *Intact*—As adult norms have not been established, the therapist should gather his or her own provisional norms by testing a few normal adults.

Validity

To improve validity, rule out aphasia, apraxia, and primary motor problems.

Reliability

Inter-rater reliability (r = 0.93) was established for this test on a sample of adult head trauma clients.[26]

Test 2 – Point to Body Parts on Command[25]

Description

The therapist asks the client to point to or indicate in some way the body parts named on himself, on the examiner, or on a human figure doll or puzzle. There is no standardized form of this test. The therapist can make up his or her own:

1. Show me your left hand.

2. Show me your right eye.

3. Show me your left foot.

4. Show me your left shoulder.

5. Show me your right elbow.

6. Show me your left knee.

7. Show me your right ear.

8. Show me your left wrist.

9. Show me your right ankle.

10. Show me your right thumb.

Scoring

Nonstandardized

Intact—Client correctly indicated all parts named within a reasonable length of time.

Validity

To improve validity, rule out aphasia, apraxia, and primary motor problems as causes of poor performance. This is similar to Test 1 under Autotopagnosia, except that the words "left" and "right" are included in the commands. The two tests could be combined by using commands with and without "left" and "right" in them. One could then compare the results. Does the client do better with commands omitting "left" and "right"? Does he indicate the correct body part but on the wrong side (ie, lift left hand when commanded to "Show me your right hand")? If so, it is a problem of right-left discrimination. If the client is totally confused and indicates the wrong body part altogether, it may be a problem of autotopagnosia.

Reliability

Inter-rater reliability (r = 0.94) was established for a variation of this test on a sample of adult clients with head trauma.[26]

Treatment for Right-Left Discrimination

Utilizing a Restorative Approach

1. Provide extra tactile and proprioceptive input during activities—for example, a weighted cuff on the dominant wrist.

Utilizing an Adaptive Approach

1. Identify what areas of occupational performance are affected by the client's difficulty with right-left discrimination. Provide adaptations for these activities to help the client compensate—for example, wearing a watch on a certain wrist consistently, or a marking on clothing, shoes, or other necessary items with colored tape or marker to distinguish right from left.

2. When giving instructions to the client, do not use the words "right" or "left." Either point or refer to the item by its location—for example, "Your comb is next to your toothbrush."

3. When the client is dressing, work side by side facing the same way. This will be easier for the client.[47]

Finger Agnosia

Finger agnosia, which is generally associated with left parietal damage, consists of doubt and hesitation concerning the fingers.[4] A fairly common occurrence, it is usually found bilaterally with more involvement of the three middle fingers of each hand. The client has confusion in naming his or her fingers on command or knowing which one was touched.[29,48] Clients with finger agnosia will often display clumsiness in using fingers, especially in tasks requiring imitation of meaningful gestures.[20,49] Deficits in finger agnosia have been found to correlate highly with poor dexterity in tasks involving movement of the fingers in relation to each other. Some theorists have questioned why the fingers have assumed an unusual significance in body scheme disorders.[12] Some theorize it is because the fingers are the principle means of touch. Others believe it is because of its importance in reaching and as a marker for fine spatial coordinates.[12] Still others focus on the key role of the hand as an executive tool for visuomotor coordination.

Finger agnosia has traditionally been linked with Gerstmann's syndrome.[1,48] This syndrome includes finger agnosia, impaired right-left discrimination, agraphia, and acalculia. Recent documentation, however, has described the component parts of the syndrome as seen independently.[1] It is assumed by others that finger agnosia is not a primary deficit but part of an associated intellectual impairment and aphasia.[1,20] Finally, some theorize that finger agnosia is a disorder of spatial orientation with respect to the actual sequence of the fingers of the hand.[48]

EVALUATION FOR FINGER AGNOSIA

Specific evaluation of finger agnosia is generally only indicated if the client exhibits clumsiness with his or her hands and primary motor and sensory problems and motor planning problems have been ruled out as causes for poor performance.

Test 1 – Finger Localization, Naming[23,26]

Description

Have the client place his or her hands palm down on the table. A picture of two hands (Figure 5-1) is placed in front of the client so that the fingers in the picture point in the same direction as the client's fingers. The therapist touches the client's fingers one at a time, saying, "I am going to touch your fingers one at a time. Name or point to the finger on the picture of the hand that is the same as the finger I touched."

This test can be given with the client watching while he or she is touched and with vision occluded. A combination of both—five items with vision and five with vision occluded—is useful to compare results. To occlude vision, the therapist can ask the client to close his eyes, shield his eyes with a file folder, or place his hands in a specially made box that has two ends open, one end covered with a curtain so that the client cannot see in. There is no standardized form of this test. The therapist can make up his or her own order—for example, "Which finger am I touching?" Touch the client with a pencil eraser on the following:

1. Right second finger
2. Left third finger
3. Right thumb
4. Left fourth finger
5. Right first finger
6. Left second finger
7. Right fourth finger
8. Left first finger
9. Right third finger
10. Left first finger

Scoring

Nonstandardized

> *Intact*—Client correctly indicates all fingers touched within a reasonable length of time.

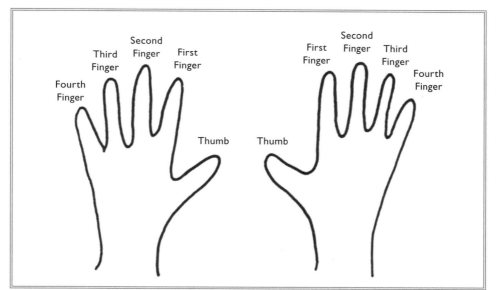

Figure 5-1. Hand chart for Tests I and 2 under Finger Agnosia (pages 146 and 147) (reduced from life size).

Validity

To improve validity, rule out impaired sensation on both hands.

Test 2 – Finger Identification by Name[23,25]

Description

The client is asked to move or point to the finger on his or her own hand named by the therapist. A variation of this test is to have the client point to the finger on his or her hand matching the one the therapist points to on the hand chart (see Figure 5-1). This test is not standardized. The therapist can make up his or her own order. Five to ten commands are probably sufficient. For an example, see Test 1 under Finger Agnosia.

Scoring

Nonstandardized

Intact—Client correctly indicates all fingers named within a reasonable length of time.

Validity

To improve validity, rule out aphasia.

Test 3 – Imitation[25]

Description

Client is instructed to imitate finger movements made by the therapist. There is no standardized form of this test. The therapist can make up his or her own movements. Five movements are sufficient. Examples follow:

1. Therapist curls right index finger forward.
2. Therapist touches left thumb to tip of left little finger.

3. Therapist touches left middle finger with tip of right index finger.

4. Therapist brings left index and middle fingers together laterally.

5. Therapist circumducts right thumb.

Scoring

Subjective

> *Intact*—Client imitates all movements correctly within a reasonable length of time.

Validity

To improve validity, rule out apraxia, abnormal muscle tone, and paralysis/paresis of affected hand.

TREATMENT FOR FINGER AGNOSIA

Utilizing a Restorative Approach

Apply the following concepts and techniques[50]:

1. Representation of the body in the cortex is use-dependent; therefore, treatment should be structured so that repeated sensory inputs are provided to those surfaces to be used for the desired task (ie, fingertips and thumb pad).

2. Repeated sensory stimulation should be high intensity for appreciation but not aversive. For example, a thin band of hook and loop fasteners is stroked across the key sensory surfaces, first with client's eyes open, then closed. The client is asked to identify which finger is being stimulated.

3. Subsequent to the stimulation, have the client perform a functional hand or ADL activity appropriate to his or her level of function (ie holding an adapted fork, dressing, etc).

4. The first skills needed are to grip an object with the appropriate amount of pressure while holding, depending on the object. If the client's finger agnosia has affected this skill, provide small lateral movements of the skin against an object (shear or friction). This type of stimulation has been found to be more effective in activating deep structures or muscle input than direct vertical pressure.

Utilizing an Adaptive Approach

1. Educate the client and his or her family as to how the finger agnosia may affect dexterity and function. Highlight areas where safety is an issue. Provide environmental adaptations as needed—for example, adaptive handles or hook and loop fasteners covered keys on a computer keyboard.

References

1. Cumming WJK. The neurobiology of the body schema. *Brit J Psychiatry.* 1988;153(2):7-11.

2. Devinsky O, D'Esposito M. The right hemisphere, interhemispheric communication and consciousness. In: *Neurology of Cognitive and Behavioral Disorders.* New York, NY: Oxford University Press; 2004.

3. Parker RS. *Concussive Brain Trauma: Neurobehavioral Impairment and Maladaptation.* Boca Raton, Fla: CRC Press; 2001.

4. Reed CL, Farah MJ. The psychological reality of the body schema: a test with normal participants. *J Exp Hum Perc Perf.* 1995;21(2):334-343.

5. Semenza C. Impairment in localization of body parts following brain damage. *Cortex.* 1988;24:443-449.

6. Zoltan B. Visual, visual perceptual and perceptual-motor deficits in brain injured adults: evaluation, treatment and functional implications. In: Kraft GH, Berrol S, eds. *Physical Medicine and Rehabilitation Clinics of North America.* Philadelphia, Pa: WB Saunders; 1992.

7. Denes G, Cappelletti JY, Zilli T, et al. A category-specific deficit of spatial representation: the case of autotopagnosia. *Neuropsychologia.* 2000;38(4):345-350.

8. Berlucchi G, Aglioti S. The body in the brain: neural bases of corporeal awareness. *Trend Neurosci.* 1997;20(12):560-564.

9. Hari R, Hanninen R, Makinen T, et al. Three hands: fragmentation of human bodily awareness. *Neurosci Lett.* 1998;240(3):131-134.

10. van Deusen J. Unilateral neglect: suggestions for research by occupational therapists. *Am J Occup Ther.* 1988;42(7):441-446.

11. Arnadottir G. Evaluation and intervention with complex perceptual impairment. In: Unsworth C, ed. *Cognitive and Perceptual Dysfunction: A Clinical Reasoning Approach to Evaluation and Intervention.* Philadelphia, Pa: FA Davis; 1999.

12. Newcombe F, Ratcliff G. Disorders of visuospatial analysis. In: Boller F, Grafman J, eds. *Handbook of Neuropsychology.* Vol 2. Amsterdam, Netherlands: Elsevier Science; 1989.

13. Zoltan B. Remediation of visual-perceptual and perceptual-motor deficits. In: Rosenthal M, Griffith ER, Bond MR, Miller JD, eds. *Rehabilitation of the Adult and Child with Traumatic Brain Injury.* Philadelphia, Pa: FA Davis; 1990.

14. Coslett HB. Evidence for a disturbance of the body schema in neglect. *Brain Cogn.* 1998;37(3):527-544.

15. Sirigu A, Grafman J, Bressler K, Sunderland T. Multiple representations contribute to body knowledge processing: evidence from a case of autotopagnosia. *Brain.* 1991;114(1B):629-642.

16. Parker RS. *Traumatic Brain Injury and Neuropsychological Impairment.* New York, NY: Springer Verlag; 1990.

17. Semenza C, Goodglass H. Localization of body parts in brain injured subjects. *Neuropsychologia.* 1985;23(2):161-175.

18. Hansen CS. Traumatic brain injury. In: Van Deusen J, ed. *Body Image and Perceptual Dysfunction in Adults.* Philadelphia, Pa: WB Saunders; 1993.

19. Semenza C. Assessing disorders of awareness and representation of body parts. In: Halligan P, Kischka U, Marshall JC, eds. *Handbook of Clinical Neuropsychology.* New York, NY: Oxford University Press; 2003.

20. Denberg N, Tranel D. Acalculia and disturbances of the body schema. In: Heilman KM, Valenstein E, eds. *Clinical Neuropsychology.* 4th ed. New York, NY: Oxford University Press; 2003.

21. Boone D, Landes B. Left-right discrimination in hemiplegic patients. *Arch Phys Med.* 1968;49(9):533-537.

22. Brown AL. Motivation to learn and understand: on taking charge of one's own learning. *Cogn Instruct.* 1988;5:311-321.

23. MacDonald J. An investigation of body scheme in adults with cerebral vascular accident. *Am J Occup Ther.* 1960;14:72-79.

24. Zoltan B, Jabri J, Panikoff L, Rychman D. *Perceptual Motor Evaluation for Head Injured and Other Neurologically Impaired Adults.* San Jose, Calif: Santa Clara Valley Medical Center, Occupational Therapy Department; 1983.

25. Sauguet J, Benton AL, Hecaen H. Disturbances of the body scheme in relation to language impairment and hemispheric locus of lesion. *J Neurol Neurosurg Psych.* 1971;34:496-501.

26. Baum B. The establishment of reliability and validity of a perceptual evaluation on a sample of adult head trauma patients. Thesis. University of Southern California; Dec 1981.

27. Taylor MM. Controlled evaluation of percept-concept—motor training therapy after stroke resulting in left hemiplegia. Research grant RD-2215-M, sponsored by Rehabilitation Institute. Detroit, Mich: Sept 1969.

28. Taylor MM. Analysis of dysfunction in the left hemiplegia following stroke. *Am J Occup Ther.* 1968;22:512-520.

29. Gregory ME, Aitkin JA. Assessment of parietal lobe function in hemiplegia. *Occup Ther.* 1971;34:9-17.

30. Maloney MP, Payne L. Validity of the draw-a-person test as a measure of body image. *Percept Motor Skills.* 1969;29:119-122.

31. Goodenough F, Harris D. *Goodenough-Harris Drawing Test.* New York, NY: Harcourt, Brace & World; 1963.

32. Frankenberg WK, Dods JB. *Denver Developmental Screening Test.* Denver, Co: Ladoca Project and Publishing; 1970.

33. Bouska MJ, Kauffman NA, Marcus SE. Disorders of the visual perceptual system. In: Umphred DA, ed. *Neurological Rehabilitation.* 2nd ed. St. Louis, Mo: CV Mosby Co.; 1990.

34. Adair JC, et al. Anosognosia. In: Heilman KM, Valenstein E, eds. *Clinical Neuropsychology.* 4th ed. New York, NY: Oxford University Press; 2003.

35. Bisiach E, Geminiani G. Anosognosia related to hemiplegia and hemianopia. In: Prigatano GP, Schacter DL, eds. *Awareness of Defects After Brain Injury.* New York, NY: Oxford University Press; 1991.

36. Weinstein EA. Anosognosia and denial of illness. In: Prigatano GP, Schacter DL, eds. *Awareness of Deficits After Injury.* New York, NY: Oxford University Press; 1991.

37. Maeshima S, Dohi N, Funahashi K, et al. Rehabilitation of patients with anosognosia for hemiplegia due to intracerebral hemorrhage. *Brain Inj.* 1997;11(9):691-697.

38. Swatell R, Martin G. Perceptual problems of the hemiplegic patient. *Lancet.* 1967;87:193-196.

39. Levine DA. Unawareness of visual and sensorimotor defects: a hypothesis. *Brain Cogn.* 1990;13:233-281.

40. Kortte, Wegener S, Chwalisz K. Anosognosia and denial: their relationship to coping and depression in acquired brain injury. *Rehabil Psychol.* 2003;48:131-136.

41. Heilman K, Barret A, Adair J. Possible mechanisms of anosognosia: a defect in self-awareness. *Philos Trans R Soc Lond B Biol Sci.* 1998;353(1377):1903-1909.

42. Ullman M. Disorder of body image after stroke. *Am J Nurs.* 1964;64:89-91.

43. Kosslyn SM, Koening O, Barrett A, Backer-Cave C, Tang J, Gabrieli JDE. Evidence for two types of spatial representations: hemispheric specialization for categorical and coordinate relations. *J Exp Psychol Hum Percept Perform.* 1989;15(4):723-735.

44. De Renzi E. *Disorders of Space Exploration and Cognition.* New York, NY: Wiley; 1982.

45. Benton A. *Right-Left Discrimination and Finger Localization.* New York, NY: Harper Bros; 1959.

46. Ayres AJ. *Southern California Sensory Integration Tests.* Los Angeles, Calif: Western Psychological Services; 1972.

47. Uomoto JM. The contribution of the neuropsychological evaluation to traumatic brain injury rehabilitation. In: Ashley M, ed. *Traumatic Brain Injury: Rehabilitative Treatment and Case Management.* Boca Raton, Fla: CRC Press; 2004.

48. Benton AL. Gerstmann's syndrome. *Arch Neurol.* 1992;49:445-447.

49. Benson DF. Disorders of visual gnosis. In: Brown JW, ed. *Neuropsychology of Visual Perception.* Mahwah, NJ: Lawrence Erlbaum Assoc; 1989.

50. Dannenbaum RM, Jones LA. The assessment and treatment of patients who have sensory loss following cortical lesions. *J Hand Ther.* 1993;6(2):130-138.

Resources

Benton AL, Sivan AB, Hamsher KD, Varney NR, Spreen O. *Contributions to Neuropsychological Assessment: A Clinical Manual.* 2nd ed. New York, NY: Oxford University Press; 1994.

Blanton S, Wolf SL. An application of upper-extremity constraint-induced movement therapy in a patient with subacute stroke. *Phys Ther.* 1999;79(9):847-853.

Brown J. *Aphasia, Apraxia and Agnosia: Clinical and Theoretical Aspects.* Springfield, Ill: Charles C. Thomas; 1972.

Damasio AR, Tranel D, Rizzo M. Disorder of complex visual processing. In: Mesulam MM, ed. *Principles of Behavioral and Cognitive Neurology.* 2nd ed. New York, NY: Oxford University Press; 2000.

Miltner WH, Bauder H, Sommer M, et al. Effects of constraint-induced movement therapy on patients with chronic motor deficits after stroke: a replication. *Stroke.* 1999;30(3):586-592.

Platz T, Winter T, Muller N, et al. Arm ability training for stroke and traumatic brain injury patients with mild arm paresis: a single-blind, randomized, controlled trial. *Arch Phys Med Rehabil.* 2001;82(7):961-968.

Schwoebel J, Coslett HB, Bradt J, et al. Pain and the body schema: effects of pain severity on mental representations of movement. *Neurology.* 2002;59(5):775-777.

Shiffman LM. Cerebral vascular accident. In: Early MB, ed. *Physical Dysfunction Practice Skills for the Occupational Therapy Assistant.* St. Louis, Mo: Mosby Year-Book; 1998.

van der Lee JH, Wagenaar RC, Lankhorst GJ, et al. Forced use of the upper extremity in chronic stroke patients: results from a single-blind randomized clinical trial. *Stroke.* 1999;30(11):2369-2375.

CHAPTER 6

VISUAL DISCRIMINATION SKILLS

Form Discrimination

The ability to distinguish different types of forms is an important ability for successful environmental interaction, and plays a primary role in human visual perception.[1,2] It plays an important role in visual recognition of objects, in visually guided manipulations, and in navigation within the environment.[3] The perception of spatial properties such as form are accomplished immediately and effortlessly. Color, orientation, edge, and motion cues are all utilized for form discrimination;[4-7] however, most common objects are recognized mainly by their shape.[2]

Difficulties with form perception have been associated with parietal and temporal lobe damage.[4,8] Within the visual system, form discrimination and processing involves cell populations in multiple visual areas.[2] Single cell recordings of the primary visual cortex indicates the possibility that some visual areas are more directly concerned with shape or form processing than others.[2] The interaction between simple and complex cells within the visual cortex may be important for form perception no matter where the form falls on the retina.[9]

Many theorists believe that form perception is accomplished by two processes with two separate systems carrying different aspects of form information.[4-6] The first system is hypothesized to perform abstract processing to recognize types of forms. The second system provides specific processing to distinguish different instances of a type of form. These two systems operate relatively independently within the brain.[6]

The Abstract Visual Form system (AVF) is utilized when visual form information should be processed and stored in an abstract, nonspecific manner.[3] For example, when an individual is scanning a cluttered desk to find a writing instrument to write a phone message, he is attempting to identify a pencil but not necessarily a particular pencil. This is accomplished by the SVF system, which distinguishes among different types of forms.

The Specific Visual Form system (SVF), on the other hand, produces specific output representations. It processes input in a manner that preserves visual details to produce output representations that distinguish different instances of the same type of form. For instance, identifying a particular, familiar pencil with which to write.

It is further hypothesized that the visual form systems process visual structure information during perception and subsequently store it in long-term "modality specific" information centers about visual form. The conceptual information associated with this structural information is not stored with it.[6] This concept of a specific center or centers that are the "form areas" exclusively has recently been challenged. Research has indicated there are a large number of cortical regions active during different form tasks.[4]

A disorder in form perception involves an inability to attend to subtle variations in form. This, in turn, will affect the client's ability to recognize common objects. For example, the client may mistake a water pitcher for a urinal or a button for a nickel.

EVALUATION FOR FORM DISCRIMINATION

Test 1 – Formboard Test[10]

Procedure

Show the client the 10 forms and test plate. Hand the client one form at a time, telling him or her to match each shape on the boards. The therapist may give a demonstration for aphasic clients. Take the form out of eyesight after the client has matched it, so that he or she cannot use the process of elimination.

Directions

Say, "Place each form on the shape that matches it."
Observe for spatial neglect, perseveration, poor planning or comprehension, and general inability to deal with objects.

Scoring

Severely impaired—Unable to match more than 1 to 4 forms

Impaired—Able to match 5 to 9 forms

Intact—Matches all 10 forms correctly

Validity

To improve validity, rule out poor vision, visual field loss, poor color discrimination, and constructional apraxia as causes of poor performance.

Reliability

Inter-rater reliability (r = 1.0) was established for this test on a sample of adult clients with head trauma.[11]

Test 2 – Functional

Description

Observe the client during various activities, and note whether he or she has difficulty distinguishing among different objects of similar forms (ie, eating utensils in the kitchen).

Scoring

Subjective
The instances when and where difficulty was observed are recorded.

Intact—Client displays no difficulty in distinguishing forms during occupational performance tasks.

TREATMENT FOR FORM DISCRIMINATION

Utilizing a Restorative Approach

1. Have the client practice sorting functional objects such as kitchen utensils. Have the client use tactile cues by feeling objects for successful task completion.

2. Place Velcro strips on elevated surfaces of specific objects with distinct edges.[12] Train the client to explore with the fingers both the location and form of the objects covered with Velcro. The client should perform the task first with his or her eyes open, then closed.

3. Inputs should be applied to have enhanced contact (ie, feeling a moving or irregular input passed through the hand).[12]

Utilizing an Adaptive Approach

1. Shapes are best recognized with an upright orientation; therefore, place items necessary to the client's function in the upright position.[7,13] For example, hang garden tools up separately instead of piled in a drawer.

2. Label important items that the client is unable to distinguish.

3. Organize items, and maintain this organization so the client can distinguish items by location.

Depth Perception (Stereopsis)

Depth perception, or stereopsis, is crucial to the individual's ability to locate objects in the visual environment, to have accurate hand movements under visual guidance, and to function safely with tasks such as navigating stairs or driving.[14-16] Impaired depth perception will affect activities that require the judgment of spatial relationships, such as threading a needle, targeting food on a plate, hammering, or putting toothpaste on a toothbrush.[1] In severe cases, the client may completely lose the ability to see any differences in depth, and a flight of stairs, for example, is seen as a number of lines on the floor.[17]

Depth perception is the third dimension beyond the two-dimensional image on the retina.[18,19] Binocular vision, along with monocular cues such as texture, shading, and linear perspective, all contribute to perception of three-dimensional shape and distance.[14,19-21] Visual acuity and ocular alignment must also be adequate for depth perception.[20,22] The parietal lobe has been associated with stereoscopic coding of three-dimensional objects, but despite recent advances in neuroimaging techniques, the neural substrates of stereopsis remain unknown.[19,23,24]

Human stereopsis is evident at about 2 months of age. The process of stereopsis, generally associated with right hemisphere dominance,[25] is considered relatively low level because "the neural mechanisms for the binocular extraction of depth occur early in the cortical hierarchy of visuospatial functions."[15] Stereopsis does not appear to depend on visual recognition and does not need to be taught. However, depth is a perceptual attribute and, therefore, cannot be arrived at without the participation of the observer.[26]

The theoretical basis of depth perception acquisition has emphasized areas such as the fusion of information from two monocular views and binocular rivalry or suppression.[15,18,27] The perception of depth has also recently been linked to the sensitivity of the visual system to spatial frequency information.[28] Classic stereopsis relies on the fact that "two physical points in space lying at different distances lead to differential retinal disparity of the two pairs of binocular image points."[27] Binocular disparity is the most important cue for depth perception.[29] More specifically, horizontal disparity is the crucial input for stereopsis. Vertical disparity does not contribute to stereopsis "although large vertical disparities must be corrected prior to stereopsis by vertical vergence eye movements."[15]

Horizontal spatial disparity is only one disparity cue for stereopsis. Temporal disparity and intraocular differences in brightness may also contribute.[15] In addition, recent research has focused on the formation of subjective occluding contours and surface resulting from unpaired points in binocular images. As Nakayama and Shimojo describe, "distant surfaces are occluded by nearer surfaces to different extents in the two eyes, leading to the existence of unpaired image points visible in one eye and not the other."[27] These researchers believe the visual system utilizes the occlusive relations in the real world to recover depth, contour, and surface from unpaired points.

The concept of binocular rivalry or suppression has also been explored. Some theorize that "when stimuli are rivalrous, one or the other may predominate in alternating fashion."[15] The "losing" image is thought to be suppressed. Due to this binocular suppression, the individual is unaware of the discordant view of the two eyes in normal viewing when fixating on a near object. Depth information related to objects in the visual environment is derived from monocular cues such as linear perspective, texture, gradients, and apparent size of familiar objects.[15] For example, when an object is farther away in depth, it will appear smaller. In addition, less detail will be evident than when it is closer in depth.[28]

As a result of acquired brain injury (ABI) it is common for the client to have fusion and no diplopia (double vision) and yet have no depth perception.[18] Stereopsis may be impaired without strabismus as a result of damage in the visual cortices through a cerebral vascular accident (CVA) or traumatic brain injury (TBI).[15]

The evaluation of depth perception has traditionally included asking the client to estimate distance in the natural environment, to judge the relative distance of real three-dimensional objects under more controlled conditions, and by measuring the acuity of stereoscopic vision.[25] An example of a functional evaluation and acuity of stereoscopic vision are subsequently described. The therapist should evaluate primary vision functions, as described in Chapter 3, prior to testing for depth perception. Visual acuity and ocular alignment, for example, are prerequisites for depth perception. Contrast sensitivity can also affect depth perception.

Test 1 – Functional Test/Observation

Description

Put a pen on the table in front of the client. Ask the client to grasp it. Hold the pen in the air in front of the client. Ask him or her to take it from you. Ask the client to perform other daily activities such as pouring water from a pitcher into a glass or positioning his or her wheelchair for a transfer. Observe the client during meals or walking up a curb or flight of stairs.

Scoring

Subjective

Intact—Client correctly follows each request without hesitation.

Validity

To improve validity, rule out apraxia, poor eye-hand coordination, ataxia, poor visual acuity, unilateral neglect, and hemianopsia.

Reliability

In a refined version of the pen test in a study of adult head trauma clients, 90% scored intact, indicating little variance in performance.[11] Additional research should indicate whether the test is appropriate for use with the adult client with brain damage.

Test 2 – Instructo Clinic, Depth Perception Test[30]

Description

The client stands 20 feet away from the testing apparatus, which contains three road signs (stop, yield, and railroad crossing). The client views four picture sets and is asked to tell which sign is nearest and which is farthest away.

Scoring

Nonstandardized

The number of correct responses is calculated and divided into categories of good, satisfactory, and marginal.

Validity

To improve validity, rule out aphasia, visual field, and other visual deficits (ie, blurred, double vision) as causes of poor performance.

TREATMENT OF DEPTH PERCEPTION DEFICITS

Utilizing a Restorative Approach

1. Provide tactile-kinesthetic guiding during activities. For example, while guiding, have the client feel the depth, distance, and size of his wheelchair before a bed-to-wheelchair transfer.[16,31]

Utilizing an Adaptive Approach

1. Alter the environment to help the client compensate. For example, place a bright colored tape at the edge of each step of stairs.

2. Have the client utilize other intact sensory systems rather than visual. For example, utilize tactile sensation in the fingers by having the client practice pouring. Put his or her finger near the inside top of a glass to feel when he or she has poured a full glass.

3. Provide verbal cuing when needed to compensate, especially when safety is an issue.

4. Generally, if the depth perception problem is related to decreased binocularity, the client's cognitive processing skills enable him or her to compensate. Even though objective testing identifies an impairment, there may be no functional problems (Mary Warren, personal communication). If the depth problem is related to acuity or contrast problems, the therapist identifies the area of function affected and teaches compensation techniques (ie, the use of cane for stairs) (Mary Warren, personal communication).

5. Educate the client and his or her family about the depth perception problem and how it will affect function. Areas for which safety is an issue should be highlighted.

Figure-Ground Perception

Figure-ground perception involves the ability to distinguish the foreground from the background. The "figure" or foreground is the part of the field of perception that is the center of an individual's attention at any given time. Those incoming stimuli not the center of attention form a dimly perceived background.[1,32,33] The separation of figures from background is accomplished by the visual system based on differences in features such as color, luminance, depth, orientation, texture, motion, and temporal information.[34] The difficulty a client with a figure-ground deficit has visually distinguishing a figure from a competing background will affect his or her ability to locate objects that are not well defined from the background.[33,35] Higher levels of perception such as figure-ground are required to organize the layout of the environment.[36] Therefore, a deficit such as this will adversely affect self-care ability. The client with a figure-ground deficit, for example, may have difficulty finding things in a cluttered drawer or shelf or finding the sleeve of an all white shirt.

Historically, theories related to the development of figure-ground perception assumed that it occurred before any object recognition.[37] It was assumed that visual processes such as figure-ground organization depend on variables related to the current stimulus and not those from memory that relate to object recognition processes. It was also assumed that object recognition would be impossible unless some prior processes sorted out or reduced the complexity of the problem. One way this is accomplished is through figure-ground organization, which differentiates between shaped and shapeless regions in the visual fields.[37]

Some theorists, however, believe that memory does play a role in figure-ground perception.[37,38] Recent research indicates that some object or shape recognition occurs before figure-ground organization is completed. This shape recognition process has been termed prefigural recognition processes and is an "edged-based" recognition process.[37] Recent research has also highlighted the importance of fixation location and attention to figure-ground organization.[13,33,37,39] In a case study of a 69-year-old male with right hemisphere damage, it was discovered that the client retained figure-ground perception despite severe left neglect, even when a stimulus appeared on the left. These researchers conclude that figures are segregated from their background preattentively. Peterson and Gibson take this concept further. They state that not only is there empirical evidence supportive of the relevance of fixation point to figure-ground, but they also suggest that "the inputs to figure-ground organization from fixation location are separate from the inputs from prefigural shape recognition processes."[37]

EVALUATION OF FIGURE-GROUND PERCEPTION

Test 1 – Ayres' Figure-Ground Test
(Subtest of the Southern California Sensory Integration Tests)[40]

Description

This is a published test requiring the client to select three pictures of objects or geometric forms from a multiple choice plate of six pictures. The three to be selected are to be found in an embedded plate (Figure 6-1). The client indicates his or her choice by naming or pointing to the picture or design. He or she has one minute to identify three embedded pictures. The test is discontinued after five errors.

Scoring

Each correctly identified picture is given a score of 1. The range of possible scores is 0 to 48. This test has been standardized only for children up to the age of 10.11 years. A score of 18 is the mean for 10.11 year olds. The following studies, however, were done with adults. Fifty-six normal adults aged 20 to 59 were studied, and the results are listed in Table 6-1.

A study was conducted with 100 adult males with the following results[38]: mean score 29.7 (considerably higher than 18.7 norm of 10.3 to 10.11 year olds); only one male obtained a perfect score of 48, indicating the test has no ceiling effect. These authors recommend its use with adults.

A study of 124 adult females indicated test results showed a normal distribution and found it to be reliable over time.[41] These authors also recommend its use with adults.

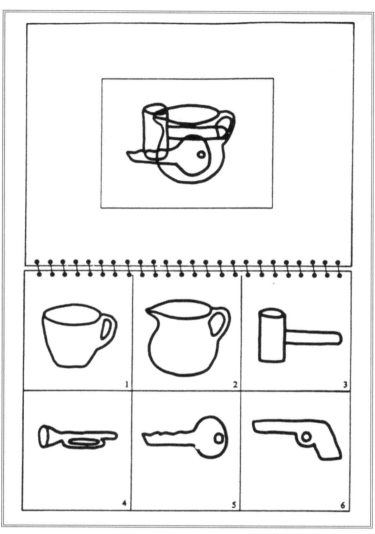

Figure 6-1. One page of the Southern California Figure-ground Perception Test.[40] (Adapted from Ayres AJ. *Southern California Sensory Integration Tests.* Los Angeles, Calif: Western Psychological Services; 1972.)

Table 6-1

Adult Normative Data on Figure-Ground Test—SCSIT

Age	Number of Subjects	Mean Score	One Standard Deviation
20 to 29	22	31.9	9.7
30 to 39	12	32.6	8.9
40 to 49	10	22.8	7.8
50 to 59	12	23.9	5.7

Intact —One standard deviation (+).

Impaired—More than minus 1 standard deviation from the mean.

Severely impaired—More than minus 2 standard deviations from the mean.

Validity

To improve validity, rule out poor visual acuity, hemianopsia, and dense aphasia. (For clients with mild aphasia who understand gestures, the test may be valid). This test has been found to discriminate between children with and without perceptual deficits (t = 5.19, p < 0.01). Its reliability test-retest coefficients of correlation range from r = 0.37 to 0.52 for children ages 4.0 to 10.11 years.

Reliability

This test has established inter-rater reliability (r = 0.87) on a sample of adult clients with head trauma.[11]

This test requires a high degree of concentration. Therefore, it may not be valid to administer it to clients who show a high degree of distractibility.

Test 2 – Overlapping Figures Subtest of the LOTCA[42]

Description

The Overlapping Figures (OF) Subtest is based on the classic embedded pictures test of figure-ground perception. The client is asked to identify six overlapping figures presented on two cards with three figures on each.

Scoring (For the Six Figures)

1 Point—Client does not identify any figures or identifies less than three figures with the aid of the board.

2 Points—Client identifies three figures with the aid of the board.

3 Points—Client identifies four figures without the board or all of the figures with the aid of the board.

4 Points—Client identifies all of the figures without the board.

Reliability

Inter-rater reliability with Spearman's rank correlation coefficient among raters ranged from 0.82 to 0.97 for the various subtests.

Validity

The majority of validity and reliability research was conducted on the remaining three subtests. The authors recommend administration of the entire test battery versus utilizing only one or two subtests.

Test 3 – Functional Test

Description

The therapist asks the client to pick out or find an object in view. There are many variations of this test. Following are some examples:

1. While in the client's bedroom, ask the client to pick up a white towel or face cloth that you have put on his white sheets.

2. While dressing, ask the client to find his sleeve, buttonholes, buttons, and bottom of the shirt.

3. While in the kitchen, ask the client to find objects that are on the counter or the knife among the unsorted cutlery in the drawer.

4. Ask the client to sort a pile of shirts into long- and short-sleeved.

Scoring

Subjective

Intact—Client does tasks within a reasonable length of time.

Validity

To improve validity, rule out poor acuity, visual object agnosia, and poor comprehension of the directions as reasons for poor performance.

Dynamic Assessment

Alter the task or environment to facilitate client performance during evaluation. For example, if the client is unable to find an item in a cluttered drawer, reduce the items one item at a time until the client is able to find the target item. Use this as a baseline measure for graded functional tasks, and alter the environment or task as the client improves.

TREATMENT FOR FIGURE-GROUND PERCEPTION

Utilizing a Restorative Approach

1. Scatter items in front of the client in a disorganized fashion. Name an object and have the client point to it. Increase the number of objects in the array as the client improves.

2. Utilize occupation-based activities that focus on the restoration of figure-ground deficits. For example, if the client was a contractor prior to the ABI, have him answer questions and interpret blue print drawings. Utilize drawings of the complexity level of the client and progress to more complex ones (ie, start with plans for enlarging a room and progress to a major kitchen remodel).

Utilizing an Adaptive Approach

1. Alter the client's environment as follows[16]:

   a) Put only a few things on the nightstand.

   b) Organize drawers, separating articles—for example, sock drawer, shirt drawer.[43]

   c) Arrange the meal tray so that it has only a few items; have the meal in several courses if necessary.

   d) Mark the wheelchair brakes with red tape so that they will be easier to distinguish from the wheel.

2. To help the client compensate, teach him or her cognitive awareness of his or her deficit; teach the client to be very systematic and examine each small area carefully by slowing down and not being impulsive. For example, in the kitchen, have the client look and even feel the countertop to find out what objects are on it.

3. Educate the client and his or her family regarding the figure-ground deficit and how it will affect function. Train them in the use of compensation techniques such as the need for uncluttered drawers, cabinets, etc.

Utilizing a Dynamic Interactional Approach

Identify what strategy for figure-ground organization the client utilizes most effectively (conceptual task characteristics). For example, does he or she sort a disorganized drawer, or does he or she utilize systematic scanning for card sorting? If possible, have the client describe to you how he or she completed the task. Once it is clear what technique or strategy the client uses, provide activities in a variety of settings or contexts that allow for application of the identified strategy (ie, the kitchen, grocery store, hardware store, etc). Do not upgrade task requirements until the client has shown some generalization of learning.

Spatial Relations

Visual perception is intrinsically spatial.[44] The individual processes descriptions of the external world that inherently contain information about spatial relations within and among objects. When the individual has a consistent point of origin through an established body scheme, continued environmental exploration leads to the perception of areas such as objects and their relationship to the individual or to each other.[45] Visual, somesthetic, proprioceptive, and auditory signals are interpreted in relation to a stored and a continually updated body scheme, which in turn, allows us to perceive spatial locations and relations among objects and events within that space.[46-48] Body-centered or egocentric information is transformed into a world framed or allocentric frame of reference.[49] In addition to the previously mentioned sensory inputs and integration, the formation of the concept of spatial relations requires the attention mechanism, memory functions, and at times, motor output for object manipulation.[50]

Spatial relations or visuospatial processing ability is the capacity to localize objects in relation to each other and understand the location of objects with respect to oneself.[1,2,48,50,51] Space perception may be dissociated from pattern perception, which gives information about what objects are and their categorization.[48] Through the ability of the perception of spatial relations, an individual can judge distances, distinguish forms, and separate objects from a surrounding background. Spatial relations are important to orienting in the environment; recognizing objects, scenes, and language; and for manipulation of objects within the hand.[19,45]

The theoretical basis for the acquisition of spatial relations has recently been explored. Some theorists focus on the importance of spatial attention.[45] They envision the apprehension of spatial relations to involve the coordination of perceptual and conceptual representations of space. The perceptual representations consist of arrays of objects and surfaces, while the conceptual component involves prepositions like above and below.[3] The acquisition process is hypothesized to involve "spatial indexing," which involves the selecting of an object in the perceptual representation and establishing a correspondence between it and a symbol it stands for in the conceptual representation. This process is accomplished through spatial attentional operations. For example, any object can be above something else. Therefore, the number of objects that can serve to relate to the reference object is infinitely large. It is impossible to relate an object to everything, so the relevant relational objects must be selected. Spatial attention is involved in this indexing process as well as in searching for targets that differ from distracters in the spatial relations.[45] These theoretical concepts related to the importance of spatial attention to spatial relations development have recently been supported by clinical research.[45]

Another recent area of focus related to spatial relations acquisition is the existence of two types of spatial relations: categorical spatial relations and coordinate spatial relations.[44,52-54] Recent research suggests that both the right and left hemispheres can compute both types of spatial relations but not equally effectively.[44,54] Theorists conceptualize a clear distinction between categorical spatial relations, such as above–below, left–right, and on–off, and coordinate spatial relations, which specify locations in a way that can be used to guide precise movements. It is further hypothesized that there are distinct subsystems that may encode the two types of spatial relations.[45] Representations are produced by processing subsystems, "with each subsystem corresponding to a set of neurons that work together to transform input into a specific type of output."[53] It is assumed that because categorical and coordinate representations are qualitatively different, separate processing subsystems produce each type of representation.[8]

Damage to the parietal lobes, predominantly the right, has been associated with visual spatial deficits.[24,51,55] Several positron emission tomography (PET) studies have indicated there is an occipitoparietal visual pathway for processing spatial location information.[48]

Spatial relations deficits can result in difficulties with tasks such as aligning buttons of a shirt, discerning which side of the shirt is the front and which is the back, or perceiving whether the arm went though the armhole or the neckhole.[50]

EVALUATION OF SPATIAL RELATIONS

Test 1 – Cross Test[56]

Description

This test requires the client to duplicate a small cross on a blank sheet of paper in the same position as it appeared on the stimulus card Figure 6-2. A blank piece of paper, the sample stimulus card, and a black felt pen are placed in front of the client, and he or she is instructed to "Draw two small crosses on this paper in the exact positions that they appear on the card. Be exact." If the client does not understand, the therapist demonstrates by drawing the crosses for him. After the client does the sample, the transparent score guide is placed over the trial so that the client can judge the extent of his or her discrepancies. Then, each of the three test cards is presented in turn with the command: "Now do the same thing with this card. Do not hurry. Be exact."

Scoring

Nonstandardized

The client's score is the total number of centimeters of discrepancy between the model and the reproduction. The transparent score guide is placed over the client's effort, and the distances between the intersection of lines on the model and the client's crosses are measured with a centimeter ruler. If there is any doubt as to which cross the client was attempting to copy, the model closest to his or her cross should be selected. If a cross is missing from a client's effort, this should be scored as one-half the width of the page.

> *Intact*—Score of 0 to 300
>
> *Impaired*—Score of 300 to 600.
>
> *Severe*—Score of 600 and above. (Scores adapted from those received by control group study of Pehoski.)[56]

Validity

To improve validity, rule out motor apraxia, poor eye-hand coordination, unilateral neglect, and hemianopsia.

Test 2 –Ayres' Space Visualization Test

(Subtest of Southern California Sensory Integration Tests)[40]

Description

This test uses two formboards, one with an egg-shaped hollow and one with a diamond shaped hollow, two pegs, four egg-shaped blocks, and four diamond-shaped blocks. The pegs are inserted

Figure 6-2. Sample and three test cards of the cross test.[56] (Adapted from Pehoski C. Analysis of perceptual dysfunction and dressing in adult hemiplegics. Thesis. Boston, Mass: Sargent College, Boston University; 1970.)

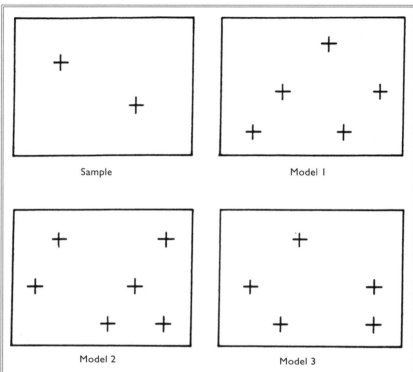

Sample   Model 1

Model 2   Model 3

Table 6-2

Adult Normative Data, Space Visualization Test—SCSIT

	Age	Number of Subjects	Mean Score	Standard Deviation
Accuracy	50 to 64	90	56.2	4.5
	65 to 74	60	56.3	4.5
Time	50 to 64	90	118.2	50.8
	65 to 74	60	158.5	74.9

Adapted from reference 57: Taylor MM. Analysis of dysfunction in the left hemiplegia following stroke. Am J Occup Ther. 1968;22:512-520.

into the formboards to create different test items. The test consists of 30 "puzzles," each consisting of one formboard and two blocks, only one of which fits the formboard. The client is asked to look at the puzzle and choose one of the two blocks. Only then is he or she allowed to try fitting his or her choice in the formboard. The test is discontinued after five errors are made.

Scoring

This test has been standardized only for children. In testing the reliability, Ayres reports the test-retest correlations range from r = 0.28 to 0.77 for children aged 4.0 to 10.0.[58] years. Using the same scoring method as Ayres, Taylor provides the adult normative data shown in Table 6-2.[57]

Until a more extensive adult normative study can be done, interpretation of scores is nonstandardized.

Intact—One standard deviation.

Impaired—More than minus 1 standard deviation from the mean.

Validity

Ayres reported a study in which she administered this test to both right and left hemiplegic adults. The left hemiplegics did better as a group than the right hemiplegics, although the difference was not significant. Because it is generally thought that left hemiplegics do significantly poorer on spatial relations test, the validity of this test with adults is in some doubt.

TREATMENT FOR SPATIAL RELATIONS

Utilizing a Restorative Approach

1. Have the client retrieve objects following verbal requests containing spatial concepts (ie, "get the brush on top of the dresser behind the bed").

2. Have the client place a variety of objects in different places around the room. The client returns to the original spot, visualizes, verbalizes, and points to where the objects are in relation to him. Once the client has localized the objects, he or she should walk (or wheel) through space to retrieve the objects in sequence.[58]

3. Have the client practice various tasks for which he or she must discriminate various spatial relations.

4. Provide tactile-kinesthetic guiding of the client to objects and among objects so the client receives tactile-kinesthetic input related to object position and distances.

5. Add reference cues and modulate task difficulty by varying the size and orientation difference among stimuli.[59]

6. Use landmarks for location. Have the client orient him- or herself in space and then from object to object.[60]

Utilizing an Adaptive Approach

1. Organize the client's environment so that necessary items are consistently in the same place. Educate the client and his or her family to the client's spatial relation deficit and the importance of maintaining a consistent environment.

2. Mark areas in drawers, cabinets, etc where key items are to be stored.

Topographical Disorientation

Topographical orientation is a complex behavior with many components. It can be defined as the ability to follow a familiar route or a new route once it has become familiar; clients generally have difficulty finding their way in space.[58,61,62] It could involve the ability to locate a public building in a city, find the kitchen in one's house, or describe verbally or with a map how to get to a specific place.[46,63] This ability requires knowledge of an ego state (where am I?), a goal (where do I need to go?), and an action (how do I get there?).[64]

Through normal development, a child acquires a perceptual ability to recognize specific locations for navigational decisions.[65] This is termed landmark or place recognition and is theorized to be the first topographic ability to develop. The child moves from developing different cognitive representations of space from the first landmark representations to egocentric route learning to metric representations of space in the exocentric world.[65,66]

Topographical orientation requires specific skills related to specialized topographical orientation as well as general visual spatial abilities and memory.[62,67] For example, in order to interact effectively with the environment, an individual requires "...an integrated viewpoint-dependent representation of the world."[68] This viewpoint preserves information about the positions of objects relative to the viewer. To establish this viewpoint, the individual must have adequate visual processing of the dimensions of visual stimuli across the visual fields, adequate depth perception and coding of forms in three dimentions, and adequate integration of form information.[68] If these processes are impaired, there can be a decreased ability to recognize visual landmarks and routes. In addition to the visual processes, the individual requires spatial working memory to hold information about where he or she is and to plan future movements. Adequate attentional processes and stored memories for previously experienced landmarks are also required.

Christianson and Raschko theorize that topographical orientation is accomplished through cognitive mapping.[69] The individual's cognitive map is a mental representation of his or her surroundings. It is the product of active information seeking and the means by which one maintains orientation within the environment by recognizing objects and landmarks.

Contemporary clinicians have observed and described several types of topographical disorientation, including egocentric disorientation, heading disorientation, landmark agnosia, and anterograde amnesia.[20,65,67] Egocentric disorientation is topographical disorientation secondary to visual disorientation.[67] These clients often sustained damage to the right or bilateral parietal lobes and cannot form egocentric spatial relationships yet have intact visual recognition abilities.[20,65] These clients are unable to learn or recall appropriate spatial directions with perceived landmarks. They suffer from a global spatial disorientation related to the relative location of objects with respect to the self.[20] These clients are severely impaired in navigating familiar and unfamiliar environments, but the impairment is not specific to topographic knowledge.[67]

The client with landmark disorientation or "landmark agnosia" is unable to use prominent, relevant environmental features for the purpose of orientation.[20] They possess a visual recognition disability that is selective or disproportionate for objects in the environment that routinely serve as landmarks yet retain or possess spatial knowledge of the environment.[67] They are, for example, able to provide good descriptions of routes or maps but are unable to apply this knowledge because of their inability to recognize landmarks. These clients may also have additional neuropsychological deficits such as prosopagnosia, achromatopsia, and some degree of visual field deficit[20] and are not assumed to have completely intact perception.[65] Landmark agnosia has been associated with bilateral lesions of the right medial tempero-occipital region.[20] The lesions are often due to a CVA involving the right posterior artery.[20]

Clients with a heading disorientation have adequate egocentric orientation and are able to recognize landmarks. They are, however, unable to generate directional information from the landmarks they recognize.[20,65] They are unable to perceive and remember the spatial relationships among landmarks in their environment.[67] This is an exocentric deficit in that they have lost a sense of exocentric direction or heading within their environment.[20,65] These clients have difficulty with both old and novel environments. This type of topographical disorientation appears to be somewhat more rare than the others and is associated with damage to the right posterior cingulate region.[20,65]

The fourth category of topographical disorientation is anterograde disorientation. These clients can find their way in environments they have known for at least 6 months before the ABI but are unable to learn new environments.[20,65] The deficit involves both spatial and landmark knowledge.[67] Lesions of the right basal temporal cortex have been associated with anterograde disorientation.[20,63]

EVALUATION OF TOPOGRAPHICAL DISORIENTATION

The test for this deficit is a functional one. If the client is unable to find his way back to his or her ward from the treatment room or from occupational therapy to physical therapy after being shown several times, this suggests a topographical disorientation problem. Through questioning the client, assess whether the difficulty is related to landmark agnosia, egocentric disorientation, heading disorientation, or anterograde disorientation. However, one must first rule out a general poor memory problem or mental confusion. Usually, topographical disorientation is not seen in isolation from the other problems of spatial relations.

TREATMENT FOR TOPOGRAPHICAL DISORIENTATION

Utilizing an Adaptive Approach

The following guidelines for environmental adaptations can be utilized to help the client compensate for this deficit[69]:

1. Identify what spaces or areas can be utilized by the client as an important landmark. How or with what type of marker should the space be identified, and where should such identification be located?

2. Provide landmarks such as pictures or objects that provide cues that give the client knowledge or feeling of where he or she is in a particular place (eg, murals, paintings).

3. Landmark designs and signs should be clear and realistic. Utilize high contrast (ie, colors that contrast with the wall for clients with visual deficits).

4. Any signs or landmarks placed for the client in a wheelchair should have the lower edge placed at 54 inches high and to the latch side of the door.

5. Signs should have contrast between the lettering and background and should avoid busy patterns.

6. Specific areas where signs facilitate topographical orientation are entries and exits, bathrooms, and eating areas.

7. If possible, the client can purchase a portable global positioning device (GPS) such as those now used in cars, for example the Navman (Navman, Auckland, New Zealand).

Additional Test Batteries of Visual Discrimination/Perception

Test 1 – Developmental Test of Visual Perception—Adolescent and Adult[70]

Description

A battery of 6 subtests (copying, figure-ground, visual-motor search, visual closure, visual-motor speed, and form constancy). It is designed for use with individuals ages 11 to 74 years old. It takes approximately 20 to 30 minutes to administer.

Scoring

Four of the subtests are administered until a ceiling is reached and the others are stopped after a designated time. Raw scores are generated which can then be converted to percentiles and standard scores using the norms contained in the user manual. The sums of standard scores can be converted into index scores and percentiles. The most reliable scores for the Developmental Test of Visual Perception-Adolescent and -Adult (DTVP-A) are the indexes.

Norms

The DTVP-A was normed on a sample of 1,664 individuals from 19 states covering all major regions of the United States. Additional measures were taken to assure representativeness and are described in the test manual.

Validity

Content validity established by 1) providing the underlying rationale for the selection of items and subtest, 2) items analysis, 3) item response theory modeling, 4) statistical procedures that detect item bias (logistic regression procedure), 5) criterion prediction validity (criterion related), and 6) factor analysis.

Reliability

Internal consistency—Measured on all but the timed subtests with Cronbach's Alpha. The internal consistency of the timed test was measured with test-retest reliability.

Subtest—100% of coefficient alphas = 0.70 or higher
      70% of coefficient alphas = 0.80 or higher

Index—64% of coefficient alpha = 0.90 or higher

Inter-rater—0.94 to 0.99

Test-retest—0.70 to 0.84

Test 2 – Motor-Free Visual Perception Test, Third Edition[71]

Description

Five visual perceptual skills (spatial relationships, visual discrimination, figure-ground, visual closure, and visual memory) are represented; however, the test is designed to provide one general, overall visual perceptual score. The test employs simple black and white line drawings, and each item is presented in a multiple choice format.

Scoring

A single row score can be converted to either a standard score, percentile ranks, and age equivalents. Scores such as scaled scores on T-scores can also be generated.

Norms

Norms were generated from a sample of 1,856 individuals representative of the demographics of the United States. Detailed information pertaining to the sample is included in the manual.

Validity

Criterion related—0.78 correlation with the total score of the DTVP-2; 0.73 with the DTVP.

Construct validity—A positive but low correlation was found with tests of general cognitive ability, which support the expectation that the Motor-Free Visual Perception Test,

Third Edition (MVPT-3) should have a low correlation with cognitive ability. Additional validity studies were conducted and described in the test manual.

Reliability

Internal consistency—Cronbach alpha = 0.86 to 0.90 with median reliability coefficient for age 11 and older = 0.89

Test-Retest—0.92

References

1. Bryan VL. Management of residual physical deficits. In: Ashley MJ, Krych DK, eds. *Traumatic Brain Injury: Rehabilitative Treatment and Case Management.* 2nd ed. Boca Raton, Fla: CRC Press; 2004.
2. Ullman S. The visual analysis of shape and form. In: Gazzaniga M, ed. *The Cognitive Neurosciences.* Cambridge, Mass: MIT Press; 1995.
3. Jolicoeur P, Ullman S, Mackay M. Curve tracing: A possible basic operation in the perception of spatial relations. *Memory Cogn.* 1986;14(2):129-140.
4. Gulyas B, Heywood CA, Popplewell DA, Roland PE, Cowey A. Visual form discrimination from color or motion cues: functional anatomy by positron emission tomography. *Proc Natl Acad Sci USA.* 1994;91(21):9965-9969.
5. Levingstone MS, Hubel DH. Psychophysical evidence for separate channels for the perception of form, color, movement, and depth. *J Neuroscience.* 1987;7(11):3416-3468.
6. Marsoleck CJ. Abstract visual-form representations in the left cerebral hemisphere. *J Exp Psychol Hum Percept Perform.* 1995;21(2):375-386.
7. Rock I, DiVita J, Barbeito R. The effect on form perception of change of orientation in the third dimension. *J Exp Psychol Hum Percept Perform.* 1991;7(4):719-732.
8. Kosslyn S, Chabis CF, Marsolek CJ, Koenig O. Categorical versus coordinate spatial relations: computational analyses and computer simulations. *J Exp Psychol Hum Percept Perform.* 1992;18(2):562-577.
9. Kandel ER. Processing of form and movement in the visual system. In: Kandel ER, Schwartz JH, eds. *Principles of Neural Science.* 2nd ed. New York, NY: Elsevier Science; 1985.
10. Zoltan B, Jabri J, Panikoff L, Ryckman D. *Perceptual Motor Evaluation for Head Injured and Other Neurologically Impaired Adults.* San Jose, Calif: Santa Clara Valley Medical Center, Occupational Therapy Department; 1983.
11. Baum B. The establishment of reliability and validity of a perceptual evaluation on a sample of adult head trauma patients. Thesis. University of Southern California, Dec 1981.
12. Dannenbaum RM, Jones LA. The assessment and treatment of patients who have sensory loss following cortical lesions. *J Hand Ther.* 1993:6(2):130-138.
13. Rock I, Mitchener K. Further evidence of failure of reversal of ambiguous figures by uninformed subjects. Perception. 1992;21:39-45.
14. Cuiffreda KJ, et al. Normal vision function. In: Gonzales EG, Myers SJ, Edelstein JE, et al, eds. *Downey and Darling's Physiological Basis of Rehabilitation Medicine.* Boston, Mass: Butterworth Heimann; 2001.
15. Rizzo M. Astereopsis. In: Boller F, Grafman J, eds. *Handbook of Neuropsychology.* Vol 2. New York, NY: Elsevier Science; 1989.
16. Zoltan B. Remediation of visual-perceptual and perceptual-motor deficits. In: Rosenthal M, Griffith ER, Bond MR, Miller JD, eds. *Rehabilitation of the Adult and Child with Traumatic Brain Injury.* Philadelphia, Pa: FA Davis; 1990.
17. Karnath HO, Zihl J. Disorders of spatial orientation. In: Brandt T, Caplan LR, Dichgans J, Diener CH, Kennard C, eds. *Neurological Disorders: Course and Treatment.* San Diego, Calif: Academic Press; 2003.
18. Neger RE. The evaluation of diplopia in head trauma. *J Head Trauma Rehabil.* 1989;4(2):27-34.
19. Sakata H, Taira M, Kusunoki M, Murata A, Tanaka Y. The TINS lecture: the parietal association cortex in depth perception and visual control of hand action. *Trends Neurosci.* 1997;20(8):350-357.
20. Devinsky O, D'Esposito M. Perception and perceptual disorders. In: *Neurology of Cognitive and Behavioral Disorders.* New York, NY: Oxford University Press; 2004.
21. Kelly JP. Anatomy of the central visual pathways. In: Kandel ER, Schwartz JH, eds. *Principles of Neural Science.* 2nd ed. New York, NY: Elsevier Science; 1985.

22. Kerkhoff G. Recovery and treatment of sensory perceptual disorders. In: Halligan P, Kischka U, Marshall JC, eds. *Handbook of Clinical Neuropsychology.* New York, NY: Oxford University Press; 2003.

23. Fortin A, Ptito A, Faubert J, Ptito M. Cortical areas mediating stereopsis in the human brain: a PET study. *Neuroreport.* 2002;13(6):895-898.

24. Kerkhoff G. Multimodal spatial orientation deficits in left-sided visual neglect. *Neuropsychologia.* 1999;37:1387-1405.

25. Newcombe F, Ratcliff G. Disorders of visuospatial analysis. In: Boller F, Grafman J, eds. *Handbook of Neuropsychology.* Vol 2. Amsterdam: Elsevier Science; 1989.

26. Westheimer G, Levi DM. Depth attraction and repulsion of disparate foveal stimuli. *Vision Res.* 1987;27(8):1361-1368.

27. Nakayama K, Shimojo S. Da Vinci stereopsis: depth and subjective occluding contours from unpaired image points. *Vis Res.* 1990;30(11):1811-1825.

28. Brown JM, Weisstein N. A spatial frequency effect on perceived depth. *Percept Psychophys.* 1988;44(2):157-166.

29. Goldberg ME, Colby CL. The neurophysiology of spatial vision. In: Boller F, Grafman J, eds. *Handbook of Neuropsychology.* Vol 2. Amsterdam: Elsevier Science; 1989.

30. Instructo-Clinic—A Psychophysical Testing Apparatus. Bumpa-Tel, Inc, PO Box 611, Cape Cir, Missouri 63701.

31. Affolter FD. *Perception, Interaction and Language: Interaction of Daily Living: The Root of Development.* Berlin: Springer-Verlag Co; 1987.

32. Craine J. The retraining of frontal lobe dysfunction. In: Trexler LE, ed. *Cognitive Rehabilitation: Conceptualization and Intervention.* New York, NY: Plenum Press; 1982.

33. Driver J, Baylis GC, Rafal RD. Preserved figure-ground segregation and symmetry perception in visual neglect. *Nature.* 1992;360:73-75.

34. Fahle M. Figure-ground discrimination from temporal information. *Proc R Soc Lond B Biol Sci.* 1993;254(1341):199-302.

35. Capitani E, Della S, Lecchelli F, Soave P, Spinnler H. Perceptual attention in aging and dementia measured by Gottschaldt's hidden figure test. *J Gerontol Psychol Sci.* 1988;43(6):157-163.

36. Bernspang B, Asplung K, Eriksson S, Fugl-Meyer AR. Motor and perceptual impairments in acute stroke patients: effects on self-care ability. *Stroke.* 1987;18(6):1081-1086.

37. Peterson MA, Gibson BS. Object recognition contributions to figure-ground organization: operations on outlines and subjective contours. *Perc Psych.* 1994;56(5):551-564.

38. Petersen P, Wikoff RL. The performance of adult males on the Southern California figure-ground visual perception test. *Am J Occup Ther.* 1983;37(8):554-560.

39. Lagreze WD, Meigen T, Bach M. Asymmetries in texture perception. *Ger J Ophthalmol.* 1994;3(4-5):220-223.

40. Ayres AJ. *Southern California Sensory Integration Tests.* Los Angeles, Calif: Western Psychological Services; 1972.

41. Petersen P, Goar D, van Deusen J. Performance of female adults on the Southern California visual figure-ground perception test. *Am J Occup Ther.* 1985;39(8):525-530.

42. Itzkovich M, Arerback S, *Belazar. Lowenstein Occupational Therapy Cognitive Assessment.* Pequanock, NJ: Maddack Inc; 1990

43. Wilson BA. Compensating for cognitive deficits following brain injury. *Neuropsychol Rev.* 2000;10(4):233-243.

44. Sergent J. Judgements of relative position and distance on representations of spatial relations. *J Exp Psych Hum Percept Perform.* 1991;91(3):762-780.

45. Logan GD. Spatial attention and the apprehension of spatial relations. *J Exp Psych Hum Percept Perform.* 1994;20(5):1015-1036.

46. Aguirre GK, Zarahn E, D'Esposito M. Neural components of topographical representation. *Proc Natl Acad Sci U S A.* 1998;95(3):839-846.

47. Mountcastle V. The parietal system and some higher brain functions. In: Gazzaniga M, ed. *Cognitive Neuroscience: A Reader.* Oxford: Blackwell Publishers; 2000.

48. Petit L, et al. Superior parietal lobule involvement in the representation of visual space: a PET review. In: Tier P, Karnath HO, eds. *Parietal Lobe Contributions to Orientation in 3D Space.* New York, NY: Springer Verlag; 1997.

49. Taube JS, Goodridge JP, Golob EJ, et al. Processing the head direction cell signal: a review and commentary. *Brain Research Bulletin.* 1996;40(5/6):477-486.

50. Arnadottir G. Evaluation and intervention with complex perceptual impairment. In: Unsworth C, ed. *Cognitive and Perceptual Dysfunction: A Clinical Reasoning Approach to Evaluation and Treatment.* Philadelphia, Pa: FA Davis; 1999.

51. Manning L. Assessment and treatment of disorders of visuospatial, imaginal, and constructional processes. In: Halligan P, Kischka U, Marshall JC, eds. *Handbook of Clinical Neuropsychology*. New York, NY: Oxford University Press; 2003.
52. Hoyer WJ, Rybash JM. Age and visual field differences in computing visual-spatial relations. *Psych Aging*. 1992;7(3):339-342.
53. Kosslyn SM, Chabris CF, Jacobs RA, Marsoleck CJ, Koenig O. On computational evidence for different types of spatial relations encoding: reply to Cook et al (1995). *J Exp Psychol Hum Percept Perform*. 1995;21(2):423-431.
54. Kosslyn SM, Koenig O, Barrett A, Backer-Cave C, Tang J, Gabrieli JDE. Evidence for two types of spatial representations: hemispheric specialization for categorical and coordinate relations. *J Exp Psych Hum Percept Perform*. 1989;15(4):723-735.
55. Shiffman LM. Cerebovascular accident. In: Early MB, ed. *Physical Dysfunction: Practice Skills for the Occupational Therapy Assistant*. St. Louis, Mo: Mosby Year-Book; 1998.
56. Pehoski C. Analysis of perceptual dysfunction and dressing in adult hemiplegics. Thesis. Boston, Mass: Sargent College, Boston University; 1970.
57. Taylor MM. Analysis of dysfunction in the left hemiplegia following stroke. *Am J Occup Ther*. 1968;22:512-520.
58. Bouska MJ, Kauffman NA, Marcus SE. Disorders of the visual perceptual system. In: Umphred DA, ed. *Neurological Rehabilitation*. 2nd ed. St. Louis, Mo: CV Mosby; 1990.
59. Kerkhoff G. Neurovisual rehabilitation: recent developments and future directions. *J Neurol Neurosurg Psychiatry*. 2005;68:691-706.
60. Scheiman M. *Understanding and Managing Vision Deficits: A Guide for Occupational Therapists*. 2nd ed. Thorofare, NJ: SLACK Incorporated; 2002.
61. Alsaadi T, Binder JR, Lazar RM, et al. Pure topographic disorientation: a distinctive Syndrome with varied localization. *Neurology*. 2000;54(9):1864-1866.
62. Golisz K, Toglia J. Perception and cognition. In: Crepeau EB, Cohn ES, Boyt Schell BA, eds. *Willard and Spackman's Occupational Therapy*. Philadelphia, Pa: Lippincott, Williams and Wilkens; 2003.
63. Damasio AR. Disorders of complex visual processing. In: Mesulam MM, ed. *Principles of Behavioral and Cognitive Neurology*. New York, NY: Oxford University Press; 2000.
64. Wickens C. Frames of references for navigation. In: Gopher D, Koriat A, eds. *Attention and Performance XVII*. Cambridge, Mass: MIT Press; 1998.
65. Aguirre GK, D'Esposito M. Topographical disorientation: a synthesis and taxonomy. *Brain*. 1999;122(9):1613-1628.
66. Boyd T, Sautter S. Route finding: a measure of everyday executive functioning in the head injured adult. *Appl Cogn Psychol*. 1993;7:171-181.
67. Farah MJ. Disorders of visual-spatial perception and cognition. In: Heilman KM, Valenstein E, eds. *Clinical Neuropsychology*. 4th ed. New York, NY: Oxford University Press; 2003.
68. Riddoch MJ, Humphreys GW. Finding the way around topographical impairments. In: Brown W, ed. *Neuropsychology of Visual Impairments*. Mahwah, NJ: Lawrence Erlbaum Assoc; 1989.
69. Christenson MA, Raschko B. Environmental cognition and age-related sensory change. *Occup Ther Pract*. 1989;1(1):28-35.
70. Reynolds CR, Pearson N, Voress J. Developmental Test of Visual Perception-Adolescent and Adult (DTVP-A). Pro Ed. 8700 Shoal Creek Blvd. Austin, Texas 78757-6897.
71. Colarusso RP, Hammill DD. *Motor-Free Visual Perception Test*. 3rd ed. Novato, CA: Academic Therapy Publications; 2003.

Resources

Arnadottir G. *The Brain and Behavior: Assessing Cortical Dysfunction Through Activities of Daily Living*. St. Louis, Mo: CV Mosby; 1990.

Benton AL, Sivan AB, Hamsher KD, et al. *Contributions to Neuropsychological Assessment: A Clinical Manual*. 2nd ed. New York, NY: Oxford University Press; 1994.

Cohen M, GrossWasser Z, Banchadske R, Appel A. Convergence insufficiency in brain-injured patients. *Brain Inj*. 1989;3(2):187-191.

Corballis PM, Funnell MG, Gazzaniga MS. Hemispheric asymmetries for simple visual judgments in the split brain. *Neuropsychologia*. 2002;42:401-410.

Driver J, Baylis GC. Attention and visual object segmentation. In: Parasuraman R, ed. *The Attentive Brain*. Cambridge, Mass: MIT Press; 1998.

Hellerstein L, Fishman B. Visual rehabilitation for patients with brain injury. In: Scheiman M, ed. *Understanding and Managing Vision Deficits: A Guide for Occupational Therapists.* 2nd ed. Thorofare, NJ: SLACK Incorporated; 2002.

Jacobs RA, Kisslyn SM. Encoding shape and spatial relations: the role of receptive field size in coordinating complementary representations. *Cogn Science.* 1994;18:361-386.

von Noordon GK. Binocular Vision and Ocular Motility 3d edition. St. Louis, Mo: CV Mosby; 1985.

Warren M. Evaluation and treatment of visual deficits. In: Pedretti L, ed. Occupational Therapy: Practice Skills for Physical Dysfunction. St. Louis, Mo: Mosby Year-Book; 1996.

Wright P, Rogers N, Hall C, et al. Comparison of pocket-computer memory aids for people with brain injury. Brain Inj. 2001;15(9):787-800.

CHAPTER 7

AGNOSIA

Agnosia, the area of deficits that deals with the client's lack of recognition of familiar objects perceived by the senses, occurs frequently in clients who have sustained an acquired brain injury (ABI). Agnosias are "...disorders of recognition specific to one sensory channel that affect either the perceptual analysis of the stimulus or the recognition of its meaning."[1] The concept of recognition includes behaviors such as attention, pattern and form perception, temporal resolution, and memory.[2] Successful object recognition is accomplished because an individual is able to distinguish depth, volume, and structure from relatively scarce two-dimensional stimuli such as photographs and line drawings.[2] As a result, "...from perceptual analysis we can derive an enormous amount of structural and semantic information about the world around us."[2]

Research has shown that the visual scene "... is parsed preattentively into candidate objects and that attention then operates on those objects to afford awareness and recognition of them and to guide subsequent action."[3] Both cerebral hemispheres work together to establish pattern recognition.[4] Warren describes the specific hemispheric function in the recognition process as follows[4]:

> The two hemispheres function together to provide efficient pattern recognition. The right hemisphere completes the initial visual processing, alerts the CNS to the presence of an object in the field, and focuses the object on the foveae of the eyes. The left hemisphere then uses the high-quality visual information received through the foveae to extract minute details regarding the critical features of the object. The advantages of both hemispheres are needed to ensure accurate identification of the object.

Devinsky and D'Esposito support this bottom-up process of object recognition utilizing visual input. They describe three stages of object recognition: visual processing, which is nonlateralized; perceptual processing, which is right hemisphere dominant; and semantic processing, which is left hemisphere dominant.[5]

Visual objects can be described through the surface features of color, motion, orientation, texture, disparity, and location.[6,7] Subsequent to this feature analysis, they are encoded into object-centered neural representations.[6] Before recognition can occur, the individual must be able to

1) construct a three-dimensional model from the two-dimensional image on the retina, 2) access the memory of previous models, and 3) associate previous models with new ones.[4]

Although vision is inarguably crucial to successful object recognition, it is by no means the only sense an individual uses. Kinesthetic and tactile input, for example, are sometimes necessary to recognize a shape or texture.[8] There are many times in life when the visual sense is not available to us for object recognition. For example, while watching a computer screen, you reach for a coffee mug, or when you reach for keys in a purse. When we are driving our car, we reach for the knob to turn on the radio without taking our eyes off the road.

Klatsky and Lederman describe the "haptic system" as the nonvisual means one can utilize to recognize an object and perform such tasks.[9-11] This system consists of two categories of receptors—cutaneous and kinesthetic—and come into play as follows[11]:

> *Objects small enough to be within a fingertip aperture can be apprehended cutaneously, whereas objects that extend beyond it require integration over multiple fingers, over time, or both, bringing in a greater contribution of kinesthesis.*

There is a two-stage model of tactile exploration that leads to object identification: 1) grasp and lift, which provides feedback on an object's features at a course level, and 2) exploratory procedures (EPs), which are guided by expectations about the objects diagnostic properties.[9] The initial grasp and lift stage generates a hypothesis about the object, and the EPs chosen confirm it.[10] Research on normal subjects has also indicated that EPs are stereotypical depending on which object properties are extracted.[9,10,12] When an appropriate EP is used, then the associated property can be used for identification.

Agnosia as the result of ABI may involve a disturbance in any one of the following sensory modes—visual, tactile, proprioceptive, and auditory—or may involve additional problems in body scheme, such as somatagnosia or anosognosia. In a category specific agnosia, ABI can cause identification deficits for some categories of objects but not for others.[13]

Visual Agnosia

Visual agnosia, or what some have described as perception without meaning, is the inability to recognize visual stimuli despite adequate primary visual function such as acuity, oculomotor function, and visual fields.[2,5,14,15] It may be restricted to a specific category, as for example, objects, faces, and colors can be disrupted separately.[1,15] For some clients, common objects such as a fork or pen may be more easily recognized than uncommon objects such as a stethoscope or city skyline.[5] Similarly, recognition may range from being able to recognize real (actual) objects but not photographs or line drawings of the object.[5] Visual object agnosia involves not only a defect in recognizing a specific object but also of the general semantic class to which it belongs.[2] Some clients with visual object agnosia may have a category specific deficit. They may have trouble with objects within a specific category (eg, manipulability tools) but otherwise can name most objects.[16] The client with visual agnosia will be able to name an object, for example, if another sensory modality such as touch is used for identification.[17]

Current theoretical information related to visual agnosia includes descriptions of two levels of deficits: apperceptive and associative agnosia.[1,2,5,15,18-21] For clients who exhibit apperceptive agnosia, the brain damage is usually diffuse and posterior.[5] These clients are unable to recognize, copy, match, or discriminate simple visual stimuli and cannot even recognize simple shapes such as a circle or square.[5] There is a failure to generate a structured description of the shape of an object.[1]

Some believe apperceptive agnosia to be the result of a disordered perception even though primary visual functions are present.[21] There is a distortion of the stimulus at the sensory-perceptual levels, which causes a failure to recognize visually presented objects.

Bauer and Demery support this concept of a defect in perceptual processing when they describe the following[2]:

> *Apperceptive agnosics fail recognition tasks because of defects in perceptual processing. They cannot draw misidentified items or match them to sample. They are generally unable to point to objects named by the examiner. The impairment most often involves elements of the visual environment that require shape and pattern perception (face, objects, letters).*

Grossman et al expand on the theoretical basis of apperceptive visual agnosia. Not only do they hypothesize that it results from the impaired appreciation of the visual perceptual features that constitute objects, as just described, but they also believe it results from "...a limitation in the cognitive resources that are available for processing demanding material within the visual modality."[20]

The second type of visual agnosia described is associative visual agnosia and is believed to be the result of disordered association. Some even view it as disorder in the highest levels of visual representations.[22] Clients with associative visual agnosia are able to describe the features and shape of an object but are unable to recognize it. When shown a picture of a car, for example, these clients are unable to state what it is, what one does with it, or what one puts in it to make it go.[5] This is different from the client with anomia who is unable to name a picture as a car but who would respond with, " It's the thing you get into and drive."[23] Unlike apperceptive visual agnosia, these clients have preserved or near preserved visual perception.[2,5,21,22] As De Renzi states, it is "...an inability to attribute meaning to a correctly perceived stimulus."[1]

The client with associative visual agnosia can copy figures or written material, match stimuli, and name objects from verbal definitions.[2,18,22,24] Many clients with visual associative agnosia do well on the majority of visual tests, such as block designs or embedded pictures. These remaining skills suggest that they have "retained the conceptual and linguistic abilities needed to demonstrate recognition."[15,24]

Associative visual agnosia does not always appear to disturb recognition of all types of stimuli equally.[19] In addition, impairment of recognition of faces (prosopagnosia), color agnosia and written material (alexia) are frequently but not always found with associative object agnosia.[2]

It is believed that the ventral or occipito–temporal pathway is important for visual object recognition.[25] A recent positron emission tomography (PET) study of normal adult males has demonstrated that the discrimination of spatial attributes of objects requires the activation of both the parietal and the temporal cortices of the right hemisphere and the right intraparietal sulcus (IPS).[26] In addition, the right occipitotemporal junction played a critical role in visuospatial recognition of objects.[26]

Functional impairments that can occur as the result of visual agnosia are diverse and potentially devastating to the client. The client can fail to recognize close relatives or precious possessions. When confronted with these deficits, clients may say they need new glasses or complain the lighting in the room is not good.[2] The following sections outline the evaluation and treatment of major types of visual agnosia that the client may exhibit.

GENERAL GUIDELINES FOR EVALUATION

1. Rule out language deficits such as anomia and primary sensory deficits as causes of poor performance.

2. Observe whether the client can describe the critical features for identification of the object.

3. Does the client know to what category of object it belongs?

4. Does the client fixate only on one feature and, as a result, miss the more important clues to identifying the object?

5. Can the client describe the functional use of the object?

6. Does placing the object in its normal context assist in object identification?

7. Does rotating the presentation of the object assist in object identification?

8. If the client is unable to identify the object from photographs or drawings, does presenting the actual object assist in identification?

Visual Object Agnosia

As previously described, visual object agnosia is the inability to recognize objects presented visually, although the primary visual skills such as acuity are intact.

EVALUATION OF VISUAL OBJECT AGNOSIA

Test 1 – Object Recognition[27]

Description

Several common objects such as a key, comb, toothbrush, or coins are placed in front of the client. Ask the client to pick up the object that is named, or demonstrate or describe its functional use.

Scoring

The examiner may assume the object is recognized if any of the following occurs:

• The client names, describes, or demonstrates the use of an object.

• The client selects the object from among a group of objects as it is named by the examiner.

Validity

To improve validity, rule out primary visual and language deficits as cause of poor performance.

Test 2 – LOTCA—Visual Identification of Objects[28]

Description

The visual identification of objects subtest (VO) is one of several subtests of the Lowenstein Occupational Therapy Cognitive Assessment (LOTCA). The remaining subtests are described in the section on orientation in Chapter 8.

Procedure

The client is shown eight cards of illustrated everyday objects—for example, chair, teapot, watch, key, shoe, bicycle, scissors, and glasses. The client is asked to name each object.

If the client is not able to name the objects because of expressive problems (eg, expressive or amnestic aphasia or severe dysarthria), he or she is shown two boards with four objects presented on each. The examiner asks the client, "Where is a chair?," "Where is a watch?," etc. This procedure is used for each of the eight objects.

If the client has receptive/expressive problems (eg, global or receptive/expressive aphasia), the examiner should show him two boards with four similar objects presented on each. The client has to match the target objects with the similar one on the boards. If the client is unable to identify similar objects, the examiner presents to him the two boards with the identical objects. The client has to do an exact matching.

Scoring

1 point—The client identifies less than four by exact matching.

2 points—The client identifies five to eight objects by exact matching.

3 points—The client identifies at least four objects by naming, understanding, or similar matching (4-7).

4 points—The client identifies all the objects by naming, understanding, or similar matching.

Validity

The authors state the Wilcoxin two-sample test was used to compare the control and client group. Results state the subtests, except the object identification subtest, differentiated the groups at the 0.0001 level of significance. This author was unable to find the measure for the object identification subtest.

Reliability

Inter-rater reliability with Spearman's rank correlation coefficient for subtest ranges from 0.82 to 0.97. Internal consistency reliability through Cronbach's alpha coefficient was calculated at 0.87 for the five subtests of perception, which includes object identification. The authors caution, however, that all parts of the battery should be given due to correlation coefficients ranging from 0.40 to 0.80 among the subtests.

TREATMENT OF VISUAL OBJECT AGNOSIA

Utilizing a Restorative Approach

1. Treatment should progress to parallel the abilities that return as the result of natural recovery from agnosia.[27] Bouska et al provide the following guidelines[27]:

   a) Common real objects should be used before line drawings.

   b) Presentation should be given in a straight on rather than at an angle or rotated.

   c) Manipulation of the object with simultaneous visual input should be attempted.

2. Averbach and Katz advocate and provide the following hierarchal order of treatment[2]:

   a) Move from simple to complex.

   b) Demonstrate for the client how to search for information. Touch and sound are used in addition to visual search.

   c) First, work with actual concrete objects. Second, with pictorial and schematic presentations (using pictures reinforces and broadens the information gathering strategy). Third, use pictures with varying degrees of ambiguity (helps the client identify objects in the presence of incomplete information). Fourth, have the client discriminate subtle differences between objects.

    d) At each stage, the client is trained to use the strategies learned in daily life—for example, identifying items according to a list in the grocery store.

3. Provide nonverbal, tactile-kinesthetic guiding through an activity. After the activity, take some of the tools used in the task and follow up the guided activity with naming the items that were used. Ask the client to recreate the steps in the task, either with words or with picture identification, sequencing cards, etc (Karen Bonfils, personal communication).

Utilizing an Adaptive Approach

1. Teach the client to consider and think critically about the verbal response before answering.[29]

2. Utilize a verbal strategy based on the description of the perceptual or functional characteristics of the object to help retrieval of the correct verbal name, and teach the client to silently verbalize these characteristics.[29]

3. Utilize intact sensory modalities other than vision for object identification.[5,30]

4. Recognition may improve when visual stimuli are moved. In the case of reading, tracing letters may help.[2]

5. Research has shown background or context may affect object recognition ability; therefore, show the object in its natural context whenever possible.[31,32]

6. Adding texture or edge orientation cues can assist in identification[9]—for example, on a car radio dial or key ring. Use this technique especially with items where safety is an issue (ie, iron or cooktop controls).

7. Organize objects in the orientation used premorbidly. For example, were shirts hanging in the closet or folded in a drawer before the ABI? Were pants folded and hung or hung on clip hangers?

8. If the client has the ability to categorize ask him or her, "What category would this object belong in?"

9. If the client does not use tactile cues, correctly guide him. Stereotypical EPs, depending on what critical features would help the most in object identification, can be facilitated.[12]

10. Encourage the client to manipulate the object with simultaneous visual and verbal input.[28]

11. Provide labels for objects as necessary to maximize independence in occupational performance. This is especially important when safety is an issue (ie, cooktop controls, gas cut off).

Prosopagnosia

Facial recognition is more orientation sensitive than the recognition of other types of objects.[22] Infants, in fact, are born with a preference to gaze at faces rather than at other objects.[22] The human face and our ability to read facial expressions are important to many of our social interactions and communication. Faces are the main key we use in everyday life to identify people we are familiar with either personally or through the media.[1] Each of us probably has around 1000 stored representations.[1]

An individual's face tells us about areas such as gender, age, race, and emotion. It also conveys information about the individual's physical uniqueness by the particular arrangement of specific features. These features provide clues to the person's identity.[33]

Prosopagnosia is a neurologically based deficit characterized by the inability to identify a known individual by his or her face. This inability is seen in the absence of severe sensory, intellectual, and visual impairments.[16,18,31,33-35] The client knows he or she is looking at a face but cannot say to whom the face belongs. The client cannot match the whole image with stored memories.[5] Clients can usually point to or name, with no difficulty, the eyes, ears, nose, or mouth either on themselves or others.[5,16] They are able to discriminate faces according to sex or race or read their emotional expression.[1,16] Semantic knowledge is intact in the prosopagnostic client, as demonstrated by the accurate retrieval of the biographical information about the individual he or she is trying to identify.[1] The severity of prosopagnosia can range from the client who cannot even identify him- or herself in a mirror, to only failing to identify a person whom he or she has known only since the onset of the ABI.[1,5] Often, staff or family members will mistakenly assume that the client has a severe memory deficit.[2] Prosopagnosia is, however, often seen with deficits in areas such as object agnosia, spatial disorientation, loss of topographical memory, constructional apraxia, and a left upper quadrant field loss.[8,33] As Bouska et al observe, "...these deficits don't cause the prosopagnosia, but rather, these functions are likely subserved by the same neurological system."[27]

Prosopagnosia is a dramatic and recognizable deficit that becomes apparent to the clinician personally or through communication with a distressed family member.[2] Clients themselves will also recognize that they have a problem and are often upset by it. Many clients train themselves to use cues other than visual to assist in recognition. For example, a spouse may be identified by his or her voice, perfume, clothes, gait, height, or body shape.[2,5,16,36]

Some theorize there are two stages of facial recognition beyond basic perception.[1] The first stage involves recognition units that store abstract representation of familiar faces from past experience with them. This stage creates a sense of familiarity, but the individual cannot identify someone at this level. The second stage involves "identity nodes," which provide information related to the individual's biography and the relationship between the familiar person and the observer. It is at this stage that identification is possible.

Two distinct categories of clients have been described: 1) clients who cannot perceive faces, which is related to a problem with structural encoding, and 2) clients who appear to have relatively intact perceptual abilities but cannot recognize or in some way process the faces they seem to perceive.[33,35] De Renzi defines two categories of prosopagnosia as follows[1]:

- *Apperceptive prosopagnosia*—Results from the disruption of the perceptual process underlying the discrimination of the external and internal face configuration.

- *Associative prosopagnosia*—The inability to identify familiar persons, which cannot be attributed to the disruption of perceptual processing or loss of semantic knowledge.

Farah conceptualizes face recognition relative to levels of visual representation. She hypothesizes that the highest levels of visual representation are subdivided into specialized systems, and prosopagnostics have lost the system that is necessary for recognizing faces and not as necessary for recognizing objects.[22] It also may be possible that faces and objects are recognized using a single recognition system and that faces are just more difficult to recognize.[22,37]

Prosopagnosia has been associated with cerebral vascular accidents (CVAs) involving the posterior cerebral arteries, posterior left hemisphere lesions, right hemisphere damage and bilateral involvement.[2,16,34,35,38] Recent functional magnetic resonance imaging (fMRI) and PET studies have linked the temporal cortex, temporofrontal cortex, and the right prefrontal cortex to prosopagnosia.[2,38-40]

To summarize, some clinicians believe the problem is perceptual in nature, while others believe it is primarily due to decreased memory.[33,34] Still others believe it is not due to perceptual or memory loss but to an impairment of the activation step of records pertinent to the face, which does not take place or takes place inefficiently.[16,41]

No matter what the hypothesized cause or associated brain activation, prosopagnosia is a common deficit particularly distressing for the client and his or her family. It can dramatically affect the client's ability to interact socially with others, therefore affecting his or her occupational roles and performance.

EVALUATION OF PROSOPAGNOSIA

Test 1 – Functional Evaluation

Although there are many tests of facial matching and identification, a functional evaluation is recommended.

Procedure

The therapist has the client identify key members of the family, friends, and coworkers. Identification is made through photographs and, whenever possible, the actual person.

Scoring

Individuals who could not be identified through facial recognition are identified.

TREATMENT OF PROSOPAGNOSIA

Utilizing an Adaptive Approach

1. Provide pictures with names; pictures of the unrecognized individual(s) in different settings, at different angles, and with other people the client is able to recognize.

2. Help the client associate the individual's face with other features and characteristics such as voice, haircut, manner of walk, height, and clothes.

3. Teach the client to make a mental list of the physical features of a person when he or she is introduced.[42] This should make the person more memorable. This technique can also be utilized with important family members or friends.[17]

4. Have the client utilize a personal data assistant (PDA) to assist in identification. An individual's picture (or pictures) can be stored with relevant personal information that will assist in identification. The client can input his or her perceptions of the individual's physical features for improved recognition.

Simultagnosia

Simultagnosia is the inability to recognize a compound visual array.[33] Clients with simultagnosia are unable to perceive more than one thing at a time, and the amount of time necessary to distinguish between two perceptual acts is excessively long. They are unable to recognize the abstract meaning of a whole stimulus array even though the details are correctly perceived. They are able to describe specific elements of a complex stimulus but cannot integrate these elements to achieve recognition of the picture.

Some clinicians believe simultagnosia is partly caused by defective short-term visual memory loss.[34] Others have observed that although these clients have normal visual field on parametric testing, they will shrink to narrow vision when concentrating on the visual environment.

In summary, simultagnosia is a disorder which involves impairment in interpreting a visual stimulus as a whole. It seems to result from an extreme reduction in visual span of apprehension.[43] Given a whole picture, the client absorbs only one aspect or part at a time. For instance, a client could point out individual letters or features but cannot give an accurate account of the whole word.[43]

Color Agnosia

ABI can result in a wide variety of problems pertaining to color, depending on whether the damage has affected discrimination, categorization, visuoverbal matching, or the imagery of color.[1] After an individual discriminates a particular color, he or she must then be able to categorize it as pertaining to a given range of hue such as red or blue. De Renzi describes as follows[1]:

Color categorization is a crucial step for any color operation carried out beyond the level of mere perceptual discrimination, such as attaching verbal labels, coloring drawings, or sorting chips according to color.

The client with color agnosia will have the inability to recognize colors such that he or she cannot pick out a color or name a color on command.[44] This client should be able to say whether two colors are the same or different if visual sensation is still intact. Color agnosia appears to occur more commonly after left hemisphere lesions; however, ventromedial occipital brain damage can result in the complete loss of color vision.[45]

Metamorphopsia

Metamorphopsia is a visual distortion of objects although the object may be recognized accurately. For instance, a chair may appear larger or smaller than it actually is.

Visual-Spatial Agnosia

Visual-spatial agnosia is a deficit in perceiving spatial relationships between objects or between objects and self, independently of visual object agnosia. Visual-spatial agnosia can include the following difficulties:

1. Difficulty with spatial relations.
2. Difficulty in judging distances such that the client may go to sit in a chair and misjudge so that he or she misses the chair.
3. Difficulty in depth perception such that the client may continue pouring water into a glass after it is filled.

Topographagnosia

Topographagnosia is an impairment in the interpretation of maps, house plans, etc.[18] The client can perform normally in real situations but cannot place himself on a map.[18] These clients are unable to draw a plan of their house or identify rooms on a plan that is drawn for them.

Environmental Agnosia

Clients with environmental agnosia will get lost in familiar places. These clients can read maps and house plans well but cannot find their way even in familiar places.[18]

Tactile Agnosia

Tactile agnosia, as compared to visual agnosia, is less understood despite the fact that it is likely as common as visual or auditory agnosia.[2] As Bohlalter et al state, "...the organization of the normal perceptual processing subserving tactile object recognition is poorly understood."[46] Tactile agnosia has traditionally been defined as a modality specific disorder evidenced by an inability to recognize objects tactually though tactile, thermal, and proprioceptive functions are still intact.[2,47-50] The client cannot associate the retrieved tactile image with other sensory images. He or she cannot recognize the object although able to recognize the tactile qualities.

Tactile agnosia, often called astereognosis, is believed by some to be a high level perceptual disorder that can occur from a failure to "integrate accurately acquired somesthetic features into a haptic mental image which can then be manipulated."[49] In a study of CVA clients, Reed and Caselli found that tactile agnosia can occur with high level faulty perceptual processes but that the ability to associate tactually defined objects and object parts can be preserved.[49] A case study described by Reed and Caselli demonstrated that tactile shape perception can be impaired independent of general spatial ability, manual shape exploration, or even precise perception of length in the tactile modality.[49]

Nakamura et al hypothesize that object recognition is accomplished when object information is processed by each sensory association cortex and is then compared with information retrieved from semantic memory.[51] Klatsky and Lederman believe structural (versus material or non-edge-based information such as color) is required for tactile object recognition.[9] Saetti et al postulate that "...the ability to assess line orientation may make a crucial contribution to the reconstruction of shapes in the tactile modality and that its impairment results in tactile morphagnosia."[50]

A case study utilizing fMRI conducted by Saetti et al indicated that once basic sensory information has been acquired, the continued processing of this information can be disrupted at different levels.[50] Their research indicated sensory outflow undergoes two independent analyses and they describe these two analyses as follows[50]:

> *One concerns the appreciation of the intermediate tactile qualities of the stimulus (its texture, weight, size, and length) by the postcentral gyrus of the hemisphere contralateral to the palpating hand. The other analysis concerns processing the orientation in space of various elements of the stimulus surface. This task is mainly accomplished by the right parieto-occipital cortex independently of the side of space where stimuli are presented. Its damage results in bilateral tactile morphagnosia.*

Stereognosis requires the integration of information related to the temperature, texture, weight, and contour of an object and involves both the cutaneous and proprioceptive (muscle and joint receptors) sensory systems.[52] The identification of objects through touch and somesthetic sensations is accomplished by the following:

1. Primary identification through recognition of texture, form, etc.
2. Secondary recognition of the significance of the object.[47]

There are four types of information processing in the tactile recognition system[47]:

1. *Ahylognosia*—Disturbance in the ability to discriminate materials
2. *Amorphagnosia*—Disturbance in the ability to discriminate forms
3. *Tactile agnosia*—Inability to recognize familiar objects
4. *Tactile aphasia*—Inability to name tactually identified objects in the absence of aphasic anomia

Tactile agnosia can occur with or without the other deficits of the tactile recognition system.

Evaluation of Tactile Agnosia

Test 1 – Stereognosis[23,53,54]

Description

Tell the client, "I'm going to put a form like one of these in your hand so that you can feel it for a little while. Then I'll show you all the forms, and you can show me the one that was in your hand." Demonstrate by putting one of the objects in the client's hand and having him or her feel it. Then put it back in the tray, and have the client show you which object he or she felt. Occlude the client's vision by having him or her close his or her eyes, shield them with a file folder, or use a box like the one described in Test 1 under Finger Agnosia. Be sure that the client does not drop objects onto the table and get auditory cues (eg, by running a finger along the teeth of a comb). Common objects often used for this test are a ball, spoon, pencil, key, penny, ring, button, block, and scissors. Test each hand alternately.

Scoring

Nonstandardized

> *Intact*—client correctly identifies all objects within a reasonable length of time. Normal subjects can name a familiar object within 5 seconds of contact.[52] The time required for recognition should be recorded as well as whether the client can identify the object.[54]

Validity

To improve validity, rule out impaired tactile sensation and paresis in the affected hand so that the client cannot feel or move the object around to feel its shape. Rule out impaired sensation in the nonaffected hand.

Test 2 – Ayres' Manual Form Perception

(Subtest of Southern California Sensory Integration Tests)[55]

Description

Procedure is the same as in Test 1. Objects used are 10 plastic geometric forms (eg, oval, triangle, circle, star, square, hexagon, octagon, diamond, cross, and trapezoid). The object is placed in the client's hand while his or her vision is occluded by a file folder shield. The client is asked to identify the object he or she is feeling from 12 geometric forms printed on a piece of cardboard placed before him or her. Hands are tested alternately. Bilateral manipulation of a form is not allowed.

Scoring

This test has been standardized for children aged 4.0 to 8.11 years. In testing reliability, Ayres reports that the test-retest correlations range from r = 0.20 to 0.64. Scoring for adults is nonstandardized.

> *Intact*—client correctly identifies all 10 forms within a reasonable length of time.

Validity

To improve validity, rule out impaired tactile sensation and paresis of the affected hand and impaired sensation of the nonaffected hand.

Test 3 – Morphognosis

Description

This is the same as the test for stereognosis except that one uses geometric shapes cut out of stiff paper only 1/32 inch thick instead of three-dimensional objects. Common shapes used are a diamond, circle, triangle, octagon, square, and egg shape.

Scoring

Nonstandardized

> *Intact*—client correctly identifies all shapes within a reasonable length of time.

Validity

To improve validity, rule out lack of tactile sensation and paresis of the affected hand and impaired sensation of the nonaffected hand.

Test 4 – Ahylognosis

Description

Same as test for stereognosis except that one uses materials of different textures. Some common materials used are rough and fine sandpaper, silk, plastic wrap, terry cloth, and corduroy.

Scoring

Nonstandardized

> *Intact*—client correctly identifies all textures within a reasonable length of time.

Validity

To improve validity, rule out impaired tactile sensation and paresis of the affected hand and impaired sensation of the nonaffected hand.

TREATMENT OF TACTILE AGNOSIA

Utilizing a Restorative Approach

1. Based on the belief that the brain has potential for recovery of sensory function through reorganization, provide sensory retraining as follows[52]:

    a) Establish some appreciation of sensory inputs from the receptors in the fingertips.

      Stage 1—A stimulus such as hooked Velcro is moved along the fingertips.

      Stage 2—When the client can appreciate the moving stimulus, then progress to the appreciation of stationary tactile inputs required for holding tasks.

Table 7-1

Exploratory Hand Movements for Object Identification

Motion	*Description*	*Use/Information Gained*
Lateral Motion	Repetitive and lateral rubbing	Texture
Pressure	Opposing forces applied normally to a surface	Hardness
Static Contact	Stationary contact on a surface without molding	Temperature
Unsupported Holding	Used to lift an object away from a supporting surface	Weight
Enclosure	Dynamic molding of the palm and/or fingers to the contours of an object	Total shape and volume
Contour Following	Hand movements following the edge	Total shape exact shape
Function Test	Hand movements in and around object	Specific function
Part Motion Test	Hand movements associated with the moving parts of an object	Function

Adapted from reference 12: Lederman SJ, Klatsky RL. Extracting object properties through haptic exploration. ACTA Psychologica. 1993;84:29-40.

Utilizing an Adaptive Approach

1. Provide the following to help the client compensate[56]:

    a) Increase the client's awareness of the problem, especially how it will affect function and personal safety (eg, kitchen).

    b) Place emphasis on sensory tasks that the client can do at the start and finish of each treatment session.

    c) Choose sensory tasks that will interest the client and which will lead to sufficient successes and failures to promote learning.

    d) Utilize other senses such as vision and use the good hand to teach tactics of perception. Utilize stereotypical exploratory procedures as appropriate (Table 7-1).[12]

    e) Train the client to focus on the specific properties of the object (ie, contour, texture, or temperature).[52]

2. Utilizing the concept that object recognition is accomplished through the interaction of top-down and bottom-up processing, facilitate object recognition through access of associated sorted personal memories.[49] In other words, provide objects for which the client can draw on experience with the object and its features.

3. Present the object within its normal context.

Auditory Agnosia

Auditory agnosia is the inability to recognize differences in sounds, including both word and nonword sounds. For example, a client may not be able to differentiate between the sound of a car engine running and the sound of a vacuum cleaner.

Evaluation and Treatment of Auditory Agnosia

Evaluation and treatment for auditory agnosia is usually done by a speech pathologist.

Apractognosia

Apractognosia consists of several different apraxic and agnostic syndromes, all centering mainly around a lack of perspective.[44] Resulting from a lesion in the nondominant hemisphere, apractognosia may include one or all of the following:

1. *Body-scheme problems*
    a) Denial of left hemiplegia
    b) Lack of awareness of left half of body or space
    c) Feelings of strangeness
    d) Right-left disorientation for both personal and extrapersonal space
2. *Apraxia for dressing*
    a) Faulty application of clothes to the body because the client cannot understand the relationship of the clothes to the body
    b) Faulty right-left manipulations used in tying a tie or a shoe
3. *Constructional apraxia due to lack of perspective*
4. *Unilateral spatial agnosia*
    a) Loss of conception of topographical relationships such that the client can no longer conceive that the bathroom is down the hall to the left of his or her room
    b) Disturbances of orientation such that the client does not know where he or she is
    c) Loss of topographical memory such that the client has forgotten his or her familiar routes from one place to another
    d) Visual coordinate problems such that the client has difficulty perceiving the vertical and horizontal correctly

Evaluation and Treatment for Apractognosia

Evaluation and treatment for the apractognosia syndrome may be found under the corresponding apraxic and agnostic deficits on the following pages:

Agnosias Related to Body-Scheme Disorders

1. *Autotopagnosia*—See this description under Body-Scheme Disorders, page 134

2. *Anosognosia*—See this description under Body-Scheme Disorders, page 142

3. *Finger Agnosia*—See this description under Body-Scheme Disorders, page 145

References

1. De Renzi E. Disorders of visual recognition. *Seminar in Neurology.* 2000;20(35): 479-485.
2. Bauer RM, Demery JA. Agnosia. In: Heilman KM, Valenstein E, eds. *Clinical Neuropsychology.* 4th ed. New York, NY: Oxford University Press; 2003.
3. Rafal R. Neglect. In: Parasuraman R, ed. *The Attentive Brain.* Cambridge, Mass: MIT Press; 1998.
4. Warren M. Providing low vision rehabilitation services with occupational therapy and ophthalmology: a program description. *Am J Occup Ther.* 1995;49(1):877-883.
5. Devinsky O, D'Esposito M. Perception and perceptual disorders. In: *Neurology of Cognitive and Behavioral Disorders.* New York, NY: Oxford University Press; 2004.
6. Corbetta M. Functional anatomy of visual attention in the human brain: studies with positron emission tomography. In: Parasuraman R, ed. *The Attentive Brain.* Cambridge, Mass: MIT Press; 1998.
7. Nakayama K, Joseph JS. Attention, pattern recognition and pop out in visual search. In: Parasuraman R, ed. *The Attentive Brain.* Cambridge, Mass: MIT Press; 1998.
8. Booth BA, Freeman RPJ. Discriminative feature integration by individuals. *ACTA Psychologica.* 1993;84:1-16.
9. Klatsky RL, Lederman SJ. Identifying objects from a haptic glance. *Percept Psychophys.* 1995;57(8):1111-1123.
10. Klatsky RL, Lederman SJ. Stages of manual exploration in haptic object identification. *Percept Psychophys.* 1992;52(6):661-670.
11. Klatsky RL, Lederman SJ. The haptic glance. In: Gopher D, Koriat A, eds. *Attention and Performance XVII.* Cambridge, Mass: MIT Press; 1998.
12. Lederman SJ, Klatsky RL. Extracting object properties through haptic exploration. *ACTA Psychologica.* 1993;84:29-40.
13. Dixon MJ. A new paradigm for investigating category-specific agnosia in the new millennium. *Brain Cogn.* 2000;42:142-145.
14. Bouska MJ, Kauffman NA, Marcus SE. Disorders of the visual perceptual system. In: Umphred DA, ed. *Neurological Rehabilitation.* St. Louis, Mo: CV Mosby; 1985.
15. Shelton PA, Bowers D, Duara R, Heilman KM. Apperceptive visual agnosia: a case study. *Brain Cogn.* 1994;25(1):1-23.
16. Damasio AR. Disorders of complex visual processing. In: Mesulam MM, ed. *Principles of Behavioral and Cognitive Neurology.* New York, NY: Oxford University Press; 2000.
17. Aloisio L. Visual dysfunction. In: Gillen G, Burkhardt A, eds. *Stroke Rehabilitation: A Function Based Approach.* St. Louis, Mo: Mosby Inc; 2004.
18. Benson DF. Disorders of visual agnosis. In: Brown JW, ed. *Neuropsychology of Visual Perception.* Mahwah, NJ: Lawrence Erlbaum Assoc; 1989.
19. Farah MJ, Feinberg TE. Consciousness of perception after brain damage. *Seminars in Neurology.* 1997;17(2):145-152.
20. Grossman M, Galetta S, D'Esposito M. Object recognition difficulty in visual apperceptive agnosia. *Brain Cogn.* 1997;33(3):306-342.
21. Schnider A, Benson F, Scharre W. Visual agnosia and optic aphasia: are they anatomically distinct? *Cortex.* 1994;30:440-457.
22. Farah MJ. Is face recognition 'special'? Evidence from neuropsychology. *Behavioral Brain Research.* 1996;76:181-189.
23. Deitz JC, Tovar VS, Thorn DW, Beeman C. The test of orientation for rehabilitation patients: inter-rater reliability. *Am J Occup Ther.* 1990;44(9):784-790.
24. Feinberg TE, Schindler RL, Ochoa E, Kwan P, Farah MP. Associative visual agnosia and alexia without prosopagnosia. *Cortex.* 1994;30(3):395-412.
25. Webster M, Ungerleider L. Neuroanatomy of visual attention. In: Parasuraman R, ed. *The Attentive Brain.* Cambridge, Mass: MIT Press; 1998.

26. Faillenot I, Decety J, Jeannerod M. Human brain activity related to the perception of spatial features of objects. *NeuroImage.* 1999;10(2):114-124.

27. Bouska MJ, Kauffman NA, Marcus SE. Disorders of the visual perceptual system. In: Umphred DA, ed. *Neurological Rehabilitation.* 2nd ed. St. Louis, Mo: CV Mosby; 1990.

28. Carlesimo GA, Casadio P, Sabbadini M, Caltagirone C. Associative visual agnosia resulting from a disconnection between intact visual memory and semantic systems. *Cortex.* 1998;34(4):563-576.

29. Katz N, Itzkovich M, Averbuch S, Elazar B. *Lowenstein Occupational Therapy Cognitive Assessment (LOTCA) Manual.* Pequannock, NJ: Maddak; 1990.

30. Rubio KB, Van Deusen J. Relation of perceptual and body image dysfunction to activities of daily living of persons after stroke. *Am J Occup Ther.* 1995;49(6):551-559.

31. Boyce S, Pollatsek A. An exploration of the effects of scene context on object identification. In: Rayner K, ed. *Eye Movements and Visual Cognition.* New York, NY: Springer-Verlag; 1992.

32. Kerkhoff G. Recovery and treatment of sensory perceptual disorders. In: Halligan P, Kischka U, Marshall JC, eds. *Handbook of Clinical Neuropsychology.* New York, NY: Oxford University Press; 2003.

33. Ellis AW, Young AW. *Human Cognitive Neuropsychology.* Mahwah, NJ: Lawrence Erlbaum Assoc; 1988.

34. Parker RS. *Traumatic Brain Injury and Neuropsychological Impairment.* New York, NY: Springer Verlag; 1990.

35. Sergent J, Villemure JG. *Prosopagnosia in a Right Hemispherectomized Patient.* New York, NY: Oxford University Press; 1989.

36. Shiffman LM. Cerebrovascular accident. In: Early MB, ed. *Physical Dysfunction Practice Skills for the Occupational Therapy Assistant.* St. Louis, Mo: Mosby Year-Book; 1998.

37. Farah MJ, Wilson KD, Drain M, Tanaka JN. What is "special" about face perception? *Psychol Rev.* 1998;105(3):482-498.

38. Haxby JV, Ungerleider LG, Horwitz B, et al. Face encoding and recognition in the human brain. *Proc Natl Acad Sci USA.* 1996;93(2):922-927.

39. Leveroni CL, Seidenberg M, Mayer AR, et al. Neural systems underlying the recognition of familiar and newly learned faces. *J Neurosci.* 2000;20(2):878-86.

40. Shah NJ, Marshall JC, Zafiris O, et al. The neural correlates of person familiarity. A functional magnetic resonance imaging study with clinical implications. *Brain.* 2001;124(4):804-815.

41. Tranel D, Damasio AR. Knowledge without awareness: an autonomic index of facial recognition by prosopagnosics. *Science.* 1985;228(4706):1453-1454.

42. Parente R, Herrmann D. *Retraining Cognition: Techniques and Applications.* 2nd ed. Austin, Tex: Pro-Ed Inc; 2003.

43. Warrington E, James M. *The Visual Object and Space Perception Battery.* Bury St. Edmunds, England: Thames Valley Test Co; 1991.

44. Hecaen H, Penfield W, Bertrand C, Malmo R. The syndrome of apractognosis due to lesions of the minor cerebral hemisphere. *Arch Neurol Psychiat.* 1956;75:400-434.

45. Heywood CA, Kentridge RW, Cowey A. Form and motion from colour in cerebral achromatopsia. *Exp Brain Res.* 1998;123(1-2):145-153.

46. Bohlhalter S, Fretz C, Weder B. Hierarchical versus parallel processing in tactile object recognition: a behavioural-neuroanatomical study of aperceptive tactile agnosia. *Brain.* 2002;125(11):2537-2548.

47. Endo K, Miyasaka M, Makishkta H, Yanagisawa N, Susihita M. Tactile agnosia and tactile aphasia: symptomatological and anatomical differences. *Cortex.* 1992;28:445-469.

48. Platz T, Winter T, Muller N, et al. Arm ability training for stroke and traumatic brain injury patients with mild arm paresis: a single-blind, randomized, controlled trial. *Arch Phys Med Rehabil.* 2001;82(7):961-968.

49. Reed C, Caselli RJ. The nature of tactile agnosia: a case study. *Neuropsychologia.* 1994;32(5):527-539.

50. Saetti M, De Renzi E, Comper M. Tactile morphagnosia secondary to spatial deficits. *Neuropsychologia.* 1999;37(9):1087-1100.

51. Nakamura J, Endo K, Sumida T, Hasegawa T. Bilateral tactile agnosia: a case report. *Cortex.* 1998;34(3):375-388.

52. Dannenbaum RM, Jones LA. The assessment and treatment of patients who have sensory loss following cortical lesions. *J Hand Ther.* 1993:6(2):130-138.

53. Cook EA, Thigpen R. Identification and management of cognitive and perceptual deficits in the rehabilitation patient. *Rehabil Nurs.* 1993;18(5):3110-3113.

54. Robertson SL, Jones LA. Tactile sensory impairments and prehensile function in subjects with left hemisphere cerebral lesions. *Arch Phys Med Rehabil.* 1994;75:1108-1117.

55. Ayres AJ. *Southern California Sensory Integration Tests.* Los Angeles, Calif: Western Psychological Services; 1972.

56. Fox JVD. Effect of cutaneous stimulation on performance of hemiplegic adults on selected tests of perception. Thesis. University of Southern California; 1963.

Resources

Averbach S, Katz N. Cognitive rehabilitation: a retraining model for clients with neurological disabilities. In: Katz N, ed. *Cognition and Occupation Across the Life Span*. Bethesda, Md: American Occupational Therapy Association Press; 2005.

Bieman-Copland S, Dywan J. Achieving rehabilitative gains in anosognosia after TBI. *Brain Cogn*. 2000;44:1-18.

Blanton S, Wolf SL. An application of upper-extremity constraint-induced movement therapy in a patient with subacute stroke. *Phys Ther*. 1999;79:847-853.

Constantinidou F, Thomas RD, Best PJ. Principles of cognitive rehabilitation: an integrative approach. In: Ashley MJ, ed. *Traumatic Brain Injury: Rehabilitative Treatment and Case Management*. 2nd ed. Boca Raton, Fla: CRC Press; 2004.

Eimer M, McCarthy RA. Prosopagnosia and structural encoding of faces: evidence from event-related potentials. *Neuroreport*. 1999; 10(2): 255-259.

Kortte KB, Wegener ST, Chwalisz K. Anosognosia and denial: their relationship to coping and depression in acquired brain injury. *Rehabil Psychol*. 2003;48(3):131-136.

Miltner WH, Bauder H, Sommer M, et al. Effects of constraint-induced movement therapy on patients with chronic motor deficits after stroke: a replication. *Stroke*. 1999;30(3):586-592.

Platz T. Tactile agnosia: caustic evidence and theoretical remarks on modality specific meaning representations and sensorimotor integration. *Brain*. 1996;119:1565-1574.

Robertson LC. Visuospatial attention and parietal function: their role in object perception. In: Parasuraman R, ed. *The Attentive Brain*. Cambridge, Mass: MIT Press; 1998.

Schwartz RL. Dissociation of gesture and object recognition. *Neurology*. 1998;50(4):1186-1188.

Seravos P, Goodale MA. Preserved visual imagery in visual form agnosia. *Neuropychologia*. 1995;33(11):1382-1394.

van der Lee JH, Wagenaar RC, Lankhorst GJ, et al. Forced use of the upper extremity in chronic stroke patients: results from a single-blind randomized clinical trial. *Stroke*. 1999;30(11):2369-2975.

CHAPTER 8

ORIENTATION AND ATTENTION

Orientation

An individual who is oriented has a recognition of one's self with regard to time, place, and person within one's personal environment.[1] An individual who is oriented can understand the self and the relationship between the self and the past and present environment.[2] This ability depends on the integration of several cognitive abilities, which are represented in different areas of the brain.[2] Some aspects of disorientation may indicate a problem with retrograde memory loss, while others reflect problems with new learning or anterograde memory.[3]

Orientation to person, for example, is a retrograde memory loss for autobiographical information. The client may also not remember his or her previous social role.[4] Orientation to date, place, and present circumstances, on the other hand, requires the ability to take in, store, and later recall new information. One study of 80 traumatic brain injury (TBI) clients indicated a quicker recovery of orientation to person.[5] The authors hypothesized that orientation to place and time may be more vulnerable because of this dependency on the retention of new information.[5] The client must also be able to monitor and store his or her internal map, which serves to assist in self-locating within the environment.

The client with acquired brain injury (ABI) who is disoriented is unsure of time, person, or place. These difficulties will cause problems in orienting oneself in space with reference to distance and to objects.[6] There can be an altered sense of time, and the client will often get lost. The client's disorientation will often lead to confusion and agitation. Disorientation, in fact, has been found to be a key factor in the severe behavior problems sometimes present in the adult client with ABI.[7] Disorientation in the adult client with ABI is consistently present in the early stages of the emergence from coma and often persists at some level throughout recovery.[8]

Deitz et al outline nine characteristics common to orientation loss[4]:

1. Disorientation may be reflected verbally or behaviorally.

2. Disorientation may be temporary or long-lasting.

3. Orientation tends to be viewed as an all-or-none phenomenon, although criteria vary from clinician to clinician.

4. Some domains of orientation appear more resistant to breakdown than others, with the dimension of time appearing to be the most vulnerable.

5. The most common sequence of recovery of orientation following brain injury is person, place, and time.

6. Temporal orientation is multidimensional.

7. Disorientation is likely to be associated with memory impairment.

8. Orientation is vulnerable to the effects of brain injury.

9. When long-lasting, disorientation requires attention because it may constitute an important obstacle to management and rehabilitation.

EVALUATION OF ORIENTATION

Test 1 – Test of Orientation for Rehabilitation Patients[4]

Description

The Test of Orientation for Rehabilitation Patients (TORP) contains 46 items and measures orientation to person and personal situation, place, time, schedule, and temporal continuity. It requires only a verbal response and is not appropriate for use with severely aphasic clients, but can be adapted for nonverbal clients. Each test item is written both as an open-ended question and as an auditory recognition task. The recognition task is used only if the client is unable to respond or responds incorrectly to the open-ended task.

Scoring

2—Client answers open-ended question.
1—Client responds to auditory recognition task.
0—Client does not respond correctly.

Validity

Content validity was established by a panel of expert judges through a specific item rating form relative to each of the five domains. Data were analyzed at the item and domain level. For all five domains, coefficient of agreement (Lu's coefficient) were statistically significant beyond the 0.05 level.

The following two items are provided as examples.*

Person and Personal Situation
"What is your first name?"

Recognition—"Is your first name …?"

Sam	Roy	George	or	(Correct) / Mike
OR				
Sheila	Amy	Judy	or	(Correct) / Harriet

Accept—Correct first name or nickname.

Place

"In what kind of place were you staying right before you came to this (hospital/rehabilitation center)?"

---

*Reprinted with permission from Therapy Skill Builders/Communication Skill Builders, reference 4: Deitz J, Tovar VS, Beeman C, Thorn DW, Trevisan MS. The test of orientation for rehabilitation patients: test-retest reliability. Occup J Res. 1992;12(3):173-185.

"What kind of place is this room in?"

Recognition—"Is this room in…?"

your home   a bank   a hotel   or   (Correct)

Accept—Correct identification of type of place (ie, hospital, rehabilitation center). If client gives more specific response such as "occupational therapy department," the examiner should rephrase the question. For example, the examiner might then ask, "What kind of place is the occupational therapy department in?"

Reliability

Test-retest reliability was established with a TBI group with correlations as follows:

0.86 person and personal situation

0.92 place

0.83 time

0.72 schedule

0.85 temporal continuity

0.95 total test

Inter-rater reliability was established through interclass correlations ranging from 0.94 to 0.99.

Test 2 – Lowenstein Occupational Therapy Cognitive Assessment Orientation Subtest[9]*

Description

The orientation subtest contains two items and is one of four subtests of the Lowenstein Occupational Therapy Cognitive Assessment (LOTCA) battery. The other areas are perception, visuomotor organization, and thinking operations. Clinical observation of attention and concentration are also included.

Procedure

Orientation for Place

Client is asked where he or she is now (ie, the name of the hospital and the name of the city in which it is located).

The examiner asks the client the following questions:

"Where are you now?"

"Where is it located?"

"Where do you live? What is your exact address?"

"Name a city that is located near your home address."

Orientation Comments

Total disorientation for place and time indicates a confusional state. Generally, orientation for place (ORP) improves before orientation for time (ORT).

Reprinted with permission from reference 9: Itzkovich M, Elazar B, Averbuch S. Lowenstein: Occupational Therapy Cognitive Assessment (LOTCA) Manual. *Pequannock, NJ: Maddack Inc; 1990.*

Scoring

Scoring is on a scale of 1 (low) to 4 (high).

For the first item, if the client answers all of the questions correctly, he gets 2 points. For partial performance or no performance, he gets 1 point. For the other two items, the client receives 1 point for each correct answer.

1 point—Minimal performance
4 points—Maximum performance

Validity

The majority of validity and reliability research was conducted on the remaining three subtests. The authors recommend administration of the entire test battery versus utilizing only one or two subtests.

Reliability

Inter-rater reliability with Spearman's rank correlation coefficient between raters ranged from 0.82 to 0.97 for the various subtests.

Dynamic Assessment[2]

Informally question the client regarding person, place, or time. Provide cuing during the questioning as needed to assess what type of cuing improves performance (ie, multiple choices, abstract versus concrete cues, or photographs). Assess what environmental factors affect orientation—for example, sundowning (ie, increased confusion in the evening due to fatigue)[10] or disorganized environment (eg, changing the location of grooming items).

TREATMENT OF ORIENTATION DEFICITS

Utilizing a Restorative Approach

1. Have the client participate in a daily orientation group. Group sessions should provide a structured setting for repetitive and consistent management of topics involved.[11,12] When designing and setting up the group, focus on members' selections, meeting frequency, meeting place, treatment, media and staff, and family education.

2. Provide daily individual reality orientation in a consistent, structured manner for areas of client disorientation. This daily reorientation can sometimes reduce clients' disorientation by making them feel less threatened by the environment when they can understand where they are and why they are there.[7]

Utilizing an Adaptive Approach

1. Provide external orientation aids such as labeled pictures of family members, friends, pets, etc. Large calendars, clocks, and orientation boards are also helpful and should be placed liberally around the treatment facility or the client's home. Have the client wear a wrist watch when he or she is able.

2. Incorporate personal items brought from home (eg, favorite possessions, radio, TV).[12]

3. The client's daily routine should be as organized, predictable, and as consistent as possible. Normalize the client's waking and bedtime while he or she is an inpatient, which will help develop a sleep-wake cycle that can continue at discharge.[13] This is also true of the client's room and personal environment. Minimize unfamiliar and unexpected changes.[14]

Table 8-1

Techniques for Redirecting the Disoriented, Confused, and/or Agitated Client

Technique	*Description/Goal*	*Type of Client*
Supportive Guidance	Orienting the client to an activity through set up and verbal intervention; guides the client's confused thinking to a desirable state without providing complex choices; the therapist will not correct every maladaptive behavior, but instead will guide the client to complete the activity.	Agitated and noncompliant
Cognitive Set Change Through Preorientation	Designed to shift the client's cognitive set gradually from what he/she is preoccupied with to the set that is considered to be desirable at that particular time; orienting the client to an activity in which he or she is going to engage a few minutes later (ie, through showing pictures or simple questioning) and answers on topics related to the upcoming activity.	In a state of severe confusion and preoccupation with non-productive activity
Focus Shift to Increase Compliance	Change the client's focus to a functionally related cognitive set which can accomplish the goal by performing the necessary task.	Severe memory impairments and is preoccupied that he/she has performed the requested task
Use Humor to Divert Attention	Nonthreatening way to remind a confused client to perform a daily routine.	Delusional thinking and non-compliance
Cognitive Re-Enactment of Premorbid Behavior	Attempts to link the client's premorbid behavior with the present request to provide a reason for the client to perform an activity.	Decreased insight
Direct Attention Through Reward and Rationale	Use of an object or an activity as a reward to direct the client to another situation or improve compliance to perform a certain task; provides a reason for the client to perform the activity.	Noncompliant

Adapted from reference 8: Yuen HK, Benzing P. Treatment methodology: guiding of behaviour through redirection in brain injury rehabilitation. Brain Inj. 1996;10(3):229-238.

4. Techniques of redirection (visually and verbally recueing or directing attention) can be used to divert the client away from the source of disorientation, confusion, and agitation. Techniques for redirecting the disoriented, confused, and/or agitated client are presented in Table 8-1.

5. Introduce yourself to the client daily if needed, and incorporate orienting information into the conversation.

6. Educate the client's family regarding the client's disorientation and explain to them the importance of a consistent daily routine and stable, consistent personal environment.

Attention

Attention is often used as a "catch all" term to describe many aspects of behavior. It is an active process that helps to determine which sensations and experiences are alerting and relevant to the individual. In essence, the stimulus that is important to an individual's needs or goals will be determined as higher priority.[15] As Lou et al state, attention "...refers to our ability to concentrate our perceptual experience on a selected portion of the available sensory information and, in doing so, to achieve a clear and vivid impression of the environment."[16] Through the mechanism of attention, an individual can closely observe objects to ascertain their features and their relationship to oneself and other objects in the environment.[17] Attention resources, in fact, can be directed and based on the properties of the stimulus itself.[18] Attention reflects an ability to narrow environmental focus as well as the ability to sustain and shift this focus.[16] It allows multiple relevant simultaneously presented environmental stimuli to be processed in a sequential manner.[18] Attention requires effort and its limited capacity can be flexibly allocated.[1] It can be generalized or focused and directed to extrapersonal or intrapersonal space.[1]

Attention is integrally involved and crucial for many cognitive functions and types of learning.[8,19-21] It is a primary step in the memory process, and without it, there can be no memory.[16,22-24] Attention involves components of consciousness, awareness, and arousal as well as affect and motivation and is the interaction between the initial information processing and the ultimate adaptive control.[1,8,20]

Historically, most theories related to attention equated it with information processing.[25] Subsequently, the concept of selectivity was developed. In other words, a target stimulus receives priority over a nontarget stimulus. This selectivity allows the individual to respond to a specific event and inhibit all simultaneous events. In recent years, in addition to the concept of selectivity, the concepts of sustained attention, vigilance, and divided attention have been incorporated into contemporary theories of attention.[21,26] In addition, the functional terms of alerting, orienting, and executive attention have been described.[27]

As just described, attentional abilities are inter-related to a number of cognitive systems and, therefore, should be viewed as a component of interconnected abilities.[28] It is a common occurrence that as attentional disorders recover, many information processing and cognitive deficits become apparent.[29,30] Parente incorporates this concept of interconnected abilities in his seven stage model of attention training.[23] The model incorporates seven related skills:

1. Basic arousal

2. Simple orientation to a visual/auditory stimulus

3. Attention with discrimination

4. Concentration and mental control

5. Distracted attention

6. Attention with immediate memory

7. Interference resistance training

There are two types of information processing that are related to attention: automatic and controlled processing. Controlled processing is utilized when new information is being considered. Automatic processing, on the other hand, occurs at a subcortical level.[28] Once a task becomes more automatic, significant attentional resources are no longer required, and attention can be directed to other more novel aspects of a particular task.[31] Many clinicians are already aware of the behavior clients exhibit relative to these two types of processing. For example, the client who has sustained an ABI requires conscious attention to complete even the simplest tasks.[32] Two disorders, focused attentional deficit and divided attentional deficit, are related to these processing concepts and can occur after an ABI.

Toglia views attention not as separate subskills that form a hierarchy but rather analyzes attentional function/dysfunction in relation to the interaction of task characteristics, environment, and the individual.[33] The complexity or familiarity of a given task, for example, will determine the extent to which particular aspects of attention are required.[33] The demands placed on each aspect of attention can differ depending on the situation. During one task, a client may exhibit good selective attention and poor attentional flexibility, while with a different task, the reverse may be true.

Often the term attention is used interchangeably with other terms such as alertness, vigilance, or effort. This creates confusion and does not assist the therapist in identifying deficits and designing treatment programs. These and other related terms, therefore, are described in an effort to clarify related concepts as follows:

1. *Alerting*—More related to the periphery, preparing the individual to mobilize to attention, and theoretically functions through different neurological systems from attention;[34] a fluctuating condition of the central nervous system (CNS);[32] phylogenically the earliest of the attentional systems;[35] associated with the frontal and parietal regions of the right hemisphere.[27]

2. *Attention*—Means by which one can orient in order to receive incoming information;[23] contains the three components of alertness, selectivity, and effort. Subcategories of attention include the following[23]:

   - Focused attention. The ability to respond to different kinds of stimulation; it involves direction and orientation, has both physical and mental components, and implies a body posture and orientation appropriate to receiving sensory information and taking motor action;[1] the mind is free of extraneous thoughts, and an effort is made to keep sensory channels open.[1]

   - Sustained attention. Vigilance; maintaining attention for a long time; the ability to self-sustain mindful conscious processing of stimuli whose repetitive, nonarousing qualities would otherwise cause habituation and distraction to other stimuli;[21,36,37] ensures that goals are maintained over time; associated with right hemisphere specialization.[21,37]

   - Selective attention. Activating and inhibiting responses selectively; involves discrimination of stimulus information and differentiating responses; helps goal directed behavior and is critical for perception;[38] ensures that an individual does not perceive a superposition of all stimuli present at a given time in our visual field by suppressing the nonattended stimuli such that only one stimulus is processed at a given time in higher cortical areas.[18] (Unilateral neglect is an illustration of a disruption of the selective attentional network.[20])

   - Alternating attention (attentional flexibility). Alternating back and forth between mental tasks (eg, chopping vegetables while periodically checking food on the stove).[39]

   - Divided attention. Ability to do several things at once; requires the ability to allocate attentional resources, switch between tasks that cannot be done simultaneously, and time-sharing of processing resources.[26]

   - Concentration. The ability to do mental work while attending, the process of active encoding in working memory.[23]

   - Vigilance. The ability to sustain attention over a period of time.[23] Thirty seconds is considered a vigilant period in a mental status examination;[40] a control process that coordinates functional components of attention (alertness, arousal, and selectivity) to direct attention to a significant feature of the environment. Note: It is this aspect of attention that appears particularly vulnerable to brain damage.[40]

Attention deficits are common after an ABI.[20,21,30,36,41-44]

Deficits can range from distractibility, difficulty focusing, or poor concentration, to difficulty with sustained or divided attention.[26,41,44,45] Clients may complain of being overly sensitive to noise and have difficulty with task completion or multitasking.[46] If there is a problem with divided attention, the client may exhibit slow processing and behavior and become "overloaded" when he or she has to deal with several alternatives.[32] For example, if there is a deficit with sustained attention, the client may not be able to attend to the relevant proprioceptive and other inputs sufficiently to relearn motor skills.[21,47] There may be complaints that when the client tries to concentrate, he or she may feel fatigued or irritable and develop a headache.[35,41] The client may take more time to complete tasks or forget what he or she was about to do.[25,26,48]

Attentional deficits have been linked to the reticular activating system, frontal and temporal lobes, and the limbic system.[20,30,44,49] Attention is accomplished by a network of anatomical areas.[50] Devinsky and D'Esposito describe the attentional functional networks as follows[20]:

> *There are at least three distinct functional networks that underlie attention, yet these networks communicate and function as a seamless unit. First, a predominantly subcortical diffuse network mediates arousal and alerting ...Second, a mixed cortical subcortical network mediates orientation to stimuli... Finally, a predominantly cortical network mediates selective attention... The interplay of these three functional networks allows us to orient, filter, and select from inputs in the complex world around us, preparing us for action or whatever is necessary to guide our behavior or achieve our goals.*

Any type of attentional deficit common to the client with ABI will impair learning and all aspects of daily functioning.[18,51] Memory, problem solving, and other higher intellectual functions all have an attentional component. Attention, therefore, should always be evaluated at the beginning of a functional cognitive evaluation.

EVALUATION OF ATTENTION

*Test 1 – Test of Everyday Attention[47]**

Description

There are eight subtests of the Test of Everyday Attention (TEA): map search, elevator counting, elevator counting with distractions, visual elevator, elevator counting with reversal, telephone search, telephone search while counting, and lottery.

Clinical Strengths[47]

1. The TEA gives a broad-based measure of the most important clinical and theoretical aspects of attention; no other existing test of attention does this.

2. The TEA has three versions that allow testing on three successive occasions with parallel material.

3. The TEA can be used analytically to identify different patterns of attentional breakdown.

4. The TEA has a very wide range of application, ranging from clients with early Alzheimer's disease to young normal subjects.

5. The TEA is the only test of attention based largely on everyday material; the real-life scenario means that most clients enjoy the test and find it relevant to their problems of adjustments in everyday life.

Reprinted with permission from Harcourt Assessment, reference 47: Robertson I, Ward T, Ridgeway Y, Nimmo-Smith I. The Test of Everyday Attention. Bury St. Edwards, England: Thames Valley Test; 1994

Table 8-2

Test of Everyday Attention Reliability—Pearson Correlations

Subtest	Normal Controls (N = 119): Version A with B	Normal Controls (N = 39): Version B with C	Stroke Clients (N = 74): Version A with B
Map Search: I Minute	0.83	0.87	0.84
Map Search: 2 Minutes	0.86	0.80	0.85
Elevator Counting	Ceiling effect	Ceiling effect	0.88
Elevator Counting With Distractions	0.71	0.68	0.83
Visual Elevator: Raw Accuracy Score	0.71	0.76	0.90
Visual Elevator: Timing Score	0.79	0.70	Not calculated
Elevator Counting With Reversal	0.66	0.68	Not administered
Telephone Search: Raw Score	0.86	0.90	0.78
Telephone Search While Counting: Dual Task Decrement	0.59	0.61	0.41 (see text)
Lottery	Ceiling effect	Ceiling effect	0.77

Reprinted with permission from Harcourt Assessment, reference 47: Robertson I, Ward T, Ridgeway Y, Nimmo-Smith I. The Test of Everyday Attention. *Bury St. Edwards, England: Thames Valley Test; 1994.*

Validity

Extensive validity measures were generated with various populations and other existing tests that purported to measure attention. Details of these studies are contained in the test manual.[47]

Reliability

Test-retest reliability coefficients are given in Table 8-2 on version A and B for 119 subjects from the normal sample and for 74 subjects of the cerebral vascular accident (CVA) sample. In addition, test-retest reliability figures are given for a subsample of the normal sample who were given version C a week after receiving version B.

Procedure

The subtest Map Search is provided as an example.*

Subjects are asked to imagine that they are on vacation (holiday) in the United States, in Philadelphia. They will carry out a number of everyday tasks during this imaginary vacation (holiday). Each task has its own scenario. The general verbatim instruction for the introduction to the test is as follows. The wording is to be followed verbatim, though the tester must judge when to re-emphasize an instruction that is unclear to the subject.

Say:

"We are interested in your concentration on a range of everyday tasks. I want you to imagine that you are on a long trip to Philadelphia (United States). I will ask you to do various tasks

*Reprinted with permission from Harcourt Assessment, reference 47: Robertson I, Ward T, Ridgeway Y, Nimmo-Smith I. The Test of Everyday Attention. *Bury St. Edwards, England: Thames Valley Test; 1994.*

such as looking at maps and looking up telephone directories while you are on this imaginary trip. Let me explain the first task."

Subtest – Map Search

This timed, visual search task involves searching a map for a total of 2 minutes and circling a particular symbol on the map when located. After 1 minute, subjects are given a different colored pen to enable the tester to count the number of targets located in 1 minute versus the total for 2 minutes.

The symbols are in the cuebook according to which version of the test (A, B, or C) is being given. There are two maps of the Philadelphia area. Each map has two types of symbols. There are 80 of each type of symbol. On each map, only one symbol is the target for a given version of the subtest. The cuebook is left open at the target symbol in front of the subject during the subtest to remind him or her of the symbol being sought.

- *For version A*—The fork and knife on version A map
- *For version B*—The screwdriver with wrench (spanner) on version B and C map
- *For version C*—The gas (petrol) pump on version B and C map

Instructions

"The symbol here (show symbol from cuebook) shows where restaurants (or garages or gas [petrol] stations) can be found in the Philadelphia area. There are many symbols like this on the map."

Point to one at the left side of map. Also, indicate to the subject that the symbols are found all over the map: left and right, top and bottom. Check that the subject can see the symbol clearly. Turn the map over so the subject cannot scan it while you give further instructions:

"Let's say you are with a family member or a friend. They are driving while you are navigating. You want to know where restaurants (or garages, or gas [petrol] stations) are located in case you decide to stop for a meal (or to get your car checked, or to fill up). What I would like you to do is to look at the map for 2 minutes and circle as many symbols as you can. I will stop you once when a minute has gone by to ask you to swap pens. OK?"

Then the subject indicates that he or she has understood (reiterate the instructions if he or she has not), turn the map over to reveal the symbols, give him or her a red pen, and begin timing. After 1 minute, ask the subject to change pens and hand him or her a blue pen. At the end of 2 minutes, ask the subject to stop.

If the subject feels that he or she has completed the task before the 2 minute time limit, or if he or she assumes that he or she has done so by reaching the right hand edge of the map, ask the subject to continue searching for any symbols that he or she might have missed until the end of the time limit.

Common Errors

Subjects usually comprehend this task very easily. Occasionally, subjects talk during the task, thereby slowing their performance. In this case, the assessor should try not to respond or simply say, "Remember to find as many as you can." In some instances, subjects stop searching after they have found only a few targets, apparently finding it difficult to persist. The assessor should make the same basic comment as above, perhaps with some encouragement: "You are doing fine so far. Keep finding as many as you can for a bit longer" or "There are quite a few symbols, can you find more?"

Scoring

Slip the version A, B, or C template into the plastic folder over the map with the printed side up. Next, count the number of target symbols circled in red. This is the 1 minute score. Then, count the number of circles in blue, and add this to the red total. This is the 2 minute score.

Test 2 – Clinical Observation and Activity Analysis

General Guidelines for Evaluation

1. Identify the components of attention (eg, alerting, selectivity, effort) that are intact and those that are impaired.

2. Observe the client in a number of settings and activities at different times during the day. Position change (lying, sitting) can also affect attention.

3. Establish functional baseline measures. Consider the frequency and severity of the problem. Select relevant functional tasks as the basis for the evaluation and reassessment.

Specific Areas or Questions to Consider and Evaluate

1. Which sensory systems are affected? Visual? Auditory?

2. What is the duration and frequency of the client's attentional abilities?

3. Under what environmental conditions can the client attend to a task? When does attention begin to break down?

4. What are some behavioral indications of the client's inattention?

5. Does the client have memory problems? Does he or she have problem solving difficulties? Decreased processing? Are these or related problems caused in part by decreased attention?

6. Are there any tasks or areas that seem to particularly interest the client and therefore, increase his or her attention?

7. Is processing occurring only at a conscious level, as opposed to a normal combination of automatic and conscious?

Scoring

Nonstandardized

The foregoing and similar questions can be incorporated into a checklist or used in conjunction with a frequency rating scale (eg, always, sometimes, rarely, or never).

Validity

To improve validity, rule out primary sensory and language problems as the causes of poor performance.

Dynamic Assessment[33,52-54]

Description

This is not a single test but is a qualitative analysis of how the client performs on a given task. Three components of the evaluation process are awareness questioning strategy, investigation and task grading, and response to cuing.

Awareness Questioning

General Questions

"Have you noticed any changes in your memory?"
"Have you noticed any changes in your attention?"
"How would you rate your ability to concentrate/remember compared to before the injury?"
(100%, 75%, 50%, 25%, 0%)

Prediction/Estimation Questions

- "On a scale of 1 to 4, how difficult do you think this task will be?"

  (1 = very difficult, 2 = difficult, 3 = easy, 4 = very easy)

- "To what extent do you feel that your ability to perform this type of task has changed?"

  (no change, slight change, definite change, big change)

- "Out of 20 items how many do you think you will remember?"

- "Do you think you would have performed any differently before the injury?"

Strategy Investigation

Observe how the individual performs a task and question the individual's responses without suggesting the answers. The client's response to strategy questions will supplement clinical observations of performance and provide the therapist with information on the client's thought process.

Task Grading Response to Cuing

If the client has trouble with 50% of the task, change one parameter.[33] Begin testing at mid level.

Procedures

Toglia has applied her theoretical concepts to five different categories of attentional tasks.[33] Table 8-3 is a sample of this application.

TREATMENT OF ATTENTION DEFICITS

Utilizing a Restorative Approach

Many believe the attentional system is one that can be modified by targeted intervention.[3,26,42] Research has indicated, however, that even in those cases where attention improved in training tasks, this improvement did not, for the most part, generalize to everyday life.[3,48,55] Perhaps the most valuable evidence that the clinician can draw upon for clinical reasoning and decision making in the treatment of attentional deficits in the adult ABI client is presented in a meta-analysis performed by Park and Ingles.[48] These clinicians conducted a 30-year meta-analysis of articles evaluating the effectiveness of interventions for attentional disorders after adult ABI. The results of their study indicated, at least for the direct intervention methods utilized in the literature, that direct training did not significantly restore damaged attentional function. The meta-analysis did reveal, however, that activities relearning skills that critically involve attention were effective, particularly if the skill being learned had a substantial attentional component. This research study validated what occupational therapists have always believed, that the most rewarding or effective programs are those which focus on training skills that are also of great functional importance to the client.[48]

As stated in Chapter 1, when utilizing a restorative approach to treatment, the activities chosen should be occupation-based and client-centered. For example, if the client's favorite pastime is

Table 8-3

Attentional Flexibility Tasks

Task Level	Sample Tasks	Response (Indicate # and letter)	Sample Cues
1. Follows one change	a) Copy the following: mmmmmnnnnnn b) Add these pairs of numbers. Now subtract these numbers: 2 4 5 6 7 3 5 5 9 3 7 2 c) Playing cards: Spread face up all over the table. Turn over the even-numbered cards. Now turn over the odd-numbered cards.	___Follows changes in task smoothly ___Occasionally (25%) errors observed following a change ___Occasionally (25%) errors observed following a change ___Errors observed following a change 50% of the time ___Errors observed following a change more than 50% of the time	*General feedback:* Are you sure you followed the sequence? *Specific feedback:* Some of the sequence is correct, but there are a few places where you ___ (eg, added instead of subtracted). *Self-initiated strategy:* Can you think of a way to make it easier to follow changes?
2. Alternates between two different sequences or responses	a) Copy the following: mnmnmnmnmnmn b) Add the first 2 pairs of numbers. Subtract the next 2 pairs of numbers and continue alternating. 2 4 7 3 6 7 9 2 12 4 11 6 13 5 15 3 c) Playing cards: Place cards in rows, face up. Turn over the odd cards, but as soon as you get to a J, Q, or K card, switch to turning over even cards. When you get to the next J, Q or K card, switch back to odd cards and so on.	Observed behaviors following change: ___No change in behavior ___Becomes distracted ___Required redirection to task ___Perseveration ___Slowness, hesitation ___Impulsive ___Remains goal-directed ___Becomes distracted (1x to 2x, 3x to 4x, >5x) but unable to redirect self back to task	*Provide strategy:* For example, this time try to say it aloud to help you. *General feedback:* Are you sure you followed the sequence? *Specific feedback:* Some of the sequence is correct, but there are a few places where you ___ (eg, added instead of subtracted). *Self-initiated strategy:* Can you think of a way to make it easier to follow changes?
3. Generates alternate responses or ideas	a) If you had $9.85, tell me all the different lunches you could order. b) Tell me all the different coin combinations that will make $1.05. c) Playing cards: Tell me all the different card combinations that add up to 21.	___Occasional redirection needed ___Frequent redirection needed ___Continual redirection needed ___Attention span is adequate ___Attention span is inadequate (indicate high) ___Fluctuations in performance ___Performance deteriorates at end of task ___Response speed modulated ___Perseverative ___Impulsive ___Slow	*Provide strategy:* For example, this time try to say it aloud to help you. *Sample task modifications:* – Change task level. – Increase saliency of cue for "change." – Decrease frequency of changes. – Decrease number of stimuli. – Eliminate time limit. – Decrease selection demands.

Adapted with permission from reference 52: Toglia J. A dynamic interactional approach to cognitive rehabilitation. In: Katz N, ed. Cognitive Rehabilitation: Models For Intervention in Occupational Therapy. *Boston, Mass: Andover Med Pub; 1992.*

sewing, activities should be provided that relate to this pastime. Research indicates that regaining this skill facilitates modification of attentional abilities as well.

During occupation-based attentional activities, the following guidelines and techniques can be utilized:

1. Identify which type or types of attention are affected, and target these areas in treatment.[25] For example, if alternating attention is impaired, provide graded kitchen activities that require different levels of alternating attention.

2. Provide cues that help the client access and use previous knowledge to organize new information.[33] This can enhance attention. For example, prior to starting an activity, describe the activity the client will be doing, and relate it to the client's past performance of it (ie, "You're going to be repairing your wife's jewelry box. Remember when you would repair things for your wife in your workshop in your garage?").

3. Provide a behavioral frame of reference to attention training.[56] For example, the client receives a token when he or she maintains attention for a predetermined time. A certain amount of tokens are exchanged for a previously agreed upon reward.

4. Motivation and the client's emotional state can alter his or her ability to attend and remember.[33] It is important, therefore, to provide training that is motivating to the client.[24]

5. Alter the task and/or environment to change the client's level of attention.[24,33,46] Identify what task level and type of environment causes decreased attention. Start activities at this stage, and progress. Tasks emphasizing the different aspects of attention can each be graded from simple to complex.[54] For example, the client may only be able to attend and sustain that attention when the activity contains a physical component,[46] or he or she may only be able to attend in a quiet environment with no auditory distractions (ie, may need ear plugs).

6. Provide training to help the client develop active listening skills as follows[57]:

    a) Maintain eye contact.

    b) As much as possible, maintain a body posture that is erect but relaxed, which indicates interest and attention.

7. In an attempt to utilize sensory input (eg, visual, tactile, auditory) in relation to motor output (eg, attention to task, participation in task), provide controlled sensory cuing with the client subsequently demonstrating active interaction with the environment. For example, placing tape on the client's finger for the client to remove can stimulate visual attention.[58] Once the client is attending to that hand (and arm), putting on the sleeve of his or her shirt can be initiated.

8. Review with the physician what medication the client is taking. Discuss what medication can help or hurt attention skills.[59] Research has shown that medication can be used to improve client's attention.[60]

9. Table top-graded activities that focus on attentional skills (ie, cancellation tasks, mazes) can be utilized as a "warm up" before occupation-based activities.

10. Teach the client to actively scan his or her environment, seek out the presence of cues, and identify them.[61,62]

11. Research has indicated that "self-alerting" procedures may be effective in improving sustained attention.[37] For example, the therapist can tap the table or clap his or her hands and say "attend" at unpredictable times while the client is performing an activity.

Utilizing an Adaptive Approach

1. Many theorists believe that the regulation of attention is largely dependent on subvocal or inner speech.[63] Verbal mediation by the client to compensate for attention deficit has been found to be an effective compensation strategy.[64,65]

   a) The client can be taught statements to prepare him- or herself to listen and ask for repetition if his or her attention strays (eg, "I must really concentrate and look at the person speaking to me").[66]

   b) Have the client vocalize step by step as he or she performs a task. Progress to subvocalization (client silently vocalizes), thereby internalizing the technique.[66]

2. If necessary, staff and family should speak slowly and in short sentences with pauses to allow time for processing.[59] Ask the client to paraphrase what he or she has just heard, and repeat information if needed. Teach the client to cue others to speak more slowly and request repetition.

3. Adapt both the external and internal client environment to reduce overload and fatigue by reducing distracters.

   a) *External*—Remove clutter and reduce noise level. Utilize ear plugs.[24] Allocate a quiet time each day to do specific tasks where there's no phone ringing, pagers, etc.[24]

   b) *Internal*—Reduce hunger, pain, anger, fatigue, etc. For example, adjust room temperature, and provide rest periods. Teach the client to shelve emotional internal distracters through techniques such as visual imagery.[57]

4. Adapt tasks in a way that information processing elements of a task are emphasized or highlighted.[67,68] For example, underline an important part of written directions, or make important elements visually bigger or a different color. This will help the client discriminate different components of the learning task.[68]

References

1. Parker RS. *Concussive Brain Trauma: Neurobehavioral Impairment and Maladaptation.* Boca Raton, Fla: CRC Press; 2001.
2. Golisz K, Toglia J. Perception and cognition. In: Crepeau E, Cohn ES, Schell BAB, eds. *Willard and Spackman's Occupational Therapy.* Philadelphia, Pa: Lippincott, Williams and Wilkins; 2003.
3. Sohlberg M, McLaughlin KA, Pavese A, et al. Evaluation of attention process training and brain injury education in persons with acquired brain injury. *J Clin Exp Neuropsychol.* 2000;22(5):656-676.
4. Deitz J, Tovar VS, Beeman C, Thorn DW, Trevisan MS. The test of orientation for rehabilitation patients: test-retest reliability. *Occup J Res.* 1992;12(3):173-185.
5. High WM, Levin HS, Gary HE. Recovery of orientation following closed head injury. *J Clin Exp Neuropsychol.* 1990;12(5):703-714.
6. Rabbit P. Changes in problem solving ability in old age. In: Birren J, Schaie K eds. *Handbook of Psychology of Aging.* New York, NY: Van Nostrand Reinhold Co; 1977.
7. Persel CS, Persel CH. The use of applied behavior analysis in traumatic brain injury rehabilitation. In: Ashley MJ, ed. *Traumatic Brain Injury: Rehabilitative Treatment and Case Management.* 2nd ed. CRC Press, 2004.
8. Yuen HK, Benzing P. Treatment methodology: guiding of behaviour through redirection in brain injury rehabilitation. *Brain Inj.* 1996;10(3):229-238.
9. Itzkovich M, Elazar B, Averbuch S. *Lowenstein: Occupational Therapy Cognitive Assessment (LOTCA) Manual.* Pequannock, NJ: Maddack Inc; 1990.
10. Filskov S, Boll T. *Handbook of Clinical Neuropsychology.* New York, NY: John Wiley & Sons, Inc; 1981.
11. McAllister TW, Saykin AJ, Flashman LA, et al. Brain activation during working memory 1 month after mild traumatic brain injury: a functional MRI study. *Neurology.* 1999;53(6):1300-1307.
12. McNeny R, Dise J. Reality orientation therapy. In: Rosenthal M, Griffith ER, Bond MR, Miller JD, eds. *Rehabilitation of the Adult with Traumatic Brain Injury.* Philadelphia, Pa: FA Davis Co; 1983.

13. McNeny R. Activities of daily living. In: Rosenthal M, Griffith ER, Kreutzer JS, Pentland B, eds. *Rehabilitation of the Adult and Child with Traumatic Brain Injury.* 3rd ed. Philadelphia, Pa: FA Davis; 1983.

14. Zoltan B. Visual, visual perceptual and perceptual-motor deficits in brain injured adults: evaluation, treatment, and functional implications. In: Kraft GH, Berrol S, eds. *Physical Medicine and Rehabilitation Clinics of North America.* Philadelphia, Pa: WB Saunders Co; 1992.

15. Heilman KM, Valenstein E, Watson RT. Neglect and related disorders. *Semin Neurol.* 2000;20(4):463-469.

16. Lou J, Lane S. Personal performance capabilities and their impact on occupational performance. In: Christiansen C, Baum C, eds. *Occupational Therapy: Performance, Participation and Well-Being.* Thorofare, NJ: SLACK Incorporated; 2005.

17. Webster J, Scott R. The effects of self-instructional training on attentional deficits following head injury. *Clin Neuropsychol.* 1983;5:69-74.

18. Nieber E, Koch C. Computational architectures for attention. In: Parasuraman R, ed. *The Attentive Brain.* Cambridge, Mass: MIT Press; 1998.

19. Averbach S, Katz N. Cognitive rehabilitation: a retraining model for clients with neurological disabilities. In: Katz N, ed. *Cognition and Occupation Across the Life Span.* Bethesda, Md: American Occupational Therapy Association Press; 2005.

20. Devinsky O, D'Esposito M. Attention and attentional disorders. In: *Neurology of Cognitive and Behavioral Disorders.* New York, NY: Oxford University Press; 2004.

21. Robertson IH. The rehabilitation of attention. In: Stuss DT, Robertson IH, eds. *Cognitive Neurorehabilitation.* New York, NY: Cambridge University Press; 1999.

22. Marrocco R, Davidson M. Neurochemistry of attention. In: Parasuraman R, ed. *The Attentive Brain.* Cambridge, Mass: MIT Press; 1998.

23. Parente R, Anderson J. *Retraining Memory: Techniques and Applications.* Houston, Tex: CSY Publishing; 1991.

24. Parente R, Herrman D. *Retraining Cognition: Techniques and Applications.* 2nd ed. Austin, Tex: PRO-ED Inc; 2003.

25. Sohlberg M, Mateer CA. Effectiveness of an attention-training program. *J Clin Exp Neuropsych.* 1987;9(2):117-130.

26. Mateer CA. Attention. In: Raskin SA, Mateer CA. *Neuropsychological Management of Mild Traumatic Brain Injury.* New York, NY: Oxford University Press; 2000.

27. Fan J, McCandliss BD, Sommer T, Raz A, Posner MI. Testing the efficiency and independence of attentional networks. *J Cogn Neurosci.* 2002;14(3):340-347.

28. Valenti C. Brain injured patients in vision therapy: perspective. *Vision Therapy: Working With The Brain Injured.* 35(1). Santa Ana, Calif: Optometric Extension Program; 1999.

29. Adamovich BLB. Cognition, language, attention, and information processing following closed head injury. In: Kreutzer JS, Wehman PH, eds. *Cognitive Rehabilitation For Persons with Traumatic Brain Injury: A Functional Approach.* Baltimore, Md: Paul H. Books Publishing Co; 1991.

30. Chan R. Attentional deficits in patients with closed head injury: a further study to the discriminative validity of the test of everyday attention. *Brain Inj.* 2000;14:227-236.

31. Schmitter-Edgecombe M, Rogers WA. Automatic process development following severe closed head injury. *Neuropsychology.* 1997;11(2):296-308.

32. Wood R, McMillan T. *Neurobehavioral Disability and Social Handicap Following Traumatic Brain Injury.* Philadelphia; Pa: Psychology Press; 2001.

33. Toglia J. *Contextual Memory Test.* San Antonio, Tex: Therapy Skill Builders; 1993.

34. Breines E. *Perception: Its Development and Recapitulation.* Princeton, NJ: Geri-Rehab; 1981.

35. Constantinidou F, Thomas RD, Best PJ. Principles of cognitive rehabilitation: an integrative approach. In: Ashley MJ, ed. *Traumatic Brain Injury: Rehabilitative Treatment and Case Management.* 2nd ed. Boca Raton, Fla: CRC Press, 2004.

36. Manly T, Hawkins K, Evans J, Woldt K, Robertson IH. Rehabilitation of executive function: facilitation of effective goal management on complex tasks using periodic auditory alerts. *Neuropsychologia.* 2002;40(3):271-281.

37. Robertson IH, Manly T, Andrade J, Baddeley BT, Yiend J. 'Oops!': performance correlates of everyday attentional failures in traumatic brain injured and normal subjects. *Neuropsychologia.* 1997;35(6):747-758.

38. Alexander M, Stuss P. Disorders of frontal lobe functioning. *Semin Neurol.* 2000;20(4):427-437.

39. Okkeman K. *Cognition and Perception in Stroke Patients.* Gaithersburg, Md: Aspen Publishers; 1993.

40. Stuss DT, Alexander MP. Executive functions and the frontal lobes: a conceptual view. *Psychol Res.* 2000;63(3-4):289-298.

41. Cicerone KD. Attention deficits and dual task demands after mild traumatic brain injury. *Brain Inj.* 1996;10(2):79-89.

42. Cicerone KD. Remediation of 'working attention' in mild traumatic brain injury. *Brain Inj.* 2002;16(3):185-195.

43. Lincoln NB, Majid MJ, Weyman N. Cognitive rehabilitation for attention deficits following stroke. _The Cochrane Collection._ Chichester, England: Wiley and Sons; 2005.

44. Stuss DT, Toth JP, Franchi D, et al. Dissociation of attentional processes in patients with focal frontal and posterior lesions. _Neuropsychologia._ 1999;37(9):1005-1027.

45. Wilson BA, Evans JJ, Emslie H, Malinek V. Evaluation of NeuroPage: a new memory aid. _J Neurol Neurosurg Psychiatry._ 1997;63(1):113-115.

46. Ashley M. Evaluation of traumatic brain injury following acute rehabilitation. In: Ashley M, ed. _Traumatic Brain Injury: Rehabilitative Treatment and Case Management._ Boca Raton, Fla: CRC Press; 2004.

47. Robertson I, Ward T, Ridgeway Y, Nimmo-Smith I. _The Test of Everyday Attention._ Bury St. Edwards, England: Thames Valley Test; 1994.

48. Park NW, Ingles JL. Effectiveness of attention rehabilitation after an acquired brain injury: a meta-analysis. _Neuropsychology._ 2001;15(2):199-210.

49. Massey EW, Coffey CE. Frontal lobe personality syndromes: ominous sequelae of head trauma. _Postgrad Med._ 1983;73(5):99-106.

50. Posner MI, Peterson SE. The attention system of the human brain. _Annu Rev Neurosci._ 1990;13:25-42.

51. Duchek J. Cognitive dimensions of performance. In: Christiansen C, Baum C, eds. _Occupational Therapy: Overcoming Human Performance Deficits._ Thorofare, NJ: SLACK Incorporated; 1991.

52. Toglia J. A dynamic interactional approach to cognitive rehabilitation. In: Katz N, ed. _Cognitive Rehabilitation: Models For Intervention in Occupational Therapy._ Boston, Mass: Andover Med Pub; 1992.

53. Toglia J. _Attention and Memory. AOTA Self Study Series: Cognitive Rehabilitation._ Bethesda, Md: American Occupational Therapy Association Press; 1994.

54. Uomoto JM. Neuropsychological assessment and rehabilitation after brain injury. In: Craft GH, Berrol S, eds. _Physical Medicine and Rehabilitation Clinics of North America._ Philadelphia, Pa: WB Saunders; 1992.

55. Ponsford JL, Kinsella G. Evaluation of a remedial programme for attentional deficits following closed-head injury. _J Clin Exp Neuropsychol._ 1988;10(6):693-708.

56. Wood RL. Attention disorders in brain injury rehabilitation. _J Learning Disabilities._ 1988;21(6):327-332.

57. Harrell M, Parente R, Bellingrath EG, Liscia KA. _Cognitive Rehabilitation of Memory._ Gaithersburg, Md: Aspen Publishers; 1992.

58. van Zomeren AH, Fasotti L. Impairments of attention in brain-damaged patients. In: von Steinbuchel N, von Cramon DY, Poppel E, eds. _Neuropsychological Rehabilitation._ Berlin: Springer-Verlag; 1992.

59. Cohen RF, Mapou RL. Neuropsychological assessment for treatment planning: a hypothesis-testing approach. _J Head Trauma Rehabil._ 1988;3(1):12-23.

60. Tankle RS. Application of neuropsychological test results to interdisciplinary cognitive rehabilitation with head-injured adults. _J Head Trauma Rehabil._ 1988;3(1):24-32.

61. Piasetsky E, Ben-Yishay Y, Weinberg J. The systematic remediation of specific disorders: selected application of methods derived in a clinical research setting. In: Trexler LE, ed. _Cognitive Rehabilitation Conceptualization and Intervention._ New York, NY: Plenum Press; 1982.

62. Rahami L. The intellectual rehabilitation of brain-damaged patients. _Clin Neuropsychol._ 1982;44:44-45.

63. Wall N, et al. _Hemiplegic Evaluation._ Boston, Mass: Massachusetts Rehabilitation Hospital; 1979.

64. McGlynn SM. Behavioral approaches to neuropsychological rehabilitation. _Psychological Bulletin._ 1990;108(3):420-4410.

65. Parente R. Executive skills training. In: Parente R, Herrmann D, eds. _Retraining Cognition: Techniques and Applications._ Gaithersburg, Md: Aspen Publications; 1996.

66. Whyte J, Polansky M, Fleming M, et al. Sustained arousal and attention after traumatic brain injury. _Neuropsychologia._ 1995;33:797-813.

67. Dougherty PM, Radomski MV. _A Dynamic Assessment Approach for Adults with Brain Injury: The Cognitive Rehabilitation Workbook._ Gaithersburg, Md: Aspen Publishers; 1993.

68. Wood RL. Management of attention disorders following brain injury. In: Wilson BA, Moffat N, eds. _Clinical Management of Attention Disorders Following Brain Injury._ Rockville, Md: Aspen Publisher; 1984.

Resources

Ayres AJ. _Sensory Integration and Learning Disorders._ Los Angeles, Calif: Western Psychological Services; 1980.

Ben-Yishay Y, Rattok I, Ross B. _Working Approaches to Remediation of Cognitive Deficits in Brain-damaged Persons: Rehabilitation Monograph 62._ New York, NY: New York University Medical Center; 1981.

Brown SC, Craik FIM. Encoding and retrieval of information. In: Tulving E, Craik FIM, eds. _The Oxford Handbook of Memory._ New York, NY: Oxford University Press; 2000.

Cabeza R. Functional neuroimaging of episodic memory retrieval. In: Tulving E, ed. *Memory, Consciousness, and the Brain.* Ann Arbor, Mich: Psychology Press; 2000.

Chronister K. The Missing link in fall-prevention programs. *OT Practice.* 2004;9:11-14.

Cook EA, Thigpen R. Identification and management of cognitive perceptual deficits in the rehabilitation patient. *Rehabil Nurs.* 1993;18(5):3110-3113.

Corbetta M. Functional anatomy of visual attention in the human brain: studies with positron emission tomography. In: Parasuraman R, ed. *The Attentive Brain.* Cambridge, Mass: MIT Press; 1998.

Craik F, Kester JD. Divided attention and memory: impairment of processing or consolidation? In: Tulving E, ed. *Memory, Consciousness and the Brain.* Ann Arbor, Mich: Psychology Press; 2000.

Crawford JR, Sommerville J, Robertson IH. Assessing the reliability and abnormality of subtest differences on the Test of Everyday Attention. *Brit J Clin Psychol.* 1997;36(Pt 4):609-617.

Daffner K, Mesulam MM, Holcomb PJ, et al. Disruption of attention to novel events after frontal lobe injury in humans. *J Neurol Neurosurg Psychiatry.* 2000;68(1):18-24.

Daffner KR, Mesulam MM, Scinto LF, et al. The central role of the prefrontal cortex in directing attention to novel events. *Brain.* 2000;123(Pt 5):927-939.

Devinsky O, D'Esposito M. Memory and memory disorders. In: *Neurology of Cognitive and Behavioral Disorders.* New York, NY: Oxford University Press; 2004.

Diller L, Weinberg J. Differential aspects of attention in brain-damaged persons. *Percept Motor Skills.* 1972;35(1):71-81.

Dimitrov M, Granetz J, Peterson M, et al. Associative learning impairments in patients with frontal lobe damage. *Brain Cogn.* 1999;41(2):213-230.

Grey JM. The remediation of attentional disorders following brain injury of acute onset. In: Wood RL, Fussey I, eds. *Cognitive Rehabilitation in Perspective.* London, England: Taylor & Frances; 1990.

Houghton G, Tipper SP, Weaver B, Shore DI. Inhibition and interference in selective attention: some tests of a neural network model. *Visual Cogn.* 1996;3:119-164.

Itzkovich M, Elazar B, Averbuch S. *Lowenstein: Occupational Therapy Cognitive Assessment (LOTCA) Manual.* Pequannock, NJ: Maddack Inc; 1990.

Katz DL, Mills VM. Traumatic brain injury: natural history and efficacy of cognitive rehabilitation. In: Stuss DT, Robertson IH, eds. *Cognitive Neurorehabilitation.* New York, NY: Cambridge University Press; 1999.

Kolb B, Gibb R. Frontal lobe plasticity and behavior. In: Stuss D, Knight R, ed. *Principles of Frontal Lobe Function.* New York, NY: Oxford University Press; 2002.

Lezak M. *Neuropsychological Assessment.* New York, NY: Oxford University Press; 1983.

Luria AR. *Higher Cortical Functions in Man.* 2nd ed. New York, NY: Basic Books, Inc; 1980.

Raskin SA. Memory. In: Raskin SA, Mateer CA, eds. *Neuropsychological Management of Mild Traumatic Brain Injury.* New York, NY: Oxford University Press; 2000.

Robertson I, Ridgeway V, Greenfield E, Parr A. Motor recovery after stroke depends on intact sustained attention: a 2-year follow-up study. *Neuropsychology.* 1997;11(2):290-295.

Roediger HL. Why retrieval is the key process in understanding memory. In: Tulving E, ed. *Memory, Consciousness and the Brain.* Ann Arbor, Mich: Psychology Press; 2000.

Schwartz SM. Adults with traumatic brain injury: three case studies of cognitive rehabilitation in the home setting. *Am J Occup Ther.* 1995;49(7):655-667.

Shiffman LM. Cerebrovascular accident. In: Early MB, ed. *Physical Dysfunction Practice Skills for the Occupational Therapy Assistant.* St. Louis, Mo: Mosby Year-Book, Inc; 1998.

Toglia J. A dynamic interactional approach to cognitive rehabilitation. In: Katz N, ed. *Cognition and Occupation Across The Life Span.* Bethesda, Md: American Occupational Therapy Association Press; 2005.

Toglia J. Approaches to cognitive assessment of the brain-injured adult: traditional methods and dynamic investigation. *Occup Ther Pract.* 1989;1(1):36-57.

Warren M. *Brain Injury Visual Assessment Battery For Adults (biVABA).* Birmingham, Ala: VisAbilities Rehab Services, Inc; 1990.

Wilson BA, Emslie HC, Quirk K, Evans JJ. Reducing everyday memory and planning problems by means of a paging system: a randomized control crossover study. *J Neurol Neurosurg Psychiatry.* 2001;70(4):477-482.

CHAPTER 9

MEMORY

Memory

Memory is not a simple function but one that relates to learning and how we perceive our world. It involves the process by which an individual encodes, stores, and retrieves information.[1] Whenever we try to remember something, we are involving many other cognitive skills.[2,3] For example, if an individual has difficulty with sustained attention, he or she will likely have memory problems as well. Personality, awareness, motivation, anxiety, depression, and lifestyle all may affect an individual's memory status and how any problems are subsequently dealt with in his or her daily life.[4,5] In addition, an individual's mood or level of motivation will affect the quality of new learning.[4] Memory is essentially perception that has been stored at an earlier time and can then be brought forward. Memory processes organize what is perceived for later retrieval.[6]

Many everyday tasks are accomplished through the retrieval of relatively standardized schema.[7] Memories are associative and are defined by networks of interconnected cortical neurons.[8] Memory has both structure and process components, which are defined by Lou et al as follows[6]:

> *The structure component is our memory store and includes what we refer to as short, long and sensory memory. The process of memory involves reproducing or recalling what has been learned, particularly through the use of associative mechanisms.*

No matter what definition one utilizes for memory, the underlying concept that it includes permanent change in the central nervous system (CNS), which can later be reproduced, appears to be universally accepted.[9] The constant interaction between an individual and the environment elicits memories, which can be retrieved in an exact or equivalent form.[9] Memory requires input from the environment (both internal and external), change within the CNS, maintenance of that change, and an output (behavioral or information) that somehow consistently relates to the input.[9]

SENSORY, PERCEPTUAL, AND WORKING MEMORY

The memory process begins with the input of sensations. The individual selectively attends to the environment depending on his or her interests at the time of a given sensory input from the environment. This process of sensory memory, which is the first phase of an individual's information processing, has the capability to process enormous amounts of information for brief duration.[4] Sensory memory is generally broken down into iconic or sensory visions and echoic or auditory sensory memory.[4] Sensory memory is very short-term memory, is modality specific, and either is transferred for further analysis or it degenerates.[6] Fuster places sensory memory at the base of a hierarchy of perceptual memory.[8] He hypothesizes that perceptual memory is acquired through the senses and comprises all that is commonly understood as personal memory.[8] The hierarchy of memory is conceptualized with the memories of elementary sensations at the bottom and the top as being comprised of abstract concepts that, though originally acquired by sensory experience, have become independent from these experiences in cognitive operations.[8] Whether one accepts the concept of a perceptual memory hierarchy or not, it is generally accepted that if information is distorted at this first stage of processing, then the encoding process in all other areas of memory will be adversely affected.[4]

The process continues from sensory memory to working memory. Some define working memory as a temporary storage and manipulation of information.[8,10] It allows for the temporary activation of data or information for quick retrieval and manipulation.[11] Working memory is the short-term storage of information that is not accessible in the environment and the process that keeps this information active for use at a later time.[12] Fletcher and Henson describe working memory as a "mental workspace" that manipulates information for complex problem solving.[13] Working memory is the ability to hold information, internalize it, and use it to guide what we do.[14] It is involved in the processing of information during the carrying out of a wide variety of daily tasks.[10]

Working memory can deal with approximately seven pieces of information at a time and is considered part of a control mechanism for higher intellectual processing and functions.[4,15-17] Microelectrode research has indicated that working memory consists of a temporary activation, for prospective action, of a wide cortical network for long-term memory.[8] In working memory, the prefrontal cortex cooperates not only with subcortical structures, such as the thalamus or basal ganglia, but also works with posterior cortices.[8]

From working memory, items are encoded and consolidated into long-term memory. Consolidation is "…the integration of new memories within the individual's existing cognitive linguistic schema or framework."[3] The consolidation process can take minutes or hours and can be stored in long-term memory—in some cases, for life.[9,15,18] The deeper working memory processes information, the better it is remembered.[4]

Encoding begins with selective attention and is the means by which information is transformed in working memory so that it can be stored efficiently in long-term memory.[4] Encoding, however, requires more than the initial selective attention. The individual must also process information or input at an abstract, schematic, and conceptual level.[19] It is this process that allows subsequent explicit (conscious) retrieval of memory.[13]

The type of rehearsal that occurs during working memory will determine the success of the encoding process. Craik and Kester describe two types of rehearsal: 1) maintenance rehearsal—when information is kept passively in mind (ie, rote repetition) and 2) elaborative rehearsal—when information is meaningfully related to other information presented either previously or currently.[19]

Retrieval is the process of recovering previously encoded information.[19] It is the final aspect of the memory process. It involves "…our ability to access the residue of past experience and (in some cases) convert it into conscious experience."[20] There are two stages of retrieval: 1) the search for available information and 2) the directing of an appropriate verbal or motor response.[21] Iconic retrieval is accomplished through a simple read-out, whereas working memory retrieval is dependent on rehearsal ability.[4] Working memory for purely visual tasks depends on the ability to sustain a visual image and scan it.[4]

Various types of memory play an important role in an individual's ability to function and communicate successfully.[22] The client with acquired brain injury (ABI) may have any aspect or type of memory impaired. The clinician, therefore, should have an understanding of the types of memory that exist. In addition to sensory, perceptual, and working memory, just described, an individual possesses implicit and explicit memory, declarative and nondeclarative (procedural) memory, prospective memory, semantic and episodic memory, and long-term memory. These categories of memory are subsequently described.

IMPLICIT AND EXPLICIT MEMORY

It is now generally accepted that an individual possesses both implicit and explicit memory and that they can be clearly dissociated.[23-26] In addition, in a meta-analysis of 36 studies of clients with memory loss, it was demonstrated that amnesiacs can have impaired implicit memory for novel events but preserved implicit memory for familiar information.[24] Explicit memory consists of information which can be consciously declared to have been learned or experienced.[23] For the client to demonstrate explicit memory, he or she must have "...explicit access to the learning experience and is aware of previous encounters with a particular set of stimuli."[25]

Implicit memory involves information whose learning is only reflected by changes in future behavior as a result of the prior experience without the client consciously remembering the experience itself.[23] The client does not need to be aware of the changes in performance that came about through a prior experience in order to have implicit memory.[25] In other words, explicit memory tasks require conscious awareness of a prior experience, whereas implicit memory tasks do not.[26]

DECLARATIVE AND NONDECLARATIVE (PROCEDURAL) MEMORY

Declarative memory enables conscious recollection of past facts and events.[1,27] Some differentiate between memory of nonpersonal events (declarative) and personal events (episodic).[28] Others define declarative memory to include episodic (events) and semantic (facts).[12,29]

Nondeclarative memory, often called procedural memory, involves nonconscious memory ability.[1,6] It refers to the information that is learned or acquired during the development of skill learning (motor skills, perceptual skills, and cognitive skills).[1,8,12]

The information related to nondeclarative memory involves a "...mixed group of abilities whereby experience alters behavior unconsciously, without providing access to any memory context."[1] Procedural memories can be motor skills or mental procedures such as performing complex math problems.[12]

PROSPECTIVE MEMORY

Prospective memory is remembering to complete an activity or carry out a task at a time in the future.[30-33] It involves remembering what one intends to do as well as remembering the context of a given task.[34-36] Prospective memory allows an individual to carry out an intended action in the future without performing continuous rehearsal of the intention until the appropriate time has occurred.[34] McDaniel et al identify two types of prospective memory: 1) event-based prospective memory—when some environmental event signals the appropriateness of the intended action (ie, giving a friend a message when you see her) and 2) time-based prospective memory—when a particular time or a particular amount of elapsed time signals the appropriateness of the intended action (ie, a 3:00 PM doctor's appointment).[37] Examples of prospective memory include activities such as remembering to buy bread when you pass the store on the way home, remembering to take medications, or remembering to make a phone call.[36,37]

SEMANTIC AND EPISODIC MEMORY

Semantic and episodic memory have many similarities. For example, the way in which information is registered in the episodic and semantic systems is similar.[38] Both depend on limbic system structures for encoding and consolidation,[39] and both appear to depend on neocortical areas of the frontal and temporal lobes for their retrieval.[39] Episodic and semantic memory both help an individual gain factual information through different sensory modalities and are capable of achieving this gain very rapidly.[38] Despite these similarities, many believe they are basically different and should, therefore, stand on their own as separate entities.[23,28,38]

Semantic memory involves general facts or knowledge about the world.[23] These facts can relate to memory for people or memory for events.[28] As Kapur states, the range of personal semantic memory can include basic autobiographical knowledge expressed in verbal form (name, age, family, schooling, etc) or a nonverbal form (ie, ability to recognize as familiar and to name the faces of family members).[28] With semantic memory, it is possible for an individual to know that he or she personally witnessed an event without actually consciously remembering the event.[38] In other words, semantic memory, in fact, is not dependent on episodic memory. Episodic memory, however, is dependent on semantic memory.[28]

Episodic memory consists of knowledge of a previously experienced event along with the awareness or understanding that the event occurred in his or her past.[12,40,41] It involves personal knowledge and can involve an autobiographical recollection of experiences.[23] It is memory for an item or event along with the spatiotemporal context in which the item was studied or an event occurred.[43] Episodic memory allows an individual to mentally travel back in time.[38,41,42] It allows the individual to re-experience events that occurred minutes ago or decades ago.[44] Some believe that the development of episodic memory depends on the acquisition of a specific kind of temporal understanding (ie, understanding and possessing the concept of particular past times).[42]

LONG-TERM MEMORY

When incoming information goes through the consolidation process previously described, that information is subsequently stored in a variety of long-term retention systems.[23] These long-term memory systems can hold an unlimited amount of information in a permanent state for hours or years.[30] It is hypothesized that different information is stored in different ways, and the system allows an individual to search only parts of this complex and vast system depending on what information he or she is trying to retrieve.[6] Fuster describes the retrieval process of long-term memory as follows[8]:

> *At any time in our daily life, the bulk of our long-term memory is dormant and out of consciousness. Presumably, the neuronal aggregates of its networks are relatively inactive. A network is reactivated when the memory it represents is retrieved by the association processes of recall or recognition. An internal or external stimulus, whose cortical representation is part of the network by prior association, will reactivate that representation and, again by association, the rest of the network. Neither the stimuli nor the activated memory need be conscious.*

Recent research supports the concept that there are two broad categories of long-term memory, which are each hierarchically organized.[8] These two categories are perceptual and executive long-term memory.[45]

Recent neuroimaging studies have begun to delineate some of the areas associated with various types of memory and stages in the memory process. PET studies indicate that networks of distributed brain regions subserve episodic and semantic memory.[32] PET studies conducted by

Wiggs et al indicated that semantic memory tasks activated the left temporal and left frontal brain regions whereas episodic memory tasks activated the medial parietal cortex, retrosplenial cortex, and the thalamus.[46] fMRI studies of normals and those with amnesia suggest the existence of the following memory system[46]:

> *These studies suggest the existence of a memory system centered in the medial temporal and frontal lobes that is dedicated to the storage and retrieval of episodes and several neocortical memory systems that are dedicated to the processing and representation of perceptual and semantic information.*

PET and fMRI studies have, in fact, consistently demonstrated activation of the frontal cortex in a number of memory tasks.[13] For example, the left frontal cortex has been associated with incidental and intentional encoding tasks.[13] Moscovitch and Winocur note that the frontal lobe uses established memories to direct other activities such as learning, problem solving, or planning.[47] Prospective memory, working memory, and episodic memory all have been associated with prefrontal systems.[37,48,49]

Neuroimaging studies have also identified subcortical structures associated with some memory functions. Procedural learning, for example, is associated with subcortical structures and spared in cases of cortically based memory impairment.[14] The hippocampus is involved in the conscious recall of events and seems to play an important role in the formation of memory networks in the association cortex.[8,50] Damage to the hippocampal system, in fact, causes deficits in the formation and retrieval of memories in virtually all explicit memory tasks.[26]

It is apparent that the memory process requires overlapping and widely distributed systems. Fuster provides the following example, which illustrates this interconnection[8]:

> *My memory of the sight and sounds of San Francisco's cable car (sensory memory) is associated with the memory of my last visit to that city (episodic memory), with the meaning of the term 'cable car' (semantic memory), and with the concept of public transportation (conceptual memory).*

The client with ABI can have any aspect of impaired memory. Even those classified as having a mild traumatic brain injury (TBI) are shown to have impaired working memory processes.[51] Memory loss, in fact, has been well documented as one of the most common sequelae of ABI.[52-55] Research has also shown that these memory deficits persist for a large number of clients a year or more after a stroke; however, the incidence may be lower than during the more acute stage.[56] The client with ABI can have any aspect of impaired memory. Memory loss can be general or relate to specific types of coded information, and any sense or combination of senses can elicit a recollection.[4,17,57,58] Wilson outlines the following common characteristics of memory loss after ABI[59]:

- Difficulty learning and remembering new information
- Immediate memory is usually normal or almost normal
- Problems arise after delay or distraction
- Frequently, there is retrograde amnesia (loss of memory for events before the ABI)

The nature of the deficit depends on the extent and location of cortical and/or subcortical damage.[12] Memory loss associated with ABI can significantly affect occupational performance. Deficits in memory processing, storage, and retrieval will affect client insight, awareness and motivation.[6] They can affect the client's ability to follow a conversation, plan activities, travel independently, and initiate use of compensatory strategies or perform activities of daily living (ADLs).[53] As Wilson states, "…if a memory impaired person tries to return to a former lifestyle, there will certainly be a mismatch between the present impoverished level of memory functioning and the demands of everyday life."[59]

EVALUATION OF MEMORY

Test 1 – Rivermead Behavioral Memory Test, Second Edition[60]

Description

This is a test of everyday memory functioning. Test items involve either remembering to carry out some everyday task or retaining the type of information needed for adequate everyday functioning. There are four parallel versions of the test, which negates any practice effect due to repeated testing. Items are presented in sequences so that early items can be recalled by the client later in testing.

Scoring

There are two scoring systems for the Rivermead Behavior Memory Test, Second Edition (RBMT-II): screening score and standardized profile score. For the screening score, each item is scored pass (1) or fail (0), with a total possible score of 12. The cut off point is three or more failures (ie, a score of 9 or less on the RBMT–II screening score is impaired).

The standardized profile score is described in the test manual.

Procedure

The following are examples of test items of version A of the RBMT-II.[60]*

Items 1 and 2—First and second name

The subject is shown a photographic portrait and asked to remember the first and second name of the person in the photograph:

> "What I want you to do is to remember this person's name (show photograph). Her name is Catherine Taylor. Can you repeat the name? Later on, I am going to ask you what her name is."

The photograph is then placed face downwards on the table.

Item 3 – Appointment

The alarm is set for 20 minutes, and the subject is required to ask a particular question relating to the near future, when the alarm sounds:

> "I am going to set this alarm to go off in 20 minutes." (Demonstrate alarm and set.) "When it rings, I want you to ask me about your next appointment. Say something like, 'Can you tell me when I have to see you again?,' or words to that effect."

Validity

1. The test was give to clients with brain damage and controls, with the clients having substantially lower scores than the control subjects.

---

*Reprinted with permission from Thames Valley Test Co, reference 60: Wilson B, Cockburn J, Baddeley AD, et al. The Rivermead Behavioral Memory Test. 2nd ed. Bury St. Edmunds: Thames Valley Test Co; 2003.

2. Performance on the RBMT-II was correlated with performance on a number of standard memory tests.*

Reliability

Inter-rater reliability was established with 40 subjects and 2 raters with 100% agreement between both raters. Parallel-form reliability was established by giving two versions of the test to 118 clients. The correlation between the two scores was 0.78 for the screening score and 0.85 for the profile score.

Rivermead Behavioral Memory Test – Extended

There is now an extended version of the Rivermead Behavioral Memory Test (RBMT-E), which is designed to assess subtle impairments of everyday memory performance.[61] This test has also been adapted for clients with restricted mobility.[62]

Rivermead Behavioral Memory Test[63]

Description

A shortened version of the Rivermead Behavioral Memory Test (RBMT) was used with 176 adults with ABI and shown to be sensitive to memory deficits and the effects of dysphagia. A subscale consisting of the following items was generated: remembering a belonging or an appointment, remembering a route around the room either immediately or after a delay, remembering to deliver a message, recognizing pictures of faces, and knowing the date.

Reliability

Standard profile scores with the full and abbreviated tests were compared for 135 clients with no language loss to determine the extent to which the two scales placed them in the same category of memory function. Cut-off points had been derived from the percentile distribution of client and control subjects.[64] Results indicated that 102 (75%) nonlanguage impaired clients fell into the same category whichever scale was used. Thirty of the 33 clients who fell into either a higher or lower category if the abbreviated scale was used were on the borderline.

Test 2 – Autobiographical Memory Interview[65]**

Description

The Autobiographical Memory Interview (AMI) Test provides an assessment of the client's personal remote memory, including identifying the pattern of any deficit and its temporal gradient. Test items require the client to recall facts from his past life relating to childhood, early adult life, and more recent facts. Each subtest is scored out of 21 points.

Procedure

The following items are examples from each section of the overall test battery.

Section A – Childhood (Period Before School)

Personal semantic questions:

• Ask the subject for the address where he or she was living before going to school.

Additional areas were examined, such as sex differences, intelligence, age, etiology, aphasia, and perceptual problems. Detailed results of these studies are contained in the test manual supplements 2 and 3.[60] A study of 119 ABI clients supported the RBMT as superior to traditional memory tests such as the Wescher Memory Scale Revised for assessing everyday memory functioning.[53]

**Reprinted with permission from Thames Valley Test Co, reference 65: Kopelman M, Wilson B, Baddeley AD. The Autobiographical Memory Interview. Bury St. Edmonds: Thames Valley Test Co; 1990.*

     2 points—Full address

     1 point—Street and town only

     0.5 points—Town or street only

- Ask the subject the names of three friends or neighbors from the period before the subject went to school.

     1 point—Each surname

     0.5 points—Each if first name only

Section B – Early Adult Life

Personal semantic questions:

- Ask the subject for the name of his or her main secondary (or high) school. If the subject attended several secondary (or high) schools, ask which one was attended when the subject was 13 years old.

     1 point—Correct name

    Note: If the subject only attended one school, it can be scored twice if correct, but separate incidents must be given for primary and secondary schools with a total of six names of friends or teachers.

Second C – Recent Life (Present Hospital or Institution)

Personal or semantic questions:

    Note: It is expected that most subjects will be seen in a hospital or institution (eg, a research institute). However, if the subject is being seen in another location (eg, own home), the questions should be rephrased to accommodate this.

- Ask the subject for the name of the hospital or place (eg, institution) where he or she is currently being seen.

     1 point—Correct name of the hospital or institution

Scoring

Scoring is computed by a "cut off," which is related to the number of standard deviations from the norm. Cut-off scores are described in the test manual.

Validity

1. Examines how well the test discriminated between amnesic clients and healthy controls
2. Examines the intercorrelation among different remote memory tasks in the total client group
3. Compares the pattern of temporal gradients across different tests of remote memory
4. Checks the authenticity of the memories produced

Reliability

Inter-rater reliability was established with three raters with correlations between 0.83 and 0.86.

Test 3 – The Subjective Memory Questionnaire[66]

Description

This self-report scale consists of 43 items relating to everyday life. These items cover areas such as people's names, facts about people, film titles, jokes, and directions to get somewhere.

Scoring

Two different 5-point rating scales are utilized. The first 36 items are answered on a "very good" to "very bad" scale. Items 37 to 43 are temporal and are answered on a "very rarely" to "very often" scale.

Validity

To improve validity, rule out attentional and language related problems as causes of poor performance.

Reliability

Test-retest reliability has been established (p < 0.001) on this questionnaire.[66] Item correlation also indicated "high positive item to test correlations."[66]

Test 4 – Self-Report Memory Questionnaire[54]

Description

A memory questionnaire was developed from a review of existing self-report questionnaires (Table 9-1).

Scoring

A score for memory problems and a score for strategy use is generated by using a 5-point scale for each item.

Validity/Reliability

The memory items chosen represented the broad areas covered by three established questionnaires (the Cognitive Failures Questionnaire,[67] Subjective Memory Questionnaire,[66] and the Inventory of Everyday Memory Experiences[68]).

The selection of specific items was based on their reported high factor loadings and item reliabilities.

Test 5 – Clinical Observation and Activity Analysis

General Guidelines for Evaluation

1. Identify the aspects of memory that are impaired and those that are relatively intact.
2. Observe the client in a number of settings.
3. Consider the amount of structure versus nonstructure within the environment.
4. Consider the time interval between stimulus and recall (ie, immediate, short-term, and long-term).
5. Establish functional baseline measures. Consider the frequency and severity of the problem as it relates to function. Select relevant functional areas or tasks as the basis for evaluation and reassessment.

Specific Areas and Questions to Consider and Evaluate

1. Which sensory system is affected? For instance, immediate recall can be tested for different sensory systems as follows[69-71]:
    a) *Visual*—The client is asked to reproduce simple geometric figures, which are presented for 5 to 10 seconds and then covered.[69-71] Note: If a person's perceptual abilities are impaired, it is likely that this will affect memory for visual material and the ability to use visually based strategies to assist in memory problems.[72]

Table 9-1

Self Report Memory Questionnaire

AGE:
SEX: M, F

The following questionnaire refers to memory problems that are common to many people. Some, however, occur more frequently for different people. Could you please read each question carefully and tick the response which most accurately shows how frequently such experiences occur in your daily living.

	≥1 time daily	2 to 6 times a week	A few times a month	A few times a year	Never
(1) How often do you forget the names of people minutes after being introduced?					
(2) When calling someone that you regularly call, do you ever have to look up his or her number?					
(3) How often would you fail to remember the address of someone you frequently write to?					
(4) Think of times when someone has given you directions to get to an unfamiliar place. How often do you forget these before you get there?					
(5) When you go out to run a few errands, how often do you forget to do at least one of them?					
(6) How often do you find at the end of a conversation that you forget to bring up a point or question that you had intended to?					
(7) How often are you unable to find something that you put down only minutes ago?					
(8) How often do you discover when you have gone out that you must return for something that you left behind?					
(9) If someone says that they have told you something earlier, how often are you unable to recall them doing so?					
(10) When someone asks you to give a friend a message, how often do you forget to do so?					
(11) How often do you find that when you want to introduce people you know, you can't remember someone's name?					
(12) How often do you forget birthdays or dates when you intended to do something special?					
(13) When you want to remember a story or an experience, how often are you unable to do so?					
(14) If you need to know what the date is, how often do you look it up or ask someone because you can't remember?					
(15) How often do you think of something a person told you but forget who said it?					
(16) Do you ever begin to tell someone a story only to learn that you have already told them?					
(17) If you go to a supermarket to buy 4 to 5 items without a list, how often do you forget at least one item?					
(18) How often do you find that you have failed to button or zip part of your clothing?					
(19) How often do you forget that you have already done something and begin to do it again (eg, set alarm clock)?					

(continued)

Table 9-1 *(continued)*

Self Report Memory Questionnaire

	≥1 time daily	2 to 6 times a week	A few times a month	A few times a year	Never
(20) How often do you make appointments that you later forget to keep?					
(21) Do you ever have trouble remembering the time for a bus or train that you regularly catch?					
(22) How often do you borrow items from others and forget to return them?					
(23) How often are you unable to recall your size for either clothing or shoes?					
(24) How often do you forget the time that daily events occur (eg, TV programs or the mail)?					
Totals	x1	x3	x2	x1	x0

Strategy use

People often use various strategies to assist their memory for everyday information. Please indicate how often you typically make use of each strategy.

	≥1 time daily	2 to 6 times a week	A few times a month	A few times a year	Never
(1) How often do you use a pen and paper to remember any of the items in the memory questions 1 to 24?					
(2) How often do you use a diary or personal organizer to remind you about these items?					
(3) Do you ever ask other people to remind you about the items mentioned?					
(4) Do you ever use strategies such as talking to yourself or thought associations to remember everyday details?					
(5) Please list any other strategies that you use to assist your memory and how often you use them.					
Totals	x4	x3	x2	x1	x0

Score for memory problems _____

Score for strategy use _____

Reprinted with permission from Taylor and Francis, Ltd, reference 54: Ownsworth TL, McFarkand K. Memory remediation in long-term acquired brain injury: two approaches in diary training. Brain Inj. 1999;13:622-623.

   b) *Kinesthetic*—The client is asked to reproduce a series of hand positions presented to him.[72] Note: If the client is apraxic, do not give this test.

   c) *Auditory*—The client is asked to reproduce a series of rhythmic taps.[69] Note: If the client is aphasic, verbal memory and the ability to use verbal memory strategies are likely to be affected.

2. Is nonverbal memory impaired? Verbal memory?

3. Is memory loss global or modality specific?

4. Is it a learning or a performance problem? Can the client improve with practice?

5. Can the client utilize identified strategies for improved memory?

6. Is it a problem of learning new information or recalling old information?

7. Is the client aware of his memory problem?

8. Which memory processes are affected? Does the client have trouble identifying as well as reproducing (recall versus recognition)?

9. Is it a semantic memory loss? Is it episodic?

10. Does the client have difficulty with free recall?

11. Does the client have difficulty with serial learning (ie, remembering sequences)?

12. Does the client have difficulty with paired associated (ie, remembering relationships)?

13. Can the client display temporal organization memory (ie, can he or she judge which stimuli were seen most recently or recreate the order in which stimuli were presented)? Impairment in this area will lead to difficulty in ordering actions in appropriate sequence, which leads to trouble with planning goal directed acts.[14]

14. Does altering the task or environment facilitate recall?

Scoring

Nonstandardized

The previous or similar questions can be incorporated into a checklist (yes/no) or used in conjunction with a frequency rating scale (eg, always/sometimes/rarely/never). These questions or checklists should be used in a variety of environments and tasks. Comparisons of performance can then be made. This information can then be incorporated into the treatment plan.

Validity

To improve validity, rule out perceptual, language, and attentional deficits as causes of poor performance.

DYNAMIC ASSESSMENT

*Test 2 – Contextual Memory Test[30,73,74]**

Description

The Contextual Memory Test (CMT) is intended as a supplement to other measures of memory and cognition. It is designed to objectively measure awareness and strategy use in adults with memory impairment and/or screen clients for memory impairment that may require further testing. Test items are functionally oriented. Areas covered are as follows:

1. *Awareness of memory capacity*—Through general questioning, prediction of memory capacity prior to task performance, and estimation of memory capacity following task performance

2. *Recall of line drawn objects*—Immediate and delayed

3. *Strategy use*—The ability to describe use of strategies and the ability to benefit from a strategy provided by the examiner

---

*The CMT actually has both static and dynamic components. Part I may be used alone to screen individuals for memory impairment and Part II provides a dynamic component to assessment.[74]

Scoring

There are three recall raw scores—immediate, delayed, and total recall—which are converted to standard scores. Prediction scores are generated through comparison with the actual recall score. The estimation score is also calculated through comparison with the actual recall score. Strategy use is examined through the effect of context, the total strategy use, and the order of recall.

Validity

Concurrent validity was determined by examining the correlation between the CMT and RBMT. Correlations ranged from 0.80 to 0.84. The Rasch analysis was used to chart the individual abilities and item difficulties of the controls and brain injury subjects. Results are described in the test manual.

Reliability

Parallel form reliability was conducted with the two forms of the test, with reliability estimates ranging from 0.73 to 0.81. Quasi (partial) test-retest reliability ranged from 0.74 to 0.87 for the control group and from 0.85 to 0.94 for the group with brain injury. The Rasch method was utilized to generate additional reliability measures, which are covered in the test manual. Parallel form reliability for prediction and strategy scores was also generated and described in the test manual.

Norms

Normative data was collected on 1) 375 adults in the New York area ages 18 to 87 with a mean age of 46 and 2) 217 adults in Israel ages 18 to 86.[74]

Note: The immediate recall score of the CMT demonstrated one of the strongest correlations ($r = 0.59$) to instrumental ADL as compared to other standardized cognitive measures.[75]

GENERAL TREATMENT GUIDELINES

1. Client-centered treatment of memory deficits has resulted in the greatest degree of generalization. Target the problems that are real and important in the client's daily life, and be flexible in combining techniques as needed for increased success.[14]

2. Identify the client's learning style. Each client's individual learning style will indicate which treatment strategies are most likely to help the client remember.[76]

3. Research has indicated that pictures are remembered much better than words; therefore, utilize pictures whenever possible to facilitate recall.[19]

4. The client with decreased attention and concentration may not be able to use internal strategies; however, these clients may benefit from strategically placed environmental cues.[76]

5. The client's participation is required for successful integration and use of memory strategies.[55]

6. Domain specific learning should be utilized with the client with diffuse memory loss.[76] Treatment for any client, no matter the severity of the memory deficit, should occur in the most naturalistic environment possible.

7. Clients with memory loss may also have trouble forgetting unnecessary information, creating unnecessary information overload.[6] During treatment, therefore, provide only information that is absolutely necessary for task completion.

8. The technique of errorless learning has been found to be successful for clients with memory loss (especially episodic memory).[5,14,62,77] Errorless learning is the process where the client is prevented from making mistakes during the learning process. In this process, no guessing or trial and error is allowed during the learning process.

9. Family/caregiver education and training is crucial to the success of any intervention for the client with memory deficits. A good working relationship with the family/caregiver will help provide continuity of intervention in the home environment.[78]

10. Intervention strategies should be practiced daily by the staff and family. Coordination of treatment efforts among team members is also crucial for consistency of procedures and opportunities for additional practice.[78]

11. Have the client keep a "Things I Forget List." Review it with the client to parse out what types of information are forgotten. This information can be used to assist in treatment planning. For example, is verbal information forgotten but not visual information; is information forgotten when presented in a distracting environment, when the client is under stress, at the end of the day, etc.[14]

Utilizing a Restorative Approach

There remains controversy among clinicians as to the effectiveness of a restorative treatment approach to memory deficits. Although there appears to be some success in improvement for specific tasks, this does not appear to generalize to other similar tasks or ADLs.[12,55] Some believe restoration of memory function is unlikely and advocate the use of the compensation approach instead.[3,59,60,77] Others believe this approach can be effective within certain guidelines. For example, mnemonics have not been found to be helpful for remembering more than a short list of materials or names; therefore, they should be used with short lists for increased chance of success.[14]

Due to the limited evidence supporting the restorative approach to memory deficits, when using the approach, the therapist should frequently monitor its effectiveness and follow the treatment principles subsequently described.

The following general treatment principles should be applied in the restorative approach to memory deficits:

1. The restoration of short-term memory will have limited effect in early stages of recovery.[4] Attentional processes and sensory memory should be addressed first.

2. Attention training results in improved memory in many clients.[79]

3. Along with attention and concentration, rehearsal is a necessary antecedent of memory retraining.

Attention	$\rightarrow$	Rehearsal
$\downarrow$		$\downarrow$
Can select information to rehearse		Maintains information to encode it and store it in long-term memory

4. The client must relearn rehearsal skills before any other form of working memory training can work. The therapist must evaluate how many rehearsals are required to bring the client's memory to average levels.

5. Teach the client to rehearse information in a manner that will ensure that it transfers to long-term memory so that it can be retrieved later.[4]

6. Effective encoding of information is required for future recall.[79] If the material is well analyzed, recall later will be easier.

7. Identify and characterize the client's preserved memory abilities, and build memory retraining strategies around them.[80]

8. Research has shown that it is possible to teach a client with severe memory loss different kinds of domain specific learning that can be applied to ADLs.[81,82] This is only accomplished if the procedure is consistent, the job is broken down into component steps, and the clients taught each component directly.

9. Organization facilitates recall.[4] The ABI client may lose the ability to organize automatically (refer to section on organization and planning).

10. Straight repetitive drills do not appear to generalize to untrained memory of functional memory outside the clinic.[3,82] Repetition with the use of vanishing cues, however, has been shown to be effective.[83] Computer software with vanishing cues built into the program are especially helpful.

11. Utilize an indirect, direct, or domain-specific approach depending on the client's awareness of memory loss, strategy use, and recall status.[84]

12. A retrieval cue will only be effective if the information in the cue was incorporated in the trace of the target event at the time of the original encoding.[19] For example, if a client first remembered an object by its color and shape, then a cue about its size will not help with recall of the object.

13. Retention after a delay in time is most successful (ie, when rehearsals are spaced out over time rather than massed together in a short period of time).[19]

14. In addition to elaboration and rehearsal, organization (grouping together of items into larger units, usually based on meaningful relationships between items) has been shown to be helpful when learning new information.[19,85]

15. Items should be encoded in terms of 1) item specific features—characteristics that are unique to a particular item, and 2) associative features—characteristics shared with other information presented either concurrently or in the past.[19,85]

Utilizing an Adaptive Approach

Unlike the restorative approach, there has been reported success with memory compensation strategies and the use of procedural learning strategies.[31] For this reason, there has been a shift in the last 10 years from attempts to restore memory function to providing methods to alleviate the consequences of impaired memory.[77] These methods can include internal aids (person related), memory strategies, external aids, and contextual or environmental adaptations. In the following section, examples of each of these methods are described. It is up to the therapist's clinical reasoning to guide decision making as to which method or combination of methods is appropriate for a particular client. The therapist should also keep in mind that some clients will resist the use of compensatory strategies or external aids because they feel it is "cheating" or will slow down or prevent recovery of memory.[59] The therapist should try to persuade the client that by using compensatory techniques as a substitute they are, in fact, being encouraged to engage in normal behavior.[59]

MEMORY STRATEGIES IN TREATMENT

Many mental strategies used in treatment of decreased memory fall under the category of mnemonics. Mnemonics involve the mental manipulation of information and are used to teach the client with memory impaired to organize, store, and retrieve information more efficiently.[5] Wilson provides the following general guidelines for the use of mnemonics with memory impaired clients[59]:

1. Mnemonics are useful for teaching new information. However, most clients with brain injury will not use them spontaneously.

2. Dual coding (ie, using two methods rather than one) will probably result in more efficient learning than the use of one method alone.

3. Information on the component skills of a new task should be taught one step at a time.

4. If visual imagery is employed (ie, transforming a name or word to be learned into a picture, such as remembering Barbara as a barber), it is better for the client with impaired memory to see a drawing of the picture on paper or card rather than to rely on a mental image.

5. Information to be learned should be realistic and relevant to the everyday needs of clients. Thus, it is better to teach people things they really need to know rather than material from a workbook.

6. Individual styles, needs, and preferences should be recognized. Not everyone will benefit from the same strategy.

7. Generalization issues need to be addressed. If a client learns to use a notebook in the department, this does not necessarily mean the book will be used outside the department unless this is specifically taught.

Specific Memory Strategies

Assist the client in developing and effectively utilizing both internal and external memory aids and strategies to compensate for memory loss. The following are examples of strategies and external aids which can be utilized.*

1. *Active listening*—Refer to the section on Treatment of Attention Deficits (page 200).

2. *Note taking*—Use lists, schedules, instructions, and directions.

3. *Audio taping*—This technique is especially useful with clients with poor motor skills, slow information processing, and decreased vision.

4. *Rehearsal*—The more sensory systems used, the more likely the information will be remembered. Use methods which are the client's best methods of encoding. This method is only effective when used in combination with other strategies.

5. *Association*—Two new pieces of information can be associated, or new information can be associated with old information. Associations can be gained from all sensory modalities. An emotional association can also assist in recall.

6. *Pegging*—This technique can be used to assist the client in remembering someone or to assist him in remembering various tasks. An example follows:

   S – shopping

   L – laundry

   E – eat lunch

   E – exercise

   P – pick up children at school

   To remember someone, pick out a key feature to associate with that person and attach a name or object to it. For example, overweight → barrel → Darryl.

   Rhyming mnemonics—A word that rhymes with the word or information to be recalled is utilized (eg, fun-sun, heaven-seven).

7. *PQRST Method*[92]

   Preview—The client skims the material to learn the general content.

   Question—The client asks him- or herself key questions about the content.

15,19,26,38,46,48,58,60,70,72,74,83,84, and 86-107

> *Read*—The client reads the information with the goal of answering the question.
>
> *State*—The client repeats or rehearses the information read.
>
> *Test*—The client tests him- or herself by answering the questions he or she posed previously.

8. *Loci*—The client forms associations between locations and the information to be remembered. The client takes an imaginary walk around his or her favorite room or neighborhood and envisions items to be recalled in various locations (ie, bread on the table, milk on the television, etc).

9. *Chunking and grouping*—This is a way to organize information to be recalled—for example, categories (grouping meat products in a grocery list), object properties (color, size, shape), function (knives in a drawer), and origin (items that grow on trees).

10. *Mental retracing*—Some research has indicated this is the most frequently utilized internal memory strategy by clients.[107]

11. *Visual imagery*—Clients with left hemisphere brain damage may find this to be an effective tool.[4] Research has shown that visual imagery works well when used for the acquisition of specific relevant items of information such as learning the names of new faces.[55]

12. *Story method*—The client forms a story about the words or phrases he or she is to remember.[16]

13. *Self-reference*—The client judges how the material relates to him or her. This has been found to assist retention more than relating it to others.[48]

14. Mnemonic cues plus the use of Polaroid pictures have been used successfully.[78] For example, to remember her physical therapist, a client with ABI used "Heather is healthy" with a photo of her physical therapist. It is interesting to note that this particular client also generalized this technique to remember her neighbor.[78]

15. Some clinicians have found that repeated exposure to the same stimuli eventually shapes the correct response from the client.[108]

16. A research study conducted with two groups of 12 clients with memory impairment demonstrated that the group who received mnemonic-based treatment (verbal elaboration and imagery) did better than the group receiving treatment utilizing the vanishing cues method.[109]

17. Whenever possible, utilize source memory (the ability to recall the time and place when a piece of information was learned) to assist with recall. A parent, for example, may be able to tell when and how the client originally learned how to balance a checkbook or cook a particular recipe. This information can then be used as cues during these activities.

18. Utilize the memory systems that remain intact.[78] For example, visual imagery can be utilized to overcome a verbal memory deficit.[55]

EXTERNAL AIDS

General principles of effective external cuing include the following:

1. Give the cuing as close as possible to the time the action is required.

2. Make it active.

3. Be specific about what is required.

4. Retrieval cues that are similar to the ones used in the original learning process can be especially helpful to recall.

5. Questioning the client during presentation appears to assist in retention.

6. If using a device:

   a) Make it portable. The device should be able to store as many cues as possible.

   b) It should have as wide a time range as possible.

   c) It should be easy to use and not be dependent on any other instrument.

   d) Training for the use of an external memory device should include the following[100]:

      • *Acquisition*—How to use the device

      • *Application*—When and where to use the device

      • *Adaptation*—Learning to use the device in novel situations

Harrell et al offer an eight-step treatment model for the application of strategies and aids as well as memory retraining tasks as follows[93]:

1. Select a task or strategy:

   a) Choose one for which the client can experience success.

   b) Follow a hierarchy of skills (ie, attention and concentration before recall of information).

   c) Make the task relevant to the client's life (ie, age, interest, etc).

   d) Make tasks measurable (ie, time to complete, percentage or number completed, number of strategies used, etc).

2. Measure the client's performance without any assistance give.

3. Set relevant goals, with the client if possible. Identify both short and long-term goals.

4. Choose and teach a strategy or way to approach the task. Use a strategy that is most applicable to the client's real world.

5. Provide the client with opportunities to practice new learning on a regular basis until the strategy is overlearned.

6. When the client has mastered the strategy, or plateaued, decide if the goal has been reached or needs to be altered.

7. Practice transfer and generalization in a hierarchical manner as follows:

   a) Transfer to a different task in therapy.

   b) Transfer to the next therapy session.

   c) Transfer to a different type of therapy or situation.

   d) Generalize to the real world.

8. Practice the strategy in different settings, especially real world settings.

The following is an example of how to apply this model to a specific recall task.[93]

Task: Immediate Recall of Short Articles

Description

The client and therapist choose a short article to read. Each presentation increases in length (eg, from 2 to 20 paragraphs), each article being exposed for the same length of time (eg, 3 to 5 minutes). After presentation, the client can respond by writing, pointing, or reciting orally.

Materials

Therapists can use articles from magazines, newspapers, short stories, books, essays, poems, and so forth.

Scoring

Percentage of information remembered from the article.

Baseline

Highest percentage of material recalled from the article.

Strategies

Chunking, highlighting, note taking, outlining, reading aloud (and audio taping for repetition).

Variations

* Types of articles can be varied from concrete to abstract, from old information that the client already knows to entirely new information, and so forth.

* This can be used as a recognition task by giving the client multiple-choice questions to answer at the end; the client can also recall information independent of cues.

* The task can be used for delayed recall by asking the client to remember information several minutes, days, or weeks later.

* Scoring can be done with the highest percentage of information recalled.

Generalizations

Manuals (car, appliances, computer), speeches, and materials for class or work

Specific External Aids

The client with ABI will generally not use external aids spontaneously. To be successful the client must be trained in their use and provided with a variety of opportunities and contexts to practice use:

1. *Datebook*—The type that has specific times to schedule activities is recommended.[14] The client can schedule a specific day and time for activities such as grocery shopping, leisure activities, or studying.

2. *Memory notebook*—Expanded from a basic datebook. The contents can be flexible depending on the client's needs. Potential sections might include orientation, transportation, things to do, feelings log, etc.[55]

3. For cooking tasks, step by step directions in a checklist format can be generated for the client. The client can check each subtask as he or she performs it. The client should be trained in the use of the checklist before discharge.

4. Parente and Herrmann advocate the use of items such as the following aids to facilitate independence in ADLs for the client with memory impairment[85]:

    * *Car finders*—A device that blinks lights or honks horn when activated by device on user's keychain

    * *Key finders*—Device can be attached to keychain and other important objects that have an auditory alarm or signal that can be activated by hand clapping, etc.

- *Smart irons*—Irons that have an automatic shut off switch activated when the iron remains flat and motionless for 30 seconds. These can be purchased at most department stores.

- *Dialing phones*—Provide single button dialing. Stores several phone numbers that can be retrieved and dialed automatically by pushing a single button that corresponds to a person's name. The therapist should work with the client to identify what numbers he or she wants programmed.

- *Digital recorders*—Better than tape recorders because the numbers mark the messages; useful for making to-do lists as the client can delete each message as he or she completes the item to do.

- *Personal data storage devices (PDA)*—For example, Texas Instruments (Dallas, Tex), Casio (Tokyo, Japan), and RadioShack (Fortworth, Tex) all make inexpensive ones. (Refer to Chapter 13 for more detailed information on PDAs.)

- *Telememo watches*—For example, Seiko (Mahwah, NJ) and Casio can store up to 50 phone numbers, names, dates, and times of appointments.

5. Use of palmtop computers has been found to be effective in assisting clients with impaired memory.[110] In a study of 12 ABI clients, 9 clients found them useful and 7 out of these 9 clients continued their use after the trial ended at 2 months, 4 months, and 4-year follow up.[110] Clinical observation during the study also indicated palmtop computer use decreased client anxiety, increased self-esteem, and facilitated improvement in role performance.[110]

6. Wilson describes the use of "Interactive Task Guidance Systems," which provide a set of cues to guide clients through sequential steps of an everyday task such as cooking or cleaning.[5] The microcomputer acts as a compensatory device, giving step by step directions.[5]

7. One recently developed product that has shown great promise for use with the ABI client is the Neuropage.[5-111] This device is especially effective for clients who have difficulty with external aids because they forget to use them, cannot program them, use them unsystematically, or are embarrassed by them.[111] This is due to the design of the pager system, which is described as follows[111]:

This system uses an arrangement of microcomputers linked to a conventional computer memory and, by telephone, to a paging company. The scheduling of reminders or cues for each person is entered into the computer, and from then on, no further human interfacing is necessary. On the appropriate date and time, Neuropage accesses the user's date files, determines the reminder to be delivered, and transmits the information.

Environmental Adaptations and Cues

1. Keys can be color coded with matching colors on locks.[14]

2. Have the client keep a central location for a family communication board, keys, wallet etc.[14]

3. Have the client utilize a 7-day medication organizer.[112]

4. Have the client utilize cookers, lights, etc, which turn themselves off after certain intervals. For example, use slow cookers.[5]

5. Label doors with pictures of what is inside the room.[14] Label drawers, cabinets, and closets as needed.[5,59]

6. Place important items where they cannot be missed (ie, neckcord for glasses, notebook on belt, briefcase by front door, etc).[5]

7. Utilize colored burner covers and coordinating stickers to cue the client as to which burner he or she will be turning on.[14]

8. Place a reminder list inside the front door (ie, what to bring, safety checklist before leaving, etc).[14]

Note: Environmental adaptations and external aids alone are not always going to be enough. For example, in social situations, the client cannot bring a memory book to remember someone's name to greet them.[5]

References

1. Giuffrida C, Neistadt M. Overview of learning theory. In: Crepeau E, Cohn ES, Schell BAB, eds. *Willard and Spackman's Occupational Therapy*. Philadelphia, Pa: Lippincott, Williams and Wilkins; 2003.
2. Averbach S, Katz N. Cognitive rehabilitation: a retraining model for clients with neurological disabilities. In: Katz N, ed. *Cognition and Occupation Across the Live Span*. Bethesda, Md: American Occupational Therapy Association Press; 2005.
3. Sohlberg MM, Mateer CA. *Introduction To Cognitive Rehabilitation: Theory and Practice*. New York, NY: The Guilford Press; 1989.
4. Parente R, Anderson J. *Retraining Memory: Techniques and Applications*. Houston, Tex: CSY Publishing; 1991.
5. Wilson B. Memory rehabilitation in brain injured people. In: Stuss DT, Robertson IH, eds. *Cognitive Neurorehabilitation*. New York, NY: Cambridge University Press; 1999.
6. Lou JQ, Lane SJ. Personal performance capabilities and their impact on occupational performance. In: Christiansen CH, Baum CM, eds. *Occupational Therapy: Performance, Participation and Well-Being*. Thorofare, NJ: SLACK Incorporated; 2005.
7. Forde EME, Humphreys GW. The role of semantic knowledge and working memory in everyday tasks. *Brain Cogn*. 2000;44:214-252.
8. Fuster JM. Network memory. *Ann Rev Psychol*. 1998;49:451-459.
9. Filskov S, Boll T. *Handbook of Clinical Neuropsychology*. New York, NY: John Wiley & Sons, Inc; 1981.
10. Logie RH. *Visuo-Spatial Working Memory*. Hillsdale, NJ: Lawrence Erlbaum Assoc; 1995.
11. Grafman J. The structured event complex and the human prefrontal cortex. In: Stuss D, Knight R. *Principles of Frontal Lobe Function*. New York, NY: Oxford University Press; 2002.
12. Devinsky O, D'Esposito M. Memory and memory disorders. In: *Neurology of Cognitive and Behavioral Disorders*. New York, NY: Oxford University Press; 2004.
13. Fletcher PC, Henson RNA. Frontal lobes and human memory: insights from functional neuroimaging. *Brain*. 2001;124:849-881.
14. Raskin SA. Memory. In: Raskin SA, Mateer CA, eds. *Neuropsychological Management of Mild Traumatic Brain Injury*. New York, NY: Oxford University Press; 2000.
15. Baddeley AD. Memory theory and memory therapy. In: Wilson BA, Moffat N, eds. *Clinical Management of Memory Problems*. Gaithersburg, Md: Aspen Publishers; 1984.
16. Gathsercole SE, Baddeley AD. *Working Memory and Language*. Mahwah, NJ: Lawrence Erlbaum Assoc; 1993.
17. Parker RS. *Traumatic Brain Injury and Neuropsychological Impairment*. New York, NY: Springer Verlag; 1990.
18. Luria AR. *Higher Cortical Functions in Man*. 2nd ed. New York, NY: Basic Books, Inc; 1980.
19. Craik F, Kester JD. Divided attention and memory: impairment of processing or consolidation? In: Tulving E, ed. *Memory, Consciousness and the Brain*. Ann Arbor, Mich: Psychology Press; 2000.
20. Roediger HL. Why retrieval is the key process in understanding memory. In: Tulving E, ed. *Memory, Consciousness and the Brain*. Ann Arbor, Mich: Psychology Press; 2000.
21. Sandler AB, Harris JL. Use of external memory aids with a head-injured patient. *Am J Occup Ther*. 1992; 46(2):163-1662.
22. Adamovich BLB. Cognition, language, attention and information processing following closed head injury. In: Kreutzer JS, Wehman PH, eds. *Cognitive Rehabilitation For Persons with Traumatic Brain Injury: A Functional Approach*. Baltimore, Md: Paul H Books Pub; 1991.

23. Constantinidou F, Thomas RD, Best P. Principles of cognitive rehabilitation: an integrative approach. In: Ashley MJ, ed. *Traumatic Brain Injury: Rehabilitative Treatment and Case Management.* 2nd ed. Boca Raton, Fla: CRC Press; 2004.

24. Gooding PA, Mayes AR, van Eijk R. A meta-analysis of indirect memory tests for novel material in organic amnesics. *Neuropsychologia.* 2000;38(5):666-676.

25. Hazeltine S, Grafton ST, Ivry R. Attention and stimulus characteristics determine the locus of motor-sequence encoding. A PET study. *Brain.* 1997;120(Pt 1):123-140.

26. Verfaellie M, Keane MM. The neural basis of aware and unaware forms of memory. *Semin Neurol.* 1997; 17(2):153-161.

27. Hamann SB, Squire LR. Intact perceptual memory in the absence of conscious memory. *Behav Neurosci.* 1997;111(4):850-851.

28. Kapur N. Syndromes of retrograde amnesia: a conceptual and empirical synthesis. *Psychol Bull.* 1999; 125(6):800-825.

29. Gabrieli JDE. Cognitive neuroscience of human memory. *Ann Rev Psychol.* 1998;49:87-115.

30. Golisz K, Toglia J. Perception and cognition. In: Crepeau E, Cohn ES, Schell BAB, eds. *Willard and Spackman's Occupational Therapy.* Philadelphia, Pa: Lippincott, Williams and Wilkins; 2003.

31. Katz DL, Mills VM. Traumatic brain injury: natural history and efficacy of cognitive rehabilitation. In: Stuss DT, Robertson IH, eds. *Cognitive Neurorehabilitation.* New York, NY: Cambridge University Press; 1999.

32. Nyberg L, McIntosh AR, Tulving E. Functional brain imaging of episodic and semantic memory with positron emission tomography. *J Mol Med.* 1998;76(1):48-53.

33. Zola SM. Memory, amnesia, and the issue of recovered memory: neurobiological aspects. *Clin Psychol Rev.* 1998;(8):915-932.

34. Burgess PW, Quayle A, Frith CD. Brain regions involved in prospective memory as determined by positron emission tomography. *Neuropsychologia.* 2001;39(6):545-555.

35. Cockburn J. Task interruption in prospective memory: a frontal lobe function? *Cortex.* 1995;31:87-97.

36. Mateer C. The rehabilitation of executive disorders. In: Stuss DT, Robertson IH, eds. *Cognitive Neurorehabilitation.* New York, NY: Cambridge University Press; 1999.

37. McDaniel MA, Glisky EL, Rubin SR, Guynn MJ, Routhieaux BC. Prospective memory: a neuropsychological study. *Neuropsychology.* 1999;13(1):103-110.

38. Wheeler MA, Stuss DT, Tulving E. Toward a theory of episodic memory: the frontal lobes and autonoetic consciousness. *Psychol Bull.* 1997;121(3):331-354.

39. Markowitsch HJ, Calabrese P, Neufeld H, et al. Retrograde amnesia for world knowledge and preserved memory for autobiographic events: a case report. *Cortex.* 1999;35(2):243-252.

40. Buckner RL, Koutstaal W, Schacter DL, et al. Functional-anatomic study of episodic retrieval using fMRI. I. Retrieval effort versus retrieval success. *Neuroimage.* 1998;7(3):151-162.

41. Klein SB, Loftus J, Kihlstrom JF. Memory and temporal experience: the effects of episodic memory loss on an amnesic patient's ability to remember the past and imagine the future. *Social Cogn.* 2002;20(5):353-379.

42. McCormack T, Hoerl C. Memory and temporal perspective: the role of temporal frameworks in memory development. *Develop Rev.* 1999;19:154-182.

43. Cansino S, Maquet P, Dolan RJ, Rugg MD. Brain activity underlying encoding and retrieval of source memory. *Cereb Cort.* 2002;12(10):1048-1056.

44. Cabeza R. Functional neuroimaging of episodic memory retrieval. In: Tulving E, ed. *Memory, Consciousness, and the Brain.* Ann Arbor, Mich: Psychology Press; 2000.

45. Fuster J. Physiology of executive functions: the perception-action cycle. In: Stuss D, Knight R, eds. *Principles of Frontal Lobe Function.* New York, NY: Oxford University Press; 2002.

46. Wiggs C, Weisberg J, Martin A. Neural correlates of semantic and episodic memory retrieval. *Neuropsychologia.* 1999;37(1):103-118.

47. Moscovitch M, Winocur G. The frontal cortex and working with memory. In: Stuss D, Knight R, eds. *Principles of Frontal Lobe Function.* New York, NY: Oxford University Press; 2002.

48. Levy R, Goldman-Rakic PS. Segregation of working memory functions within the dorsolateral prefrontal cortex. *Exp Brain Res.* 2000;133:23-32.

49. Schacter DL, Norman KA, Koutstaal W. The cognitive neuroscience of constructive memory. *Annu Rev Psychol.* 1998;49:289-318.

50. Maquire E. Neuroimaging studies of autobiographical event memory. *Phil Trans R Soc Lond B.* 2001;356:1441-1451.

51. McAllister TW, Saykin AJ, Flashman LA, et al. Brain activation during working memory 1 month after mild traumatic brain injury: a functional MRI study. *Neurology.* 1999;53(6):1300-1307.

52. Giles GM, Shore M. The effectiveness of an electronic memory aid for a memory-impaired adult of normal intelligence. *Am J Occup Ther.* 1988;43(6):409-411.

53. Makatura TJ, Lam CS, Leahy BJ, et al. Standardized memory tests and the appraisal of everyday memory. _Brain Inj._ 1999;13(5):355-367.

54. Ownsworth TL, McFarkand K. Memory remediation in long-term acquired brain injury: two approaches in diary training. _Brain Inj._ 1999;13:605-626.

55. Tate RL. Beyond one-bun, two shoe: recent advances in the psychological rehabilitation of memory disorders after acquired brain injury. _Brain Inj._ 1997;11(12):907-918.

56. Stewart FM, Sunderland A, Sluman SM. The nature and prevalence of memory disorder late after stroke. _Br J Clin Psychol._ 1996;35(Pt 3):369-379.

57. Christiansen C. Occupational therapy: intervention for life performance. In: Christiansen C, Baum C, eds. _Occupational Therapy: Overcoming Human Performance Deficits._ Thorofare, NJ: SLACK Incorporated; 1991.

58. Labowie-Vief G, Gonda J. Cognitive strategy training and intellectual performance in the elderly. _J Gereontol._ 1967;31(3):327-332.

59. Wilson BA. Memory rehabilitation: compensating for memory problems. In: Dixon R, Backman L, eds. _Compensating for Psychological Deficits and Declines._ Mahwah, NJ: Lawrence Erlbaum Assoc; 1995.

60. Wilson B, Cockburn J, Baddeley AD, et al. _The Rivermead Behavioral Memory Test._ 2nd ed. Bury St. Edmunds: Thames Valley Test Co; 2003.

61. Wilson BA, Clare L, Baddeley A, et al. _The Rivermead Behavioral Memory Test-Extended Version (RBMT-E)._ Bury St. Edmunds: Thames Valley Test Co; 1999.

62. Clare L, Wilson BA, Emslie H, Tate R, Watson P. Adapting the Rivermead Behavioral Memory Test Extended Version (RBMT-E) for people with restricted mobility. _Br J Clin Psychol._ 2000;39(Pt 4):363-369.

63. Cockburn J, Wilson B, Baddeley A, Hiorns R. Assessing everyday memory in patients with dysphasia. _Br J Clin Psychol._ 1990;29:353-360.

64. Wilson B, Cockburn J, Baddeley A, Hiorns R. The development and validation of a test battery for detecting and monitoring everyday memory problems. _J Clin Exp Neuropsychol._ 1989;11(6):855-870.

65. Kopelman M, Wilson B, Baddeley AD. _The Autobiographical Memory Interview._ Bury St. Edmonds: Thames Valley Test Co; 1990.

66. Bennet-Levy J, Powell GE. The subjective memory questionnaire. An investigation into the self-reporting of "real life" memory skills. _Br J Social Clin Psychol._ 1980;19:177-188.

67. Broadbent DE, Cooper PF, FitzGerald P, Parkes KR. The Cognitive Failures Questionnaire (CFQ) and its correlates. _Br J Clin Psychol._ 1982;21:1-16.

68. Herrmann DJ, Neisser U. An inventory of everyday memory experiences. In: Gruenberg MM, Morris P, Sykes R, eds. _Practical Aspects of Memory._ London: Academic Press; 1978:35-51.

69. Christenson AL. _Luria's Neuropsychological Investigation._ New York, NY: Spectrum Publications; 1975.

70. Wall N, et al. _Hemiplegic Evaluation._ Boston, Mass: Rehabilitation Hospital; 1979.

71. Zoltan B. Visual, visual perceptual and perceptual-motor deficits in brain injured adults: evaluation, treatment and functional implications. In: Craft GH, Berrol S, eds. _Physical Medicine and Rehabilitation Clinics of North America._ Philadelphia, Pa: WB Saunders Co; 1992.

72. Brooks N, Lincoln NB. Assessment for rehabilitation. In: Wilson BA, Moffat N, eds. _Clinical Management of Memory Problems._ Rockville, Md: Aspen Publishers; 1984.

73. Toglia JP. _Attention and Memory. AOTA Self Study Series: Cognitive Rehabilitation._ Bethesda, Md: The American Occupational Therapy Association; 1994.

74. Toglia J. A dynamic interactional approach to cognitive rehabilitation. In: Katz N, ed. _Cognition and Occupation Across The Life Span._ Bethesda, Md: American Occupational Therapy Association Press; 2005.

75. Kizony R, Katz N. Relationships between cognitive abilities and the process scale and skills of the assessment of motor and process skills (AMPS) in patients with stroke. _OTJR: Occupation, Participation, and Health._ 2002;22:82-92.

76. Pedretti L, et al. Evaluation of sensation, perception and cognition. In: Early MB, ed. _Physical Dysfunction: Practice Skills for the Occupational Therapy Assistant._ St. Louis, Mo: CV Mosby; 1998.

77. Hunkin NM, Squires EJ, Parkin AJ, Tidy JA. Are the benefits of errorless learning dependent on implicit memory? _Neuropsychologia._ 1998;36(1):25-36.

78. Kime SK, Lamb DG, Wilson BA. Use of a comprehensive programme of external cueing to enhance procedural memory in a patient with dense amnesia. _Brain Inj._ 1996;10(1):17-25.

79. Sohlberg M, Mateer CA. Effectiveness of an attention-training program. _J Clin Exper Neuropsych._ 1987;9(2):117-130.

80. Salmon DP, Butters N. Recent developments in learning and memory: implications for the rehabilitation of the amnesic patient. In: Meir MJ, Benton AL, Diller L, eds. _Neuropsychological Rehabilitation._ New York, NY: Guilford Press; 1987.

81. Freeman MR, Mittenberg W, Dicowden M, Bat-Ami M. Executive and compensatory memory retraining in traumatic brain injury. _Brain Inj._ 1992;6(1):65-70.

82. Zencius A, Wesolwski MD, Burke WH. A comparison of four memory strategies with traumatically brain-injured clients. *Brain Inj.* 1990;4(1):33-38.

83. Glisky EL, Schacter DL. Acquisition of domain-specific knowledge in patients with organic memory disorders. *J Learning Disabil.* 1988;21(6):333-351.

84. Toglia JP. *Contextual Memory Test.* San Antonio, Tex: Therapy Skill Builders; 1993.

85. Parente R, Herrmann D. External aids to cognition. In: Parente R, Herrmann D, eds. *Retraining Cognition: Techniques and Applications.* 2nd ed. Austin, Tex: PRO-ED; 2003.

86. Atkinson RC, Shiffrin RM. The control of short-term memory. *Sci Am.* 1971;225(2):82-89.

87. Baum B, Hall K. Relationship between constructional praxis and dressing in the head-injured adult. *Am J Occup Ther.* 1981;35(7):438-442.

88. Ben-Yishay Y. *Working Approaches to Remediation of Cognitive Deficits in Brain-damaged Persons. Rehabilitation Monograph 62.* New York, NY: University Medical Center; 1981.

89. Bourne LE, Dominowski RL, Loftus EF. *Cognitive Processes.* Englewood Cliffs, NJ: Prentice-Hall; 1979.

90. Craik F. Human memory. *Ann Rev Psychol.* 1970;30:63-102.

91. Crovitz H. Memory retraining in brain-damaged patients: the airplane list. *Cortex.* 1979;15:131-134.

92. Glasgow RE, Zeizz RA, Barrera JR, Lewinsohn PM. Case studies on remediating memory deficits in brain-damaged individuals. *J Clin Psychol.* 1977;33(4):1049-1054.

93. Harrell M, Parente F, Bellingrath EG, Liscia KA. *Cognitive Rehabilitation of Memory.* Gaithersburg, Md: Aspen Publishers; 1992.

94. Harris J. Methods of improving memory. In: Wilson BA, Moffat N, eds. *Clinical Management of Memory Problems.* Rockville, Md: Aspen Publishers; 1984.

95. Lewinsohn PM, Danaher BG, Kikel S. Visual imagery as a mnemonic aid for brain-injured persons. *J Consult Clin Psychol.* 1977;5(5):717-723.

96. Lezak M. *Neuropsychological Assessment.* New York, Oxford University Press; 1983.

97. Malec J, Questad K. Rehabilitation of memory after craniocerebral trauma: case report. *Arch Phys Med Rehab.* 1983;64:436-438.

98. Moffat N. Strategies of memory therapy. In: Wilson BA, Moffat N, eds. *Clinical Management of Memory Problems.* Rockville, Md: Aspen Publishers; 1984.

99. Parente R. Executive skills training. In: Parente R, Herrmann D, eds. *Retraining Cognition: Techniques and Applications.* Gaithersburg, Md: Aspen Publications; 1996.

100. Schwartz SM. Adults with traumatic brain injury: three case studies of cognitive rehabilitation in the home setting. *Am J Occup Ther.* 1995;49(7):655-667.

101. Uomoto JM. Neuropsychological assessment and rehabilitation after brain injury. In: Craft GH, Berrol S, eds. *Physical Medicine and Rehabilitation Clinics of North America.* Philadelphia, Pa: WB Saunders; 1992.

102. van Zomeren AH, Fasotti L. Impairments of attention in brain-damaged patients. In: von Steinbuckel N, von Cramon D, Poppel, eds. *Neuropsychological Rehabilitation.* Berlin: Springer-Verlag; 1992.

103. Webser J, Scott R. The effects of self-instructional training on attentional deficits following head injury. *Clin Neuropsychol.* 1983;5:69-74.

104. Weintraub S. Neuropsychological assessment of mental state. In: Mesulam MM, ed. *Principles of Behavioral and Cognitive Neurology.* 2nd ed. New York, NY: Oxford University Press; 2000.

105. Wills P, Clare L, Shiel A, Wilson BA. Assessing subtle memory impairments in the everyday memory performance of brain injured people: exploring the potential of the Extended Rivermead Behavioral Memory Test. *Brain Inj.* 2000;14(8):693-704.

106. Wilson B. Memory therapy in practice. In: Wilson BA, Moffat N, eds. *Clinical Management of Memory Problems.* Rockville, Md: Aspen Publishers; 1984.

107. Wilson B. Recovery and compensatory strategies in head injured memory impaired people several years after insult. *J Neurol Neurosurg Psychiatry.* 1992;55(3):177-1.

108. Cermak LS, Hill R, Wong B. Effects of spacing and repetition on amnesic patients' performance during Perceptual identification, stem completion, and category exemplar production. *Neuropsychology.* 1998;12(1):65-77.

109. Thoene AIT, Glisky EL. Learning of name-face associations in memory impaired patients: a comparison of different training procedures. *J Intern Neuropsychol Soc.* 1995;1:29-38.

110. Kim HJ, Burke DT, Dowds MM Jr, Boone KA, Park GJ. Electronic memory aids for outpatient brain injury: follow-up findings. *Brain Inj.* 2000;14(2):187-196.

111. Wilson B, Evans JJ, Emslie H, Malinek V. Evaluation of Neuropage: a new memory aid. *J Neurol Neurosurg Psychiatry.* 1997;63(1):113-115.

112. Glitsky EL, Glitsky ML. Memory rehabilitation in the elderly. In: Stuss DT, Robertson IH, eds. *Cognitive Neurorehabilitation.* New York, NY: Cambridge University Press; 1999.

Resources

Ayres AJ. *Sensory Integration and Learning Disorders.* Los Angeles, Western Psychological Services; 1980.

Balota DA, Dolan PO, Duchek JM. Memory changes in healthy young and older adults. In: Tulving E, Craik FIM, eds. *Oxford Handbook of Memory.* New York, NY: Oxford University Press; 2000.

Breines E. *Perception: Its Development and Recapitulation.* Princeton, NJ: Geri-Rehab; 1981.

Clare L, Wilson BA, Carter G, et al. Intervening with everyday memory problems in dementia of Alzheimer type: an errorless learning approach. *J Clin Exper Neuropsychol.* 2000;22(1):132-146.

Cook EA, Thigpen R. Identification and management of cognitive perceptual deficits in the rehabilitation patient. *Rehabil Nurs.* 1993;18(5):3110-3113.

Deitz J, Tovar VS, Beeman C, Thorn DW, Trevisan MS. The test of orientation for rehabilitation patients: test-retest reliability. *Occup J Res.* 1992;12(3):173-185.

Diller L, Weinberg J. Differential aspects of attention in brain-damaged persons. *Percept Motor Skills.* 1972;35:71-81.

Dimitrov M, Granetz J, Peterson M, et al. Associative learning impairments in patients with frontal lobe damage. *Brain Cogn.* 1999;41(2):213-230.

Dougherty PM, Radomski MV. *A Dynamic Assessment Approach for Adults with Brain Injury: The Cognitive Rehabilitation Workbook.* Gaithersburg, Md: Aspen Publishers; 1993.

Duchek J. Cognitive dimensions of performance. In: Christiansen C, Baum C, eds. *Occupational Therapy: Overcoming Human Performance Deficits.* Thorofare, NJ: SLACK Incorporated; 1991.

Efklides A, et al. Wechsler memory scale, rivermead behavioral memory test, and everyday memory questionnaire in healthy adults and Alzheimer patients. *Eur J Psychol Assess.* 2002;18:63-77.

Gilewski MJ, Zelinski EM, Schaie KW. The Memory Functioning Questionnaire for assessment of memory complaints in adulthood and old age. *Psychol Aging.* 1990;5(4):482-490.

Gomez Beldarrain M, Grafman J, Pascual-Leone A, Garcia-Monco JC. Procedural learning is impaired in patients with prefrontal lesions. *Neurology.* 1999;52(9):1853-1860.

High WM, Levin HS, Gary HE. Recovery of orientation following closed head injury. *J Clin Exp Neuropsychol.* 1990;12(5):703-714.

Hunkin NM, Parkin AJ. The method of vanishing cues: an evaluation of its effectiveness in teaching memory-impaired individuals. *Neuropsychologia.* 1995;33(10):1255-1279.

Itzkovich M, Elazar B, Averbuch S. *Lowenstein Occupational Therapy Cognitive Assessment (LOTCA) Manual.* Pequannock, NJ: Maddack Inc; 1990.

Kim HJ, Burke DT, Dowds MM, George J. Utility of a microcomputer as an external memory aid for a memory-impaired head injury patient during in-patient rehabilitation. *Brain Inj.* 1999;13(2):147-150.

Maguire EA. Neuroimaging studies of autobiographical event memory. *The Royal Society.* 2001;1441-1451.

Majid MJ, Lincoln NB, Weyman N. *Cognitive Rehabilitation for Memory Deficits Following Stroke. The Cochrane Collaboration.* Hoboken, NJ: John Wiley and Sons; 2005.

McNeny R, Dise J. Reality orientation therapy. In: Rosenthal M, Griffith ER, Bond MR, Miller JD, eds. *Rehabilitation of the Adult with Traumatic Brain Injury.* Philadelphia, Pa: FA Davis; 1983.

McGlynn SM. Behavioral approaches to neuropsychological rehabilitation. *Psychological Bulletin.* 1990;108(3):420-4410.

Nieber E, Koch C. Computational architectures for attention. In: Tulving E, Craik F, eds. *The Oxford Handbook of Memory.* New York, NY: Oxford University Press; 2000.

Okkeman K. *Cognition and Perception in the Stroke Patient.* Gaithersburg, Md: Aspen Publishers; 1993.

Rabbit P. Changes in problem solving ability in old age. In: Birren J, Schaie K, eds. *Handbook of Psychology of Aging.* New York, NY: Van Nostrand Reinhold Co; 1977.

Robertson I, Ward T, Ridgeway Y, Nimmo-Smith I. *The Test of Everyday Attention.* Bury St. Edwards: Thames Valley Test Co; 1994.

Schmitter-Edgecombe M, Fahy JF, Whelan JP, Long CJ. Memory remediation after severe closed head injury: notebook training versus supportive therapy. *J Consult Clin Psychol.* 1995;63(3):484-489.

Shiffman LM. Cerebro vascular accident. In: Early MB, ed. *Physical Dysfunction Practice Skills for the Occupational Therapy Assistant.* St. Louis, Mo: Mosby Year-Book; 1998.

Skilleck C. Computer assistance in the management of memory and cognitive impairment. In: Wilson BA, Moffat N, eds. *Clinical Management of Memory Problems.* Rockville, Md: Aspen Publishers; 1984.

Strub RL, Black RW. *The Mental Status Examination in Neurology.* Philadelphia, Pa: FA Davis; 1977.

Tankle RS. Application of neuropsychological test results to interdisciplinary cognitive rehabilitation with head-injured adults. *J Head Trauma Rehabil.* 1988;3(1):24-32.

Toglia JP. Approaches to cognitive assessment of the brain-injured adult: traditional methods and dynamic investigation. *Occup Ther Pract.* 1989;1(1):36-57.

Toglia JP. A dynamic interactional approach to cognitive rehabilitation. In: Katz N, ed. *Cognitive Rehabilitation: Models For Intervention in Occupational Therapy*. Boston, Mass: Andover Med Pub; 1992.

Wilson B, Emslie HC, Quirk K, Evans JJ. Reducing everyday memory and planning problems by means of a paging system: a randomized control crossover study. *J Neurol Neurosurg Psychiatry*. 2001;70(4):477-482.

Wood RL, Fussey I. *Cognitive Rehabilitation in Perspective*. London: Taylor and Francis; 1990.

CHAPTER 10

EXECUTIVE FUNCTION

Executive Function

Executive function is crucial to everyday success. The term "executive function" refers to a variety of skills which govern the bulk of cognitive processing, come into play primarily during nonroutine activity, and generally govern an individual's performance.[1-4] Disorders of executive ability are most apparent in novel and unstructured situations.[5] Impairments are sometimes called "dysexecutive syndrome" and are common following acquired brain injury (ABI).[4,6,7]

Some theorists have conceptualized executive function as a supervisory control system or central executive responsible for planning, error correction, directing attention, information processing, and inhibition of habitual responses.[1,8-10] Others link executive function to the ability to select, manipulate, and update retrieved memories.[11] Research to support this link has shown that autobiographical memory retrieval and memory retrieval within an specific context is indeed associated with impaired executive function.[11,12]

Ylvisaker and Szekeres describe two categories of executive function.[13] The first category is knowledge base, which is an organized system of general information, learned skills or routines, rules, and procedures. Without this knowledge base, new information is difficult to interpret, organize, and remember. The second system is the executive system, which deals with the mental functions related to forming, planning, and achieving goals. Component areas of this system are "...realistic goal setting (based on an awareness of one's strengths and weaknesses), planning, self-directing and initiating, self-inhibiting, self-monitoring, self-evaluating, self-correcting, and flexible problem solving."[13]

The consensus of experts within the field would describe problems with the following skills as reflective of impaired executive function: initiation, planning and organization, problem solving, mental flexibility, concept formation or abstraction, categorization, and decision making.[1,14-17] In addition, many include self-error correction, self-monitoring, and behavioral regulation.[1,14,15,17] Some theorists hypothesize self-monitoring and self-awareness as part of "metacognition," or a person's understanding and manipulation of their own cognitive and perceptual processes.[18] The ability to evaluate a task's level of difficulty in relation to an individual's strengths or weaknesses and the ability to predict success have been described as metacognitive skills.[19] These self-regulating processes are thought to develop during early childhood and are thought to be dependent on the maturation and integrity of the prefrontal cortex.[1] Parente and Herrmann describe two categories of metacognition: 1) *static*, which refers to a person's awareness of the state of his or her processes and the appropriate methods for improving performance or directing behavior toward a goal, and 2) *dynamic*, which refers to an individual's ability to exercise control over his or her cognition and initiate appropriate action.[20]

Metacognition has also been described as involving higher order integrative processes.[19] Metacognitive processes are believed to be engaged in tasks such as self-checking arithmetic or determining the amount of studying that is enough to pass an examination.[21] Metacognitive abilities have been viewed as critical components in the transfer and generalization process.[3,19] Executive functions have been described as the dynamic "doing" aspect of metacognition.[19] At this time, this author believes that the term "metacognition" is an evolving concept that has not been completely refined or operationalized. The concepts of executive function, therefore, will be utilized in the subsequent material presented in this chapter. Although many have conceptualized self-awareness and self-monitoring as executive skills, this author feels due to its overall importance in daily function, it should be parsed out as a separate entity that interrelates with the components of executive function subsequently described. This author believes that executive abilities combined with accurate self-awareness and self-monitoring, attention, and memory are all the basis for generalization of skills to daily functioning.

Impaired executive function has been associated with frontal lobe and subcortical limbic damage.[22-25] Recent neuroimaging studies have shown that executive functions are subsumed by distributed circuitry rather than discrete structures.[26] In addition, it is believed that different regions within the prefrontal cortex are associated with different aspects of executive control.[27,28] The dorsolateral prefrontal cortex, for example, has been associated with problems in planning, organizing, sequencing, and abstracting.[26]

It has been theorized that the adult level of executive function is reached in three stages. Simple planning and organized visual search develop by age 6, hypothesis testing and impulse control by age 10, and complex motor sequencing and verbal fluency during adolescence.[29] Others have observed that between the ages of 1.5 and 5 years old and again between ages 5 and 10 years old, a sequence of changes takes place related to a reorganization of attentional, executive, and self-reflexive processes.[22]

Adequate executive function allows for effective adaptation and accommodation to changing environmental demands. Decreased executive function leads to functional impairment, even with mild traumatic brain injury (TBI), and these deficits are often the most persistent.[25] In a study of 90 TBI clients, executive functioning, along with memory and premorbid intelligence, were predictors of functional dependence after discharge.[30] Executive function has also played a key role in the level of social and vocational recovery in clients with ABI.[6,17,31]

Executive function is critical to activities ranging from meal preparation to driving a car to vocational functioning and social independence.[25,32] Duran and Fisher link executive function to functional abilities through the concept of executive abilities and state executive abilities "…pertain to the behavioral manifestations of executive functions in the context of daily life task performances, including personal or instrumental activities of daily living (IADLs)."[33] In other words, disorders of executive function, when they are manifest as disability, become disorders of occupational performance.[33] Clients with poor executive function are often impulsive, show tangential conversations, make perseverative comments, and are socially inappropriate. They often cannot adequately monitor their social situation or relations with others. These clients will often judge their own performance in general or global terms rather than looking specifically and objectively at what they have done. When trying to solve a problem, they will only consider one possible solution to a problem and will fail to consider relevant information in choosing the best solutions.

Activities that previously required little or no effort may now require deliberate control and effort, which results in decreased efficiency.[2]

EVALUATION OF EXECUTIVE FUNCTION

Often, traditional tests of executive function will not pick up a deficit despite severe problems that show up in activities of daily living (ADL).[34] This may be due to the fact that executive problems generally do not affect well-structured tasks.[4] Traditional tests, in fact, are often structured to actually prevent clients from needing to apply executive abilities for successful test performance.

Many clinicians now believe nonspecific, open-ended tasks are especially useful in evaluating a client's executive function.[35] Burgess et al advocates for assessment to include multi-tasking, as this reflects what most everyday activities entail.[34] Burgess et al outlines the following characteristics of everyday activities[34]:

1. *Many tasks*

2. *Interleaving—Performance on these tasks needs to be dovetailed in order to be time effective.*

3. *One task at a time—Due to cognitive or physical constraints, only one task can be performed at a time.*

4. *Interruptions and unexpected outcomes—Unexpected, sometimes high priority, interruptions occur, and things will not always go as planned.*

5. *Delayed intentions—The time to return to a task that is already in progress is not signaled directly by the situation.*

6. *Differing tasks characteristics—Tasks usually differ in terms of priority, difficulty, and the length of time they will occupy.*

7. *Self-determined targets—People decide for themselves what constitutes adequate performance.*

8. *No immediate feedback—No minute-to-minute performance feedback. Failures are not signaled at the time they occur.*

The evaluation and treatment of self-awareness and self-monitoring as a separate entity strongly related to and affecting executive skills is subsequently described in Section I of this chapter. This is followed by Section II, which contains information pertaining to the evaluation and treatment of the component executive function skills of initiation, planning and organization, problem solving, decision making, categorization, mental flexibility, and abstraction. Finally, Section III provides detailed information related to several occupation-based executive function evaluations.

Although some associated behavioral issues are discussed, it is not within the scope of this book to cover these areas in detail. The reader is encouraged to search out this information and is referred to the references.

SECTION I

EVALUATION AND TREATMENT OF SELF-AWARENESS AND MONITORING

Effective self-awareness and self-monitoring are crucial in everyday life and have been shown to have a strong relationship to functional outcome.[22,36,37] Decreased self-awareness is not a global deficit but rather the degree of impairment can vary depending on the area of function that is assessed and the method used to make this assessment.[38] Self-awareness involves both "...knowledge of one's cognitive abilities and an ability to monitor performance of cognitive activities through recognizing and correcting errors and regulating activity performance."[5] An individual must be able to make judgments that relate to objective information concerning interactions with the environment as well as with subjective inner experiences.[39,40] An individual's experience must be monitored over the past and present and anticipated in the future.[28] Self-monitoring is an individual's ability to evaluate and regulate the quality and quantity of his or her behavior."[20] An individual constantly monitors his or her behavior so that incorrect responses can be identified and corrected.[28] The individual who can apply self-monitoring can manage his or her own learning "...by acknowledging the requirement of effort in success, applying the correct means to utilize these efforts, and regulating activities so that plans can be accomplished."[41]

The convergence of emotional states and memory of abstract mental states that allow the development for the future, allows for the emergence of self-awareness.[28] An individual's emotional state can reduce his and her ability to process new information and constrain opportunities to gain knowledge of him- or herself and the world.[18] Indeed, as Abreu et al state, "...a brain injured person's ability to benefit from rehabilitation services requires a more complete understanding of the client's self-awareness of disability and how it affects motivation and participation in therapeutic activities."[42]

One can view decreased awareness at two levels: 1) unawareness of the deficit itself and 2) unawareness of the consequences of the deficit. Prigatano has identified two types of deficits depending on the location of brain damage. Prefrontal brain damage can cause the client to exhibit poor self-awareness about social judgment, the ability to anticipate change, or decreased interpersonal awareness, as well as decreased awareness for the consequences of his or her actions.[43] Decreased awareness exhibited by parietal lobe damage, on the other hand, involves awareness of body image as well as awareness of perceptual, sensory, and motor abilities. Different evaluation tools may help delineate these different aspects of decreased awareness.

Stuss and Alexander describe a four-level hierarchal model related to self-awareness. The four levels are as follows: 1) arousal-attention, 2) perceptual-motor, 3) executive mediation, and 4) self-awareness.[28] Each level feeds forward to the higher level, and each level also feeds backwards to the lower level. Direct contact with the external environment is restricted to the perceptual-motor level.[28] The two highest levels are associated with frontal lobe function.

Barco et al identify three levels of awareness that can serve as a basis for evaluation and treatment. These areas are defined by Barco et al as follows[44]:

1. *Intellectual awareness*—The cognitive capacity of the client to understand to some degree that a particular function is diminished from premorbid levels

2. *Emergent awareness*—The ability of clients to recognize a problem when it is actually occurring

3. *Anticipatory awareness*—The ability to anticipate that a problem is going to happen because of some deficit

Some degree of intellectual awareness is considered a prerequisite for both emergent and anticipatory awareness. Clients with poor emergent awareness can describe their deficit and what they should do for it; however, because they do not recognize that a problem is occurring, they cannot compensate when necessary. The complete understanding of the implications of one's deficits is the highest level of intellectual awareness and is closely linked with anticipatory awareness.[44]

Golisz and Toglia observe that clients at the stage of intellectual awareness are a safety risk because they do not perform within their limitations.[5] The clients at this level may realize they have a memory problem, for example, but will not make lists or use mnemonics to help them remember.[5] Clients with emergent awareness may be a safety risk if they try to perform tasks outside their ability.[47] Clients with anticipatory awareness are generally not a safety risk.[5]

Knight describes two classes of cognitive function that are related to self-awareness.[45] These are simulation, which is the process of generating internal models of external reality, and reality checking, which are the processes that monitor information gained from the external world in an effort to accurately represent their spatio-temporal context.[45] These cognitive functions are considered supervisory or executive. Reality checking is necessary for an individual to discriminate between internally generated possibilities and the model of the external world as it currently exits.[45] It is also essential for simulation processes to be carried out without compromising the ability to interact with the environment. Knight elaborates on the cognitive processes of simulation and reality testing[45]:

> *Simulation processes generate an alternative reality that must be evaluated in relation to its divergence from the current reality. Reality checking involves a continual assessment of the relationship between behavior and environment. As an individual acts on the environment, the consequences of the action must be incorporated into existing plans. If the environment deviates from expectations, one needs to detect this change, and plans must be reassessed. Reality monitoring has also been proposed as a major mechanism underlying different disturbances of self-awareness.*

Clients with moderate to severe ABI often exhibit some degree of decreased awareness of the changes in their physical, cognitive, and behavioral function.[40] They have a poor conscious picture of their functional disabilities. They may show limited or poor interpersonal boundaries and interactions as well as poor self-care, manners, and grooming.[25] This is different from psychological denial in that they simply do not perceive the extent of their impairments or associated disability.[43] Some of the differences between impaired self-awareness and psychological denial have been described by Prigatano and Klonoff and are summarized in Table 10-1.

The client with decreased awareness may be completely unaware of blatant deficits that are obvious to those around him or her. Some clients deny that they have a problem, to the point of becoming hostile to those who attempt to point deficits out. Still others may be indifferent to their limitations. Some clients are perfectly fine with abandoning a task even though it is clearly incomplete.[47] Some are completely satisfied even after it is pointed out that the task is not finished. Other clients may exhibit complete denial and resort to fabrication when someone is pointing out a deficit area. These fabrications are an attempt to provide a verbal rendering for their altered competencies.[18] These fabrications are an erroneous account for which the client is not willfully lying.[18] Clients may also exhibit actual delusions. For example, they may be quite convinced that their

Table 10-1

Characteristics of Impaired Self-Awareness Versus Psychological Denial

Impaired Self-Awareness

Clients lack information about themselves.

Clients experience confusion when given feedback regarding their behavioral or functional limitations.

Clients exhibit a cautious willingness or indifference when asked to work with this new information about themselves.

Psychological Denial

Clients show partial or implicit knowledge about themselves.

Clients resist or become angry when given feedback regarding their behavior or functional limitations.

Clients display an active struggle to work with "new information" about themselves.

Adapted from reference 46: Prigatano G, Klonoff PS. A clinician's rating scale for evaluating impaired self-awareness and denial of disability after brain injury. Clin Neuropsychol. *1998;12(1):56-67.*

hemiplegic arm is not theirs. As partial awareness emerges, the client may be unable to describe exactly how their abilities have changed.[43]

As just described, decreased awareness is an inability to recognize deficits or problem circumstances caused by neurological injury.[44] There is a failure to acknowledge impairments of cognitive and/or motor function when questioned.[48,49] Since the client does not acknowledge impairments, he or she often is not motivated to compensate for them.[5] Recent research has indicated that an unawareness of cognitive deficits does not always coincide with unawareness of motor deficits.[48,49] Areas that have been found to influence awareness include memory or intellectual impairments, decreased sensory and perceptual abilities, decreased inhibition, and impulsivity or inability to plan for the future.[44]

Decreased awareness of deficits can have a profound effect on the client's behavior as well as his or her ability to participate in rehabilitation. In some cases, the individual will not seek out or accept treatment.[50,51] Prigatano et al, in study of clients with ABI, discovered that clients underestimated their abilities in emotional and social interactions.[50] These clients had difficulty in handling arguments, adjusting to unexpected changes, and controlling their temper. These skills are all required for social competence.

Just as decreased awareness can affect behavior, so can the stage when the client begins to understand the changes in his or her function. At this time, a psychological denial of deficits may be apparent. Results of one study of 23 clients with ABI indicated that the better the insight the clients demonstrated, the worse their emotional dysfunction.[52] During this first stage of adjustment, the client rejects any information that points out his or her limitations and claims there is nothing wrong.[18] This is different from the denial previously described when the client is unaware. Following an initial stage of denial, the client will begin to come to terms with the changes in his or her function and begin to develop a new self-concept.[18] Finally, the client will not only recognize his problems but will actively try to develop ways to change or adapt to his or her new level of function.[18] It is important that the occupational therapist assist the client in moving through these stages of adjustments.

Functional implications of decreased awareness include impulsiveness and poor safety awareness. Many studies report that clients consistently overrate their abilities.[42] The client must be taught to control and monitor his or her performance and how to use feedback effectively.[53] The client often has low frustration tolerance, often resulting in anger. The client will be unable to correct any errors or mistakes because he or she is unable to perceive them. As previously noted, some clients may be able to perceive their errors but are unable to self-correct and regulate the quality of their behavior and performance. This deficit of poor self-monitoring is the inability to evaluate and regulate the quality of behavior.[54] This inability to control and monitor behavior will, in turn, affect judgment in all functional tasks. The client, for example, may impulsively try to get out of bed and walk to the bathroom despite paralysis, or he or she may be unsafe around the stove.

Due to the documented occurrence of decreased awareness in clients with ABI and the associated functional implications, evaluation is crucial to client treatment planning decisions. Its evaluation can assist in providing the client's family with necessary education, support, management strategies, and assistance in the development of realistic goals.[55]

EVALUATION OF SELF-AWARENESS AND MONITORING

Test 1 – Clinical Observation and Activity Analysis

General Guidelines for Evaluation

1. Determine whether the client is aware of and responsive to his or her environment. One measure of the client's awareness is his or her ability to utilize feedback.[56]

2. Observe if the client requests clarification of instructions appropriately and attempts to self-correct. Try to elicit this response by giving unclear or hasty directions or by giving too much information.

3. Observe the client in a number of settings and activities during the day. Limited insight, poor safety awareness, and impulsiveness can vary depending on the setting and the task. Define what types of conditions (including specific instructions to inhibit a certain behavior) improve or worsen disinhibited or socially inappropriate behavior.[13]

4. Establish functional baseline measures. Consider the degree and frequency of the problem. Select relevant occupation-based tasks as the basis of evaluation and reassessment.

Specific Areas and Questions to Consider and Evaluate

1. Can the client perceive and verbalize (or somehow communicate) the extent and type of problems he or she is having?

2. Is the client willing to try to understand and accept his or her problems when they are pointed out?

3. Once the client admits that he or she has a specific problem, can he or she then perceive how it will affect his or her overall function beyond a specific task?

4. How does the environment affect the client's awareness and behavior? Does a quiet, structured environment decrease impulsivity and increase insight? In which environment does safety become an issue (eg, kitchen, community)?

5. Does verbal, visual, or tactile cuing improve insight or decrease impulsiveness?

6. What is the duration and frequency of the client's impulsiveness and decreased insight or safety awareness?

7. Is there a task or tasks that are particularly helpful in illustrating a specific problem to the client?

Scoring

Nonstandardized

These and similar questions can be incorporated into a checklist or used in conjunction with a frequency rating scale (eg, always/sometimes/rarely/never).

Validity

To improve validity, rule out decreased attention, poor memory, and aphasia as causes of poor performance.

Test 2 – Self-Awareness of Deficits Interview[57]

Description

The self-awareness of deficits interview (SADI) is an interviewer-scored, structured interview used to obtain qualitative and quantitative data on the status of self-awareness following ABI. It contains three areas of questioning: 1) self-awareness of deficits, 2) self-awareness of functional implications of deficits, and 3) ability to set realistic goals. The specific interview questions (which can be adapted or reworded by the interviewer within the context of the interview) for each of these areas is presented in Table 10-2.

Scoring

Responses are rated on a four-point scale with 0 indicating no disorder of self-awareness and a score of 3 indicating a severe disorder of self-awareness. Specific scoring criteria for each of the three interview categories are summarized in Table 10-3.

Reliability

Inter-rater reliability among five interviewers and 25 TBI clients was established through analysis of variance (ANOVA) and intra-class agreement (0.78, 0.57, and 0.78) on the three sections respectively. The scores for the three subsections combined had an acceptable level of intraclass correlation (ICC) of 0.82.

Test 2 – Awareness Questionaire[58]

Description

There are three forms of the questionnaire: 1) the client rates his or her functioning in physical, cognitive, behavioral, and community areas, 2) a family member (or significant other) who has been familiar with the client both before and after ABI rates the client's functioning on the same items, and 3) a clinician who is familiar with the client after the ABI rates the client on the same items. The clinician form also includes an item for which the clinician rates the extent to which the client has accurate awareness of his or her deficits.

Scoring

Decreased awareness is measured by discrepancy scores between 1) family member ratings and client self-ratings, 2) clinician ratings and client self-ratings, and 3) client self-ratings and standardized tests of cognitive abilities.

Validity

Several validity studies have been conducted, and the reader is referred to the references for additional information.[38,58-60]

Reliability

Internal Consistency Cronbach Coefficient Alphas were high and are presented in the test manual.[38]

Table 10-2

Self-Awareness of Deficits Interview

Self-Awareness of Deficits

1. Are you any different now compared to what you were like before your accident? In what way? Do you feel that anything about you or your abilities has changed?
2. Do people who know you well notice that anything is different about you since the accident? What might they notice?
3. What do you see as your problems, if any, resulting from your injury? What is the main thing you need to work on/would like to get better?

Prompts

Physical abilities (eg, movement of arms and legs, balance, vision, endurance)?

Memory/confusion?

Concentration?

Problem-solving, decision-making, organizing, and planning things?

Controlling behavior?

Communication?

Getting along with other people?

Has your personality changed?

Are there any other problems that I haven't mentioned?

Self-Awareness of Functional Implications of Deficits

1. Does your head injury have any affect on your everyday life? In what way?

Prompts

Ability to live independently?

Managing finances?

Look after family/manage home?

Driving?

Work/study?

Leisure/social life?

Are there any other areas of life that you feel have changed/may change?

Ability to Set Realistic Goals

1. What do you hope to achieve in the next 6 months? Do you have any goals? What are they?
2. In 6 months time, what do you think you will be doing? Where do you think you will be?
3. Do you think your head injury will still be having an effect on your life in 6 months time?
   If yes: How?
   If no: Are you sure?

Reprinted with permission from Taylor and Francis, Ltd (http://www.tandf.co.uk/journals), reference 57: Fleming JM, Strong J, Ashton R. Self-awareness of deficits in adults with traumatic brain injury: how best to measure? Brain Inj. 1996;10(1):14.

Table 10-3

Scoring Criteria for the Self-Awareness of Deficits Interview

Self-Awareness of Deficits

0   Cognitive/psychological problems (where relevant) reported by the client in response to general questioning or readily acknowledged in response to specific questioning.

1   Some cognitive/psychological problems reported, but others denied or minimized. Client may have a tendency to focus on relatively minor physical changes (eg, scars) and acknowledge cognitive/psychological problems only on specific questioning about deficits.

2   Physical deficits only acknowledged; denies, minimizes, or is unsure of cognitive/psychological changes. Client may recognize problems that occurred at an earlier stage but denies existence of persisting deficits or may state that other people think there are deficits but he or she does not think so.

3   No acknowledgement of deficits (other than obvious physical deficits) can be obtained, or client will only acknowledge problems that have been imposed on him or her (eg, not allowed to drive, not allowed to drink alcohol).

Self-Awareness of Functional Implications of Deficits

0   Client accurately describes current functional status (independent living, work/study, leisure, home management, driving) and specifies how his or her head injury problems limit function (where relevant) and/or any compensatory measures adopted to overcome problems.

1   Some functional implications reported following questions or examples of problems in independent living, work, driving, leisure, etc. Client may not be sure of other likely functional problems (eg, is unable to say because he or she has not tried an activity yet).

2   Client may acknowledge some functional implications of deficits but minimizes the importance of identified problems. Other likely functional implications may be actively denied by the client.

3   Little acknowledgement of functional consequences can be obtained; the client will not acknowledge problems, except that he or she is not allowed to perform certain tasks. The client may actively ignore medical advice and may engage in risk-taking behaviors (eg, drinking and driving).

Ability to Set Realistic Goals

0   Client sets reasonably realistic goals and (where relevant) identifies that the head injury will probably continue to have an impact on some areas of functioning (ie, goals for the future have been modified in some way since the injury).

1   Client sets goals that are somewhat unrealistic or is unable to specify a goal but recognizes that he or she will still have problems in some areas of function in the future (ie, sees that goals for the future may need some modification even if he or she has not yet done so).

2   Client sets unrealistic goals, or is unable to specify a goal, and does not know how he or she will be functioning in 6 months time but hopes he or she will return to pretrauma (ie, no modification of goals has occurred).

3   Client expects without uncertainty that in 6 months time he or she will be functioning at pretrauma level (or at a higher level).

Reprinted with permission from Taylor and Francis, Ltd (http://www.tandf.co.uk/journals), reference 57: Fleming JM, Strong J, Ashton R. Self-awareness of deficits in adults with traumatic brain injury: how best to measure? Brain Inj. 1996;10(1):15.

Test 3 – Self-Awareness Questionnaire[55]

Description

This is a 27-item orientation and awareness questionnaire.

All orientation questions and three of the four awareness-of-brain-injury questions have a three-choice format. Present verbally all three choices and then repeat all choices until one response is affirmed. All other items are yes/no questions.

The Self-Awareness Questionnaire can be found in Table 10-4.

Table 10-4
Self-Awareness Questionnaire

Orientation to Time and Place
(Three choice format.)

Day:

Month:

Date:

Year:

Town:

What is this place?
(army) (school) (rehabilitation center)

What is the name of this place?

Awareness of Brain Injury
(Personalize these items for each survivor.)

What happened to you to bring you here?
(parents/relatives sent you here) (car accident/fall/blow) (volunteered to come)

Why are you here?
(to receive therapy) (punishment) (unsure)

Has your brain been injured?	(Yes)	(No)

When were you injured?
(at birth) (I have not been injured) (actual year)

Awareness of Physical Impairment

Can you walk?	(Yes)	(No)
Do you have difficulty moving your legs?	(Yes)	(No)
Can you move both your arms normally?	(Yes)	(No)
Do you have difficulty moving your fingers?	(Yes)	(No)

Awareness of Communication Impairment

Can you speak normally?	(Yes)	(No)
Can you understand what people say to you?	(Yes)	(No)
Do you have difficulty reading?	(Yes)	(No)
Do you have difficulty writing?	(Yes)	(No)

Activities of Daily Living

Do you need help to feed yourself?	(Yes)	(No)
Can you dress yourself?	(Yes)	(No)
Do you need help to bathe yourself?	(Yes)	(No)
Can you shave/apply makeup yourself?	(Yes)	(No)

Awareness of Sensory/Cognitive Deficits

Do you have a good memory?	(Yes)	(No)
Do you have good vision?	(Yes)	(No)
Do you get fatigued/tired easily?	(Yes)	(No)
Do you have trouble thinking clearly?	(Yes)	(No)

Reprinted with permission from Lippincott, Williams and Wilkins, reference 55: Gasquoine PG, Gibbons TA. Lack of aware-ness of impairment in institutionalized, severely and chronically disabled survivors of traumatic brain injury: a preliminary investigation. J Head Trauma Rehab. 1994;9(4):16-24.

Test 4 – Patient Competency Rating Scale[57,61]

Description

The client and family member or significant other rate the client's abilities for performing functional activities (30 different behavioral tasks). The client and family member rate how they think the client would perform the task (the client does not actually perform the task). The Patient Competency Rating Scale (PCRS) includes items covering functional abilities, interpersonal skills, and emotional status.

Scoring

Several methods of scoring have been utilized with the PCRS and are described in the following references.[50,57] The simplest method described is to calculate the average perceived competency score across all 30 items for both the client and family member.

Reliability

Test-Retest Reliability

For 17 clients (r = 0.97) and their family members (r = 0.92), test-retest correlations using Pearson's individual items were significant for 27 out of 30 items for clients (p < 0.05) and 28 out of 30 items for family members (p < 0.05).

Test 5 – Evaluation of Three Levels of Awareness

General Guidelines for Evaluation

1. *Intellectual awareness*—Evaluated through informal interview. Ask the client to describe what difficulties he or her is having since the injury or the onset of disease. Can the client describe the functional implications these deficits have on his or her life?

2. *Emergent awareness*—Evaluated through clinical observation during a cognitive task or functional activity. Does the client recognize and correct problems? Does the client become frustrated with the task but is unable to understand what is causing the frustration? Upon questioning, is the client accurately able to reflect on how he or she is doing?

3. *Anticipatory awareness*—Evaluated through clinical observation combined with timed questions. For example, ask what types of problems, if any, the client might expect to have in a variety of situations and why the client thinks he or she will have a problem in that situation. Therapists should not provide cuing or assistance to clients during clinical observation of anticipatory awareness because therapists have to observe what the client initiates on his or her own to see if anticipatory awareness does exist.

Test 6 – Interviewing[4,5]

1. *Family, employer, caregiver, etc*—The goal of the interview is to gather information regarding the likely existence of deficits and the real impact they are having on life at home and at work.

2. *Client*—In an informal manner, the therapist can question the client on why he or she is in the hospital and what type of cognitive or physical deficits he or she may be experiencing. If the client cannot answer, questions should move from awareness of limitation to more specific questions.[5]

Test 7 – Inpatient Awareness Rating Scale[62]

The Inpatient Awareness Rating Scale (IARS) is a brief 11-item questionnaire that is used to examine congruence between the client's perception of functional abilities and that of the clinician.

Part I asks the person to rate how much help or reminders that he or she may need for everyday memory or for routine ADL activities typically performed within an inpatient hospital setting. Part II asks the client to predict how much help he or she would require upon discharge. The discrepancy between client and clinician ratings is used as a measure of awareness. A pilot study with 77 inpatients on a TBI inpatient unit indicated that the scale has acceptable internal reliability/consistency (Cronbach Alpha = 0.84). Comparison of the IARS and other awareness measures has provided preliminary validation as a measure of awareness.

DYNAMIC ASSESSMENT

Test 1 – Toglia Category Assessment and Contextual Memory Test[63,64]

As described in the sections pertaining to categorization (Toglia Category Assessment [TCA]) and memory (Contextual Memory Test [CMT]), these tests also investigate awareness by asking the client standard questions before and after task performance. The questions relate to predicting performance and estimating actual performance. Two awareness scores are calculated by comparing the prediction and estimation to the client's actual performance.[19] Test results are interpreted by looking at the client's response to awareness questions along with his or her response to cues.[63,64] The degree to which awareness can be facilitated during task performance and the client's ability to benefit from cues and show learning are analyzed.[63,64]

TREATMENT OF DECREASED SELF-AWARENESS AND MONITORING

Utilizing a Restorative Approach

1. *Intellectual awareness*—Without at least a minimal amount of intellectual awareness, a restorative approach is not appropriate. If there is a minimal amount of intellectual awareness, provide immediate, objective, and concrete feedback to the client during activities. Have the client make a strengths and weaknesses list and show it to the therapist.

2. *Emergent awareness*—Provide feedback to the client during and after a task. Use consistent cuing or terminology, and be direct and very specific. Feedback should specify the problem as it occurs and explain what the observable signs are of how the problem is affecting performance. Have the client do a self-rating scale for specific problems. The client and therapist (or family) can do the rating concurrently. The goal over time is for the client and therapist ratings to be similar. Use the rating after the treatment session is over, and discuss the results with the client.

3. *Anticipatory awareness*—Guide the client into planning for deficits. In other words, cue the client to plan and anticipate what deficits may affect performance before starting a task. Reduce cuing as the client becomes more aware.

4. Use role reversal, where the client watches the therapist perform a task with the therapist making errors and the client identifying them.[64,65] The client can also hypothesize why the errors occurred.[63] For example, the therapist was not attending to detail, scanning to the left, etc.

5. Train the client to predict his or her performance and to re-evaluate the accuracy of these predictions.[18,64]

6. Utilize the method of "Vanishing Cues."[4] The maximum cues for impaired performance are provided as it occurs (or in advance if increased anticipatory awareness is the goal). Slowly, the amount of active cuing is withdrawn until the client can develop his or her own ability to monitor performance.

7. Katz and Hartman–Maeir outline guidelines for the selection of training tasks as follows.[19] Provide tasks that target deficits so that the client can recognize deficits but not be overwhelmed, tasks that allow the client to experience improvement with practice, and tasks that allow the therapist and client to explore strategies for improving performance once the client's level of performance has reached a plateau.

Provide feedback that addresses the following:

a) Discrepancies between expected and actual performance

b) The benefits and limitations of compensatory strategies used

c) The variability of performance

d) The degree of cuing they needed to complete the task

e) The potential impact of residual difficulties on everyday functioning

8. Utilize videotaping, role playing, and group treatment techniques as appropriate to the client's level of awareness.[41] For example, use simulated social situations when teaching the client social skills.[64] Teach the client strategies for dealing with anger. Conduct practice sessions in dealing with a hierarchy of anger situations.[53] Have the client practice positive self-verbalizations.

9. Reward the client not just for completing a goal but for accurate prediction of how and if he or she can complete the goal.[13]

10. Utilize "activity processing" as follows[67]:

a) Reiterate the purpose of what you are doing.

b) Identify with the client the performance boundaries, skills, and limitations of performance. Discuss successful strategies as well as performance barriers.

c) Relate the treatment experience to relevant home or work tasks.

d) Collaborate with the client on new goals based on performance and activity processing discussion.

11. Utilize self-evaluation forms.* For example, when working on social awareness, the following could be used with the client:

Self-Evaluation

Social Interaction Incident

a) What happened?

b) How did it make me feel?

c) What did I do?

d) How did that make _____ feel?

e) Could I have behaved differently?

f) Could _____ have behaved differently?

g) Could I have avoided the situation?

h) What might be another way to handle the situation in the future?

Self-evaluation forms should be used in incidents when the client handled an interaction well, not just when there was a problem. Reward the client for the self-evaluation process even if the original need for filling out the form was due to inappropriate behavior.

---

*Self-monitoring improves with self-instruction because the auditory feedback allows the client to monitor errors more frequently.[68]

12. Provide reality testing. The client is asked to perform an activity that requires skills the client does not possess, and the therapist observes whether the client becomes aware of the difficulty he or she is experiencing.[5]

13. Have clients state each action they are about to do and then state what they are doing while they are doing it. As the client progresses, have him or her whisper it and, finally, "talk to himself" or think through what he or she is doing.[6] This approach has been shown to generalize to untrained tasks as well as to improvements in general behavior. It helps the client slow his or her approach and develop a habit of thinking through actions rather than responding impulsively.[6]

14. Identify behaviors that are a problem in a nonjudgmental way.[18]

15. Some therapists believe that simply increasing the client's awareness is not enough to change behavior.[69] They believe that clients with decreased awareness have to practice to the point where they will chose the desired response automatically.[69]

16. Some clinicians feel the traditional use of direct feedback and education are too confrontational and cause clients to increase their confabulation, which in turn, makes them more resistant to change.[36] These clinicians utilize behavior therapy techniques with a supportive, collaborative partnership. Their research has indicated removing the 'self' from the (self-awareness) problem has led to dramatic gains in all areas where it has been applied.[36] They found that when confrontation was removed, the clients no longer had to defend their position.

17. Some clinicians treat decreased awareness in a nonconfrontational approach through the use of an instructional game format called "Road to Awareness."[70] These researchers combined the game format with awareness training and found it was effective for increasing application of this knowledge to real life.

Utilizing an Adaptive Approach

1. *Intellectual awareness*—Provide repetitive education to the client and his or her family regarding the client's decreased awareness and how it will affect function. Focus also on brain function and types of damage that can occur. Provide external environmental modifications and cuing as needed. Special care should be taken for activities where safety is an issue (ie, kitchen, ambulation, driving).

2. *Emergent awareness*—Utilize "situational compensation."[44] This is compensation that is triggered by a particular situation. The therapist identifies the situation, develops an appropriate compensation plan, and trains the client in its use through practice and repetition. For example, the client has the intellectual awareness to know the house needs cleaning but not sufficient emergent awareness of how to go about cleaning it. A checklist of household tasks may be developed and provided to the client to help him or her compensate.

3. *Anticipatory awareness*—Provide recognition compensations.[44] When the client recognizes a problem is occurring, this recognition cues him or her to initiate a compensation strategy. The therapist helps the client to develop a strategy. If the client is already using a strategy, the therapist should evaluate its effectiveness and modify it as needed. Utilize the client's strengths when teaching the compensation strategy.

4. Help the client develop a mental checklist for what he or she is doing (ie, Am I on track? Am I doing what I'm supposed to be doing?).

5. Teach the client to verify he or she understands what someone is saying or asking him or her to do (ie, Do I have this right?).

6. Use role reversal. Instead of the therapist making mistakes while performing an activity (restorative), the therapist should perform the activity without making mistakes. This will teach the client how the activity should be performed.

7. Therapists should establish a good working relationship with clients so clients will trust them and sense that they will guide the clients. As clients trust their therapists, they will begin to slowly accept and recognize limitations.[43]

8. Educate the family/caregivers that without the awareness of whether a task is being performed safely, the client will always need supervision. Also, remind them that the client will not be motivated to change if he or she does not recognize that there is a problem.[65]

9. Structured journals can be generated by the client as a means of self-reflection.[64] Included in the journal is what was done, how the client performed, what was learned from the experience, and what might be done next time.[5]

10. For those clients who are unsafe in the kitchen with cooking, even with adaptations, use a microwave instead of an oven or cooktop.[33]

SECTION II
EVALUATION AND TREATMENT OF EXECUTIVE FUNCTION

Initiation

The client with ABI may have difficulty in starting a task or activity. The client may be sitting with a schedule in hand; can give the time, place, and name of a therapy; but will remain in his or her room without cues such as "Go to your therapy" or "Get started."[40] Many clients will have good language skills to engage in active conversation but will not initiate it and remain silent until a conversational topic is proposed for them.[13] The client may lack spontaneity, be slow to respond, and generally show little or no initiative.[71] The client may be able to plan, organize, and carry out complex tasks but only when instructed to do so.[71] They may repeatedly voice a plan yet never actually carry it out.[25] Oftentimes, these behaviors are misinterpreted as intentional lack of motivation or drive. This decreased ability to initiate has been linked with frontal lobe damage.[40,47,72]

Recent research has provided hope for the remediation of initiation deficits through incentive training. It is theorized that there are two types of learning: strategy learning and incentive learning.[73] Strategy learning relates to the acquisition and development of "...compensatory behaviors, memory techniques, or problem solving methods that the client can learn in therapy."[73] Incentive learning on the other hand, is the understanding that the use of a particular strategy in everyday life will result in getting something in return. The client must apply a given strategy to a real life situation and get rewarded for using it in order for incentive learning to occur.[73] In three experiments with 24 clients with TBI, it was demonstrated that cognitive skills improved immediately and dramatically with the use of incentive training as long as the therapist created a relevant incentive to activate the client's performance or initiate the activity.[73] Continued research should indicate what type of incentive is the most effective in eliciting client initiation.

Treatment techniques for decreased initiation generally focus on providing external cues and prompts. As the client improves, more internally generated strategies and self-monitoring are utilized.[41] Many therapists have found that developing a daily routine with certain routine tasks performed at the same time and in the same order is helpful.[4] When developing a routine, establish how the end of one part of a routine may act as a trigger for the next part.[6] This will help with maintaining attention through the entire task.[6]

EVALUATION OF INITIATION

Test 1 – Clinical Observation and Activity Analysis

General Guidelines for Evaluation

1. Observe the client in a number of settings.

2. Consider the amount of structure and cuing required for initiation of activity by the client.

3. Establish functional baseline measures. Consider the frequency and severity of the problem as it relates to function. Select relevant functional areas or tasks as the basis for evaluation and reassessment.

Specific Areas and Questions to Consider and Evaluate

1. Are there any associated behavioral problems such as flat or blunted affect, behavioral outbursts, or disinhibition?

2. Is the client's behavior generally passive? Does he or she respond passively to questions or suggestions?

3. What does the client do during the day? Does someone have to organize his or her activity?

4. What, if any, activities can the client initiate by him- or herself without cuing or structure?

5. What cuing method or sensory modality appears to be the most effective (ie, visual, auditory, tactile, or kinesthetic cues)?

6. Is the client aware that he or she has an initiation problem? Does he or she accept it when it is pointed out?

7. Is an associated attentional or memory problem affecting initiation abilities?

Validity

To improve validity, rule out decreased attention, processing, language, apraxia, and psychologically based (versus organic) depression as causes of poor performance.

TREATMENT FOR INITIATION DEFICITS

Utilizing a Restorative Approach

1. Provide incentive training as follows[73]:

   a) Monitor the client's needs and interests in order to identify the most appropriate incentive. Find out the client's premorbid interests and motivators.

   b) Make incentives available on an ongoing basis.

   c) Create a training environment where the incentive value is sufficient to elicit appropriate levels of interest and performance.

   d) Teach strategies to the point where they become habitual.

   e) Provide an opportunity for incentive learning by allowing the client to use newly learned strategies in a context that will provide rewards (ie, money, social praise, movie, dinner out, etc).

2. Provide sensory input (visual, auditory, kinesthetic, and tactile) to elicit a motor output (initiation). For example, tactile and kinesthetic stimulation of the client's arm combined with verbal cuing may be utilized to cue the client to initiate upper extremity dressing.

3. Provide nonverbal tactile-kinesthetic guiding to assist the client in initiating the activity.

Utilizing an Adaptive Approach

1. Provide signals such as alarm watches to trigger an activity.[4]

2. Utilize a calendar system or cue card with a list of daily activities.[4]

3. Provide an "attentional kick" such as "Just do it" or "Get going."[14] Have the client come up with his or her own "attentional kick." As the client improves, move from external to internal cuing.

4. Utilize an audio cassette that can be turned on by someone else with step-by-step instructions to follow—for example, "Take your medicine, open the little one with the white cap, take two white pills, drink some water, etc."

5. Utilize a system such as the Neuropage (Hersh and Treadgold Inc, San Jose, Calif), which is described in detail in the section on treatment for memory deficits. This system was used with a client who had an attentional-arousal problem that caused her to not initiate activities.[74] The system worked for her when a regular pager did not because in addition to the beeping there was a text message, which helped her carry out the action.

Planning and Organization

Planning can be defined as the attainment of a goal through a series of intermediate steps that do not necessarily lead directly toward that goal.[75] Planning, some argue, is not a discrete initial stage within problem solving, but an ongoing process that takes place opportunistically.[7] This could be when a task is finished, when an "impasse" in goal achievement is reached, or when novel, unexpected events happen.[7] This concept was tested in research conducted with 10 TBI clients who were provided with brief interruptions to a current activity.[7] These interruptions were used as a reminder to the client to consider current behavior and goals. The study results indicated that relatively intense, unexpected, short-lived alerts, which were accounted for in the activity instructions, can allow a window of opportunity during which the evaluation of actions against the goal can take place. These researchers concluded, "...if one aspect of executive function can be environmentally supported, other elements of problem solving and organization may stand a better chance of expression."[7]

McDonald et al state that planning includes the ability to organize steps to complete an action, prepare for setbacks in carrying out the plan, assemble needed materials, and the skills to carry out the plan.[25] They further identify seven prerequisites for planning as follows: adequate memory, motivation, sustained attention, volition, impulse control, ability to consider and weigh options, and the ability to perform complex actions.[25] Indeed, it has been shown that attention and memory can affect planning ability. For example, Golisz and Toglia note that while performing a sorting task, a client may sort items incorrectly because of an inability to recall the sorting principle."[5] In addition, if the client has volition and planning skills but an inability to carry out purposeful actions, even a well-conceived plan can be affected.[25]

In order to formulate a goal, the individual must be able to determine what he or she needs and wants and foresee the future realization of these needs.[67,76] The determination and organization of the steps needed to achieve a goal involve several component skills of planning. In order to plan, the individual must be able to conceptualize change from the present situation, relate objectively to the environment, conceive alternatives, weigh alternatives and make a choice, and develop a structure or framework to give direction to the carrying out of the plan.[71] In addition, goal-directed behavior requires the selection of new actions when previously selected actions do not achieve the goal.[39] Finally, planning and organization require the ability to identify flexible strategies, to complete a task, and determine the logical sequence of activities necessary to complete the task.[15]

Processing strategies are also crucial to effective planning and organization. These strategies can be defined as "...organized approaches, routines, or tactics that operate to select and guide the processing of information."[63] In order to develop good processing strategies, the client must be able to estimate the degree of task difficulty. If the client understands and realistically interprets task difficulty, then an appropriate plan or strategy can be developed. If this understanding or awareness is lacking, then the client's strategies will be ineffective.

The client with a planning deficit may, in fact, lack the foresight and sustained attention necessary for achieving a desired goal. Often, the client can describe in detail the elements in planning and organizing personal events but show poor, unrealistic, or illogical plans for him- or herself.[71,77] If asked to write a description of a familiar activity, for example, the client may list a series of unrelated features because he or she neglected to create a plan for the description from the beginning. The client with poor planning and organization will tend to develop unrealistic goals and underestimate the time necessary to complete a task.[5,34,78]

The client may have difficulty prioritizing several errands that have to be completed in a certain time frame.[54] Clients may also tend to perseverate in their actions and follow familiar routines even when these routines are not working instead of generating a new action plan.[25] They will also often display fragmented sequences of actions, omit relevant parts of actions, and use irrelevant parts.[79]

Disorders of planning and organization should be distinguished from memory, attentional, and mental flexibility deficits.[80,81] The ability to form and shift concepts allows for flexible planning. Impaired abstraction and mental flexibility, therefore, will adversely affect planning ability.[81] In addition, if the client is unable to organize information in order to facilitate learning and recall, the information may be stored but in a scattered manner.[80] If the information is less accessible for retrieval, then the client's problems may be erroneously interpreted as a memory problem.

Historically, planning and organization abilities have been associated with frontal lobe function.[75,80-82] A recent positron emission tomography (PET) scan study of six normal subjects, however, showed planning activated not only the frontal lobe but also the posterior parietal cortices.[83]

In recent years, some individuals working with clients who have planning and organization deficits have identified what they term "goal neglect."[10] Goal neglect occurs when the client with ABI "...is able to identify what he or she needs to achieve and may be able to derive a plan, but during the course of the operation of the plan, the main goals may become neglected and actions no longer lead to achieving the goal."[14] Goal neglect or poor goal management occurs in nonstructured, naturalistic situations in which behavior is not controlled by environmental structure.[10,83]

In answer to this problem with goal management or goal neglect, a system of Goal Management Training (GMT) has been developed.[10,14] GMT is based on the adult with ABI's inability to generate goal lists of how to solve problems and achieve goals, as well as an inability to monitor progress towards achieving goals.[14] The training is designed for the rehabilitation of clients who have impaired self-regulation that affects the organization of everyday behavior.[10]

GMT "...emphasizes a top-down approach by training broadly applicable stages of goal management and applying them to a variety of situations."[10] It can either be applied to a variety of everyday situations or to behavior in a single domain such as meal preparation.[10] Two studies of clients with ABI utilizing GMT showed improved meal preparation performance. Results were generated from both naturalistic observations and self-report measures.

The five stages of GMT are illustrated in Figure 10-1 and described as follows[10]:

> *Stage 1. Orienting*—What am I doing?
>
> *Stage 2. Defining*—The main task
>
> *Stage 3. List the steps*—Subgoals
>
> *Stage 4. Learn*—Do I know the steps? (Encoding and retention of goals and subgoals)
>
> *Stage 5. Check*—Am I doing what I planned to do? – Outcome is compared to the stated goal (monitoring).

Research conducted with 30 clients with ABI supported experimentally and clinically that GMT is an effective treatment of executive function deficits that affect independence.[10]

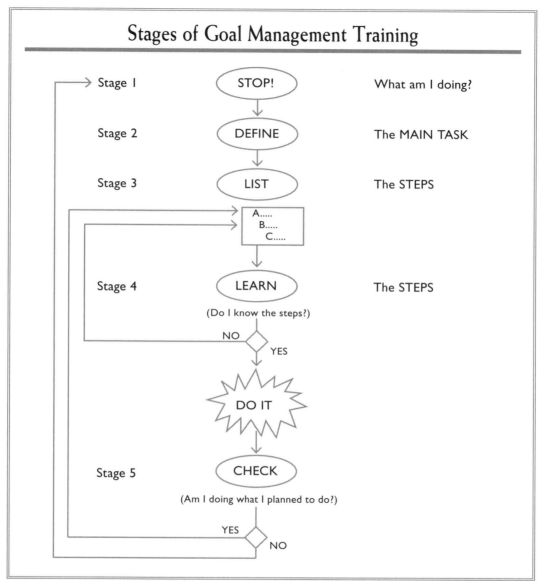

Stages of Goal Management Training

Stage 1	STOP!	What am I doing?
Stage 2	DEFINE	The MAIN TASK
Stage 3	LIST	The STEPS
	A..... B..... C.....	
Stage 4	LEARN	The STEPS
	(Do I know the steps?)	
	NO / YES	
	DO IT	
Stage 5	CHECK	
	(Am I doing what I planned to do?)	
	YES / NO	

Figure 10-1. Stages of GMT.[39] (Reprinted with permission from Cambridge University Press, Levine B, Robertson IH, Clare L, et al. Rehabilitation of executive functioning: an experimental-clinical validation of goal management training. *J Int Neuropsychol Soc.* 2000;6(3):299-312.)

EVALUATION OF PLANNING AND ORGANIZATION

Test 1 – Clinical Observation and Activity Analysis

General Guidelines for Evaluation

1. Determine whether the client is aware that he or she has a planning deficit. Defective planning often can be revealed by asking the client what he or she intends to do.

2. Observe the client in a number of settings and activities during the day. Can the client plan for activities requiring two step, three step, or more complex operations?

3. Give the client a complex task without instruction. If the client begins the task without a plan, ask him or her to create one and begin the task again. The client's plan can then be evaluated for organization and completeness.

4. Establish functional baseline measures. Consider the duration and frequency of the problem. Select relevant functional tasks as the basis of evaluation and reassessment.

Specific Areas and Questions to Consider and Evaluate

1. Is the client logical and consistent in his or her approach to the task?

2. How reliable is the client's chosen method?

3. Is there a common problem or consistently faulty planning strategy that is generalized to several activities?

4. Can the client conceptualize change (as evidenced through verbal or other means of communication) from the present?

5. Can the client present alternatives to an established plan?

6. Can the client weigh these alternatives and make a choice based on his or her judgments?

7. Does the client appear to have a framework for the plan or direction he or she is demonstrating for task completion?

8. Can the client accurately estimate task difficulty?

   Note: Questions and observations such as these can be applied to both unstructured functional and cognitive perceptual motor tasks. For example, inability to complete block designs (refer to Test 1 in the section on Problem Solving on page 260) and layout of graphic designs can be indicative or poor planning and task organization.

Scoring

Nonstandardized

These and similar questions can be incorporated into a checklist or used in conjunction with a frequency rating scale (eg, always/sometimes/rarely/never).

Validity

To improve validity, rule out decreased attention, poor memory, decreased mental flexibility and abstraction, impaired problem solving, and aphasia as causes of poor performance.

Test 2 – Occupation-Based Evaluations of Executive Functions

Refer to Section III of this chapter, starting on page 277.

TREATMENT OF PLANNING AND ORGANIZATION DEFICITS

Utilizing a Restorative Approach

1. Teach the client to relate novel information into a meaningful structure[54]—for example, to outline prose material and divide into categories when learning it.[80]

2. Teach the client that recognizing and rehearsing organizational strategies is important and that if he or she can remember elements of an organization, the individual components of the larger memory will fall into place.[54] For example, spread a variety of objects on the table, and ask the client to rehearse the types of objects he or she sees rather than rehearse each individual object.[54] The client can ask himself "how do these objects relate to each other?"

3. Increase the client's responsibility in planning the treatment session. Raskin outlines the following three stages, which can be used as a guideline for progressing the client[4]:

   Stage 1—A traditional model is used where the therapist plans and monitors the treatment session.

   Stage 2—The client is asked to sequence and monitor the tasks to be completed within the session. This includes keeping track of the time spent on each task so everything is completed within the allowed time.

   Stage 3—The client is given the full responsibility for planning and carrying out the full treatment session.

   This progression provides a structured model that could be used in all of the client's ADLs and IADLs and allows feedback from the therapist, family, and/or caregiver on the progress of the client's planning and organizational skills.[4]

4. Have the client verbalize, if possible, a plan before, during, and after a given activity. Gradually fade out overt verbalizations.[84] Also, have the client estimate task difficulty and predict the outcome of his or her identified plan. Have the client evaluate the accuracy of predictions.[54]

5. Research has indicated that training in plan-ahead and self-verbalization strategies is effective in remediating planning disorders following a TBI or cerebral vascular accident (CVA).[68,84,85] Self-verbalization requires the client to sequence each step of the task before beginning.

   Three examples of self-questioning techniques are described as follows:

   a) What do I need to do?

      I need to...

      What do I need to do now?

      I need to...

      What do I need to do now?

      I need to...

   b) What is it I want to accomplish?

      What changes need to occur to move from the present situation to my desired goal?

      What are the possible ways to make the necessary changes?

      What is the sequence or order of steps required to make the changes?

      Are there any alternatives to my plan? Which is the best alternative to use to reach my goal?

      How will I know that I have reached my goal and that my plan was successful?

   c) What is my goal?

      What is the purpose of my goal?

      Where will I perform the activity?

      How long will it take?

      What materials do I need?

      What is the order of the steps I need to take?

      Will I be able to reach my goal?

      How will I track my progress?

As the client asks these questions of himself, he can jot down his ideas or thought processes as an additional cuing mechanism. Analysis of this written plan by the therapist can then be utilized to identify any faulty planning or judgments. The client then is encouraged to develop alternative strategies:

Incorporate questioning techniques in a variety of tasks and settings. For example, searching tasks can be utilized.[13] Establish a search plan with the client by asking the following questions[13]:

a) What are we looking for? (object of the search)

Where do you suppose it is? (location, goal)

How can we find it? (plan)

How much time do we have to look? (time frame)

Do you think we can find it? (prediction of success)

Figure 10-2 illustrates a checklist for the client to use in the kitchen that utilizes the stages of GMT.[39] Checklists such as these, which incorporate the different stages of GMT, can be generated for other ADLs or IADLs—for example, brushing your teeth, dressing, or a specific community or vocational activity.

Utilizing an Adaptive Approach

1. To prevent a more impulsive style of responding to situations and to facilitate the generation of pros and cons of generated solutions, have the client write things down.[14] Progress the client, whenever possible, to mentally rehearsing a plan before doing it. This will encourage the client to process more options or consequences before settling on a plan.[54]

2. Organize reading material for comprehension.[54] The client can ask him- or herself questions after each paragraph (eg, Who is discussed? What is it about? Where did it occur?)

3. Research with clients with TBI utilizing simple, open-ended tasks (ie, carrying out arithmetic problems or dictating a route) showed that the clients "...were unable to reactivate after a delay in previously generated intentions when they were not directly signaled by the stimulus situation."[86] These researchers found the following to improve performance: 1) verbal cuing back to the task and 2) written cards with step-by-step instructions and a periodic cue card that states the original intentions or goal.

4. Provide external aids such as daily reminders, appointment calendars, and to do lists for the client. Provide not just what the client needs to do but what he or she needs to do to complete the task.[54]

5. The use of the Neuropage has been found effective with clients.[87] Results of a study of 143 TBI or CVA clients who used the Neuropage system indicated that 80% were significantly more successful in carrying out everyday activities (such as self-care, self-medication, and keeping appointments) when using the Neuropage in comparison with the baseline period.[87] Clients had one or more of the following deficits: decreased memory, decreased planning and organization, and/or decreased attention.

6. Teach the client to arrange items according to the sequence of use before starting a task.[64] He or she should place items in a linear manner with spaces between objects.[64]

7. The external and/or organizational strategy used should be comfortable for the client. Interview the client and/or his family as to what systems the client used premorbidly (ie, palm pilot, checklists, computer). Use those methods now, as the client is more likely to be comfortable with them and may have retained at least some memory for how to use them.

Goal-Management-Training-Based Recipe Checklist

Recipe: _____

PREPARATION TIME: TOTAL TIME:

COOKING TIME:

SET OVEN TEMPERATURE:

COLLECT THE INGREDIENTS: TIME NEEDED: _____

CHECK   Have I got everything I need?

PREPARE THE INGREDIENTS: TIME NEEDED: _____

CHECK   Is everything ready to start?

COMPLETE THE STEPS ONE AT A TIME: TIME NEEDED: _____

CHECK   Have I followed all the steps?

COOKING INSTRUCTIONS: TIME NEEDED: _____

CHECK   Have I written the cooking times on the blackboard?

Figure 10-2. GMT-based recipe checklist.[39] (Reprinted with permission from Cambridge University Press. Levine B, Robertson IH, Clare L, et al. Rehabilitation of executive functioning: an experimental-clinical validation of goal management training. *J Int Neuropsychol Soc.* 2000;6(3):308.)

8. Reorganize the client's living and workplace as needed. Parente and Herrmann outline the following principles for reorganizing the client's environment[20]:

a) *Accessibility*—Keep items the client uses a lot close by.

b) *Consistency*—Have a specific place for items.

c) *Grouping*—Place items commonly used together in the same place.

d) *Separation*—Keep things in distinct locations or categories (eg, clothes in a closet, pants on one rack, shirts on another).

e) *Proximity*—Items that are used together should be kept together where they are used (eg, computer paper kept near the printer).

Problem Solving

Problem solving is not a single function but rather the integration of several cognitive skills. Whenever an individual is unable to develop a means to achieve a goal, a problem arises.[20] Problem solving requires attention, the ability to devise and initiate a plan, information access (both sensory from the environment and memory), and a feedback system that gives information on the effectiveness of the solution and the need for revision.[72,88-92] Additional prerequisites for problem solving include good impulse control, the ability to organize and categorize, mental flexibility, and reasoning skills.[93] Problem solving is an active process, and breakdown can occur at any stage. In addition, the client's reasoning ability can determine the quality of the manner in which a problem will be formulated and the strategies applied for problem solutions.[93]

Effective problem solving involves some initial understanding of the problem. How good this initial representation is will determine how quickly an accurate solution can be formulated. Motivation can affect both the perception of a problem and whether or not a solution is attempted. Motivation problems can originate from depression and/or decreased self-awareness of deficits.[93] Problem solving can vary, depending on whether the client has access to and utilizes a memory aid.[89] Approaching a problem and comparing past and present experiences through memory skills enable an individual to think in an orderly manner.[94,95] The individual must be able to screen out and discard irrelevant information.[96,97] Problem solving ability will be affected if adequate attention is not taken to analyze the stimulus problem or situation completely.[2] Once the information is registered and screened, the individual must be able to modify, transform, and organize it to come up with a solution.[89,90] Problem solving requires mental flexibility. The individual needs to be able to reformulate initial ideas when a solution is incorrect or fails to solve the problem.[72] Finally, the individual must be able to make judgments about the quality of potential solutions.[89]

Adamovich describes four theoretical thinking processes involved in problem solving.[98] The client must first recognize and analyze relevant and missing information (convergent thinking). Next, he or she must draw conclusions about a given situation based on certain principles and in a systematic manner (deductive reasoning). The client must then formulate a solution based on details that lead to a standard conclusion (inductive reasoning). Finally, the client must be able to generate abstract concepts that deviate from standard concepts.

Lezak identifies four stages of executive function in problem solving as follows[71]:

> *Stage 1. Goal formation*—What do I want or need?
>
> *Stage 2. Planning*—How will I get what I need?
>
> *Stage 3. Carrying out activities*—Am I doing things to reach my goal?
>
> *Stage 4. Effective performance*—Are my activities fulfilling my objective?

Ben-Yishay and Diller support both Adamovich and Lezak in their model of problem solving.[99] They describe an eight-stage model of problem solving, which incorporates some convergent, divergent, and executive stages. The eight stages are outlined as follows:

> *Stage 1. Formulate problem*
>
> *Stage 2. Analyze conditions of problem*
>
> *Stage 3. Formulate strategy and plan of action*
>
> *Stage 4. Choose the relevant tactics (apply skills, prioritize)*
>
> *Stage 5. Execute plan—self-monitor operation*

Stage 6. Compare solution against problem

Stage 7. Satisfaction and closure

Stage 8. Integration into attitudes and skills, and personalization—What does it mean to me?

Ben-Yishay and Diller also include in their theoretical framework for treatment the concept of two domains of skills in the problem solving process[99]: 1) the core skills, which include skills such as attention, sensation, tone, language, or memory; and 2) the two higher domains of problem solving/rational processes and emotive, imaginative, and emphatic processes. They theorize that disorders of high domains can be caused by the core deficits and that effective problem solving depends on the interaction between the two domains. Evaluation and treatment, they believe, should address all aspects of the eight-stage process and two domains of skills.

Evans describes problem solving to be dependent on three broad areas.[6] The first area is the ability to be aware that a problem exists and to monitor what has been implemented as a solution. The second is the development of an action plan, and the third is the translation of intention into the action, or initiation.

Some theorists relate the concept of problem solving to that of novelty or novel activities.[6,45] They describe how the individual needs the ability to detect novelty from both external sensory events and internal thought combined with an ability to produce novel behaviors. These abilities are crucial to new learning, creativity, and environmental adaptation. These abilities allow the individual to be able to solve new problems. Whenever problem solving breaks down, the individual will be unable to deal effectively with novel situations.[6]

Golisz and Toglia divide problem solving into two categories: basic and complex problem solving.[5] Basic problem solving is utilized when the problem is clear, and easily identified information to solve the problem is available. Basic problem solving is usually one to three steps, and if the client does something incorrectly, it is immediately apparent.[5] For example, the client would notice right away if coffee grinds were coming through on a drip machine because the client did not put the filter in before scooping coffee into the machine. Complex problem solving, on the other hand, involves a situation when the client must sort out information to identify the problem—for example, why a car will not start or why a check bounced.[5]

Golisz and Toglia describe the skills necessary for complex problem solving as follows[5]:

> *Solving the complex problem requires the ability to plan, test, and reject different hypotheses and the skill to formulate alternatives to the problem. Execution of the plan entails carrying out several steps, and incorrect solutions are not readily apparent. Verification that the problem has been solved involves actively comparing the solution with the original problem.*

An important concept related to problem solving that most believe is a requisite skill for successful problem solving is that of deductive reasoning. Goverover and Hinojosa define deductive reasoning as the capacity to formulate and test hypotheses and state that deductive reasoning depends on the ability to form and manipulate mental representations of relations between objects and events.[31] It is the ability to generate and test hypotheses based on available information.[3] When utilizing deductive reasoning "…a person develops hypotheses, makes inferences, and rationalizes a conclusion."[31] This process involves decision making and judging or evaluating information and is accomplished by available information, perceptual observations, memory, beliefs, and imagination.[3,100] The importance of reasoning is described well by Parsons and Osherson as follows[101]: "…As much as perception, language and motor behavior, it is reason that allows us to interact successfully with the physical and social environment."

Clients with problem solving deficits may exhibit concrete thinking, impulsivity, confusion as to where to start solving a problem, difficulty sequencing information, and trouble learning from mistakes as well as successes.[61,102] They may have difficulty organizing and structuring their problem space and difficulty allocating adequate effort to each step, analyzing the problem, and omitting critical details.[5]

Unless the client has some degree of problem solving skills, he or she will be unable to apply newly learned skills to new situations.[103] The clinical manifestations of poor problem solving can reflect a breakdown in any aspect or stage of the overall process previously outlined. The evaluation of problem solving, therefore, can be accomplished by administering a variety of traditional and nontraditional measures as well as a detailed process analysis of the underlying deficit.[93]

EVALUATION OF PROBLEM SOLVING

Many standard traditional tests of problem solving present problems directly to the client, thereby not requiring the client to define the problem or self-initiate for task completion.[6] The tests included in this section, therefore, are felt to place problem solving demands on the client for task completion.

*Test 1 – Clinical Observations and Activity Analysis[89]**

Description

Provide an unstructured task without guidance from the therapist. Observation during functional settings and tasks is best. Observe for the following abilities. Problem solving is divided into three stages: preparation, production, and judgment. Clinical observations in selected activities are based on questions related to these three stages:

1. *Preparation and understanding the problem*—Problem analysis

   a) Can the client identify any or all elements of the problem?

   b) Can the client identify solution criteria?

   c) Can the client identify any limitations or constraints related to potential attempts at problem solving?

   d) Can the client describe or indicate how the problem compares with those he or she has already solved?

   e) Can the client divide the problem into parts or components?

   f) Can the client construct a simple problem by ignoring some information?

2. *Production*—Generating possible solutions

   a) Can the client retrieve necessary information from long-term memory?

   b) Can or does the client scan the environment for available information?

   c) Can or does the client operate or act on the content in short-term memory?

   d) Can or does the client store information in long-term memory for later use?

   e) Can the client generate a potential solution?

3. *Judgment*—Evaluating the solution generated

   a) Does the client compare the generated solution with the initial solution criteria?

---

*Adapted with permission from Prentice-Hall Inc, reference 89: Bourne LE, Dominowski RL, Loftus EF. Cognitive Processes. *Englewood Cliffs, NJ: Prentice-Hall; 1979.*

b) Does the client decide either that the problem has been solved or that more work is needed?

Scoring

Nonstandardized

The preceding or similar questions can be incorporated into a yes/no checklist or related to a frequency rating scale.

Validity

To improve validity, rule out poor attention, memory, impulsiveness, or other factors as causes of poor performance.

DYNAMIC ASSESSMENT

Test 1 – The Deductive Reasoning Test[63,64]

Equipment

Utensils from the TCA[63,64]

Description

A question game is used to assess the client's ability to formulate and test different hypotheses. The examiner tells the client that he or she has to determine which utensil the examiner is thinking of with the least amount of guessing and the fewest number of questions as possible. The client asks only "yes" or "no" questions. The examiner does not actually think of an item but answers "no" to all the questions (whenever possible) until there is only one possibility left.

If 18 utensils of different colors (red, yellow, green), size (big, small), and type (fork, spoon, knife) are used, then the answer is attainable with five questions.

If the client does not solve the problem with questions, another trial is given with a maximum of up to three trials. The examiner gives the standard sequence of prompts when the client is unable to solve the problem with 4 questions.

Scoring

Ranges from 0 (cannot obtain the right answer with maximum cues and task modification) to 7 (is able to get the correct answer with 5 questions) (maximum score = 21)[31]

Validity

Construct validity has been established.[3] A significant main effect for age was obtained (F [5, 213] = 12.35, p < 0.001).

Research has also shown this test to be significantly correlated with education (r = 0.670, p < 0.01) and age (r = –0.661, p < 0.01).[31] The results of this study also indicated that deductive reasoning (as well as categorization) are significantly related to important predictors of IADLs in persons with brain injury.[31]

Reliability

Inter-rater reliability was established with a sample of 43 individuals with brain injury and 51 people without disability.

TREATMENT OF PROBLEM SOLVING DEFICITS

*Utilizing a Restorative Approach**

There is some evidence that retraining approaches that focus on teaching problem solving skills to clients with ABI can be effective and have practical benefits.[14] The specific objectives of retraining are to improve the client's ability to perform each of the separate stages of problem solving. This is accomplished through tasks that are designed to use the skills required for each of the separate stages.[6] If utilizing the restorative approach, it is important to use occupation-based activities whenever possible. The therapist should design the activities to the client's level (ie, basic or complex problem solving).

1. Train the client in developing the following skills[104]*:

    a) The ability to recognize at a general level that a given task or situation is a problem for which a solution is not yet available.

    b) Have the client read and reread directions and ask questions to help his or her understanding of the problem.

    c) Have the client describe in his or her own words the main points, discriminating between the facts and opinions or assumptions.

    d) Train the client to identify problem solving goals, restraints, and circumstances that cause the task to be problematic.

    e) Train the client to generate alternatives or potential solutions to the problem.

    f) Teach the client to evaluate the alternative solutions and to select the most effective one. Ask the client why he or she came up with a given solution, and decide the potential consequences.

    g) Train the client to recognize "faulty" paths, correct errors, and return to the original hypothesis.

2. Utilize problem solving worksheets such as the following[105]:

Activity
Yellow Pages**

Purpose
1. Improve problem-solving skills.
2. Improve ability to make logical deductions.
3. Improve speed in decision making.

Supplies

Trial/Score Sheets #1 to #5, a copy of the written instructions for these Trials, pencil, Yellow Pages, Answer Key, Therapist Observation Sheet, Weekly Performance Summary, White Self-Assessment Quiz, stopwatch (optional).

Activity Description and Session Strategies

For each Trial, the client is given 10 hypothetical problems or situations that might require contacting local places of business. Using the Yellow Pages, the client must record in the space provided on the Trial Sheet the name of the business and telephone number

---

Research utilizing this specific restorative approach indicated improved problem solving after 3 months.
**Reprinted with permission from PRO-ED, reference 105: Dougherty PM, Radomski MV. A Dynamic Assessment Approach for Adults with Brain Injury: The Cognitive Rehabilitation Workbook. *Gaithersburg, Md: Aspen Publishers; 1993.*

that logically address each situation. The client receives verbal instructions supplemented by written instructions. A Demonstration Item is included in each Trial to be used at the therapist's discretion.

The client should be instructed to review his or her work with the therapist after finishing each Trial. The Answer Key provides possible headings under which appropriate businesses might be located for each item and is intended to be used by the client and therapist during the review process. After reviewing the Trial, the client completes the White Self-Assessment Quiz and compares it with the therapist's version. The client and therapist discuss and determine strategy modifications for subsequent Trials.

Speed in decision making is an important component in this exercise and should be emphasized. Some clients may waste time reading advertisements, or for example, looking unnecessarily for the dry cleaner closest to their home rather than recording the answer that they locate first. When it is evident that the client is becoming distracted by components of the task itself, the therapist may opt to time each Trial in order to demonstrate graphically the effect of this problem on performance.

Written Instructions

1. Before you begin work, you will need to make sure that you have a pencil, Yellow Pages directory, and Trial Sheet and that you know where to locate the Answer Key.

2. Beginning with item "A," you are to read the hypothetical problem or situation that might require you to contact a local place of business.

3. Using the Yellow Pages, you are to record (in the space provided) the name of a business and telephone number that logically address the situation.

4. After completion of item "J," bring your Trial Sheet to the therapist. Using the Answer Key, discuss your answers with him or her, and together, determine whether you have made errors.

5. Next, request the White Self-Assessment Quiz and fill it out.

6. After filling out the Quiz, be prepared to discuss the results with the therapist.

Resources: the telephone

Yellow Pages – Trial #2

Date:

Name:

Demonstration Task

Your carpet needs to be cleaned.

Answer: Carpet & Rug Cleaners: (Therapist provides example).

A. You have some money to invest.

Answer: _____

B. You are hungry for a chocolate-covered doughnut.

Answer: _____

C. You want to have your hair colored.

Answer: _____

D. You want to buy a baseball bat.

Answer: _____

E. Your toilet is backed up.

Answer: _____

F. You would like to have someone answer your telephone calls.

Answer: _____

G. Your need a water softener.
Answer: _____

H. Your washing machine needs to be repaired.
Answer: _____

I. Your lawn needs to be fertilized.
Answer: _____

J. You want to have a picture framed.
Answer: _____

Accuracy (number of errors): _____

3. If the client is trying to achieve a major goal (eg, return to work), identify with the client the specific tasks the client is required to do. Support the client in learning to perform the tasks depending on the deficits. What begins as a novel task requiring appropriate problem solving skills eventually becomes a routine task.[6]

4. Teach the client to utilize "chaining" of the activity (ie, breaking it down into functional components):

   a) Have the client describe how he or she would define and carry out a given problem.[95] Have the client continue the process by describing how he or she is doing something as he or she is doing it.[77] Progress from external environmental cues to internal cues by subvocalization (ie, the client tells him- or herself what he or she is doing as he or she is doing it).

   b) Have the client plan the step in problem solution before doing it.

   c) Have the client label the steps of the task to make them more meaningful, thus increasing his or her memory of them.[77]

5. Research has shown that client use of verbalizations assists in slowing the client down and facilitating the processes involved in producing explanations for solving the problem.[106]

6. Help the client develop internal strategies for approaching new tasks.[6] The client should be comfortable with the strategies utilized.

7. The computer game Mastermind (Invicta Plastics, Ltd, Leicester, England) has been programmed so that the level of difficulty and type of stimuli can be tailored to the individual and made progressively more difficult. This game requires problem solving and uses feedback to guide performance with no memory component.[4]

8. Have the client perform a variety of tasks in a number of settings, utilizing the remedial techniques just described.

Treatment could focus both on tabletop and functional activities. For example, try cognitive flexibility worksheets that alternate between subtraction and addition and link these with counting change and money handling. Combining the approaches could improve motivation because the client learns the relevance of the skills to ADLs.

Utilizing an Adaptive Approach

1. Monitor how the task or environment can be altered in order to improve problem solving skills. For example, depending on the client's level, limit irrelevant information, and present only what is relevant to solving the problem. Provide adaptations as needed.

   a) Provide external cues to reduce the client's use of inappropriate strategies.[102]

   b) Instruct the client to check for errors before proceeding.

When giving external cues, therapists should remember that they know how to solve the problem and the client may not.[89] Make sure that the connection between the cue and the solution is clear. Ask, "How will the client use this cue?"

2. Identify key areas of occupational performance that are affected by impaired problem solving. For the targeted areas, provide step-by-step instructions for task completion.

3. Teach the client the importance of asking for help when he or she is unable to solve a given problem. Practice this skill with the client through role playing and community reintegration treatment.

4. Parente and Herrmann describe an "Action-Goal Strategy" for solving problems and the following example to illustrate the technique.[20] This involves providing questioning techniques that break down the problem into subgoals. For example, if the client discovers his television does not work, the client would first ask, "Is the television getting electricity?" This may lead the client to check whether the television will function with other wall outlets, to check the plug, or to see if there is a blown fuse. If the television is getting electricity, the client moves to the next step: Will it work on any channel? With or without cable hook up? As the client answers each question at each stage, the possible cause of the problem and range of solutions decrease.[20]

Utilizing a Dynamic Interactional Approach

Through dynamic interactional assessment (DIA), underlying processes that affect the client's problem solving ability will be identified. These processes are also common to other cognitive domains such as memory, mental flexibility, etc. The underlying processes common to the most areas and most likely to respond to treatment are addressed.[63,64] For example, the client's decreased problem solving skills (or memory, mental flexibility, etc) may all be affected by the client's inattention to detail. Problem solving tasks should, therefore, address this underlying process. The therapist would identify the task variables—for example, how the information required to complete the problem solving task is presented or what environmental factors (limiting distracters) could be altered to facilitate performance. The activity is structured at the client's level (which has been identified during DIA) and graded as the client improves. The techniques are utilized in a number of contexts or settings.

Decision Making

Some therapists find it helpful to differentiate between problem solving and decision making. Decision making is viewed as a form of problem solving for which the problem is to choose from several options to make a decision.[20,107] In this view, problem solving is "...a more general activity in which the goal is to rectify an unacceptable situation."[20] Although problem solving involves decision making, the options in decision making are often known, and the client's task is to make a choice among these options.[20]

Factors which influence decision making are both conscious and unconscious.[108,109] Goldberg and Podell identify two types of decision making.[107] The first is veridical decision making, which is finding the correct response intrinsic to external situations.[107] Veridical decision making is client independent. This is the type of decision making based on a right or wrong answer and is the traditional type test stimulus for executive function tests.[107] The second type of decision making is called adaptive decision making and is client-centered and priority-based.[107] These types of decisions are not based on the external environment alone and are the types of decisions made in real life situations.

Clients with ABI who have impaired decision making ability may have a difficult time identifying various options and determining which options are best.[20] They have difficulty learning from their mistakes and may continuously engage in decisions that lead to negative consequences.[109] The underlying problem is thought to be that the client with ABI does not have a systematic method for making decisions.[20]

The orbitofrontal cortex as well as other large scale cortical and subcortical systems are thought to subserve decision making.[109]

Parente and Herrmann provide the following treatment guidelines for clients with impaired decision making abilities[20]:

Instruct the client (and assist as needed) to do as follows:

1. Collect all the information about the decision to be made and do not make the decision until all the facts are collected.

2. Identify all available options and choose one that he or she can control.

3. List all the positives and negatives of each option (make a two column list column 1 = benefits, column 2 = problems).

4. Identify how he or she feels about the identified options.

Parente and Herrmann also describe the Seven Question Method, which assists the client with ABI in decision making.[20] These clinicians feel the value of methods such as this system is that it forces the client to follow a structured thinking process before making a decision.[20]

Seven Question Method[20]

1. Can I define the decision? For example, which restaurant to go to dinner.

2. Does the decision involve a problem or an opportunity?

3. Is there an existing policy that dictates the decision or that otherwise overrides any decision the person may make? For example, driving after ABI, the law often requires a medical exam and clearance and to retake the written exam.

4. Can the decision be classified? For example, go/no go, right/wrong, evaluation decision (evaluate which of several options is best), discovery decision (identifying potential options in situations where none are known)

5. Is the problem real or imagined? For example, a client with no high school diploma deciding whether or not to apply for a PhD program in the fall

6. Does the decision involve money, people, or a combination of both?

7. What would happen if the client decided to do nothing?

Categorization

Categorization allows an individual to process large amounts of information and is thought to be a crucial component to all cognitive skills or ability.[110] When an individual categorizes, he or she finds commonalities and assigns objects or events into groups.[2,20] Categorization is not subserved by a single brain area, and in fact, research has indicated that visual recognition and categorization of everyday objects involve two anatomically and functionally distinct pathways.[2,110] These pathways specialize in different types of information. The first pathway is the ventral pathway, which involves the temporal lobes.[2] This pathway ". . . subserves passive recognition in which the object is perceived as a kind of thing that the observer has seen before. This recognition includes all aspects of visual memory, such as form, function, the object's typical location, and many other associated memories."[2] The second pathway, or dorsal pathway, involves the parietal lobes and mediates visually guided behavior such as reaching and grasping objects.[2] Frontal lobe function has also been associated with certain aspects of categorization abilities (ie, rule application).[110] Recent neuroimaging studies have also shown how highly differentiated cortical structures are for processes related to categorization.[110]

Recent theories pertaining to categorization suggest that there are two primary types. The first is recognition and categorization of everyday objects, and the second is recognition and categorization of novel situations as well as category learning.[2] Ashley identifies three systems utilized to create categories.[110] The first is the rule-based or rule-governed category system, which relies heavily on executive functions. The second involves the ability to recall previously experienced category members that are similar to the present novel object. This system relies on episodic memory. The third system is an implicit system, which relies on processes similar to those related to motor learning.

Perceptual features play a crucial role in basic categorization of objects. Utilization of perceptual features in categorization is referred to as the "featural approach."[110] An individual needs to be able to perceive and utilize perceptual features in order to be able to categorize.[110] Evidence has shown that in vision, there is a hierarchal process of recognition that begins with early perceptual feature processing.[110] This includes features such as color, shape, orientation, and motion. This processing leads to the processing and representation of objects and object classes.

Perceptual features become category descriptors.[110] Ashley describes three types of perceptual features used in categorization. These features are iconic, which are descriptive of physical characteristics; symbolic, which describe symbolic characteristics; and a general characteristics category, which would include descriptors such as pretty or fast. In essence, every noun, verb, preposition, adjective, and adverb can be a potential feature.[110]

As a category is defined through perceptual features, objects or members within a category may vary in degree to which they are representative of the given category.[110] A core group of perceptual features, however, is required by all category members. Some category members will have additional features not required for inclusion in the category.

The client with ABI may have underlying deficits in any aspect of categorization. Many clients are unable to use attributes to describe objects. Others can categorize utilizing iconic or physical features but are unable to use symbolic features. For example, the client may be able to recognize and categorize an apple as red but unable to categorize it as a fruit.

EVALUATION OF CATEGORIZATION: DYNAMIC ASSESSMENT

Test 1 – Toglia Category Assessment[63,64]

Description

The TCA was designed to examine the ability to establish categories or switch conceptual sets. The test uses 18 utensils that can be sorted according to size (small or large), color (red, green, or yellow), and utensil type (knife, fork, or spoon). The client is asked to sort the 18 utensils into different groups so that the items in one group are different in one way from those of the other groups. Once the client sorts the items in one way, he or she is then asked to sort them in a different way and then again in a third way. Strategy use is investigated by asking the client to explain how the groups are different after each classification. If the client has trouble, standard sequences of cues are provided. Awareness is investigated by asking the client standard questions designed to investigate awareness before and after test performance. Administration takes approximately 25 minutes.

Scoring

Scores range from 1 (unable to sort after reduction of amount) to 11 (independent sort no cues given). A separate score is assigned for each sort (ie, size, color, type), and a total score combines all three scores (maximum score = 33).[31]

Validity

Concurrent validity (r = 0.52, p < 0.001)[111]

Additional research conducted by Goverover and Hinojosa indicated that results of the TCA of clients with brain injury may be good predictors of functional performance.[31] Use of standard cues during assessment helps differentiate the underlying problem affecting performance—for example, a tendency to become stuck in one category, a concrete approach such as grouping utensils according to use or function, etc. These researchers state that study results indicate categorization (and deductive reasoning) abilities are fundamental to the performance of IADLs.

Reliability

Inter-rater reliability (0.87) internal consistency ranging from 0.74 to 0.80 (p < 0.001)[111]

TREATMENT OF CATEGORIZATION

Utilizing a Restorative Approach

Restorative techniques, such as those subsequently described, can be incorporated into the occupation-based treatment program. For example, during meal preparation, when the client is using a knife to chop vegetables, the therapist can ask the client to describe the perceptual features of the knife as he or she is working. Or, when the client is pulling up a chair to sit down to eat, the therapist could ask for what else a chair could be used (ie, as an object to stand on to reach high places, an object to place items on, etc).

1. Have the client identify iconic and symbolic features of objects that are grouped together.[110] Begin with three rows of objects (ie, row 1 – red objects, row 2 – yellow objects, row 3 – blue objects). The client should recognize the common feature as color. Create three new rows of objects that require the client to identify three different perceptual features. Each row should target different perceptual features—for example, row 1 – all objects are round, row 2 – all objects are the same color, row 3 – all objects have the same function.

2. Ashley outlines a three-level training program that helps the client identify different perceptual features of objects.[110]

Level 1

Perceptual features can include seven iconic or physical features (color, construction, size, shape, weight, texture, and detail) and one symbolic feature (function of the object). During the initial training, a checklist of the eight features may be used. Once the client begins to learn the features in an organized manner, the checklist can be faded.

Level 2

The client expands from the eight feature identification skills from Level 1 and provides an extended feature. For example, "...when describing a stop sign, the individual must identify that the stop sign is red and must identify another object that is red, such as an apple."[110]

Level 3

Level 3 is termed "abstract negation."[110] The client is asked to identify eight perceptual features of what the object is not. For example "...the stop sign is not blue, and another object which is not blue is the sun."[110]

Utilizing an Adaptive Approach

Reorganize the client's living and workspace as needed (refer to #7 under Adaptive Approach for Planning and Reorganization). This will help cue the client as to object categories and the functional use of the objects he or she sees—for example, if all eating utensils are together in one bin or all cleaning supplies are in one cabinet.

Utilizing a Dynamic Interactional Approach

As previously described, the TCA includes standard cuing to help differentiate the underlying causes of poor performance on the categorization task. Categorization tasks used in treatment will address specific deficits in the underlying processes that have been identified through DIA. Activities are structured at the client's level and are graded as the client improves. The techniques, or processing strategies, are utilized in a number of contexts or settings.

Mental Flexibility

The ability to carry out a given plan requires the ability to initiate, stop, and switch actions, depending on feedback from the environment related to these actions.[25,31,81] The client with ABI will often have difficulty with these mental shifts and will exhibit rigid, inflexible, or perseverative behavior. A client is said to show perseverative behavior in "...any situation when events of prior behavior find their way maladaptively in the ongoing behavior."[112] This occurs because the client continues to respond to prior cues that are no longer relevant.[77,113] The client has difficulty releasing a particular stimulus from his or her attention. The client may show poor association ability and have difficulty in evaluating the relevance of the result obtained from a given problem. This stimulus-bound or perseverative behavior makes it difficult for the client to generalize knowledge for future problem solution.[11,40,114] Some clients are unable to shift response strategies, at times, even while verbalizing that they know their response is wrong.[25] They have lost "...the capacity to respond to unanticipated environmental contingencies."[112] They may continuously give the same response across a variety of situations despite changes in the environmental demands. This may occur even when their responses are inappropriate or even dangerous.[25]

This inability to mentally shift between criteria or tasks is the difference between concrete and flexible, abstract thinking.[115] It will affect the client's ability to perform ADLs or IADLs ranging from meal preparation, to driving, to financial planning.[21]

EVALUATION OF MENTAL FLEXIBILITY

Test 1 – Odd-Even Cross-Out[80]

Description

This task tests the client's ability to shift from one task to another. The client is provided with a visual search worksheet with a series of numbers on it. He or she is asked to begin crossing out all the even numbers and, partially through the task, is asked to cross out only the odd numbers. This instruction is subsequently reversed back to the even numbers, then back to the odd, and so on.

Scoring

Nonstandardized

> *Intact*—The client is able to shift back and forth (odd-even) on all occasions as requested by the therapist.
>
> *Impaired*—The client is able to shift back and forth (odd-even) for only a portion of the task.
>
> *Unable*—The client is unable to successfully make the switch.

Validity

To improve validity, rule out decreased attention, decreased comprehension, visual neglect, visual field deficits, and decreased visual scanning as causes of poor performance.

Dynamic Assessment

Please refer to Test 2 for Attention in Chapter 8 (page 199) and Table 8-3 (page 201) for a description of Dynamic Assessment of Attention, which includes the concept of mental shifting and the ability to generate alternate responses or ideas.

TREATMENT FOR MENTAL FLEXIBILITY

Utilizing a Restorative Approach

1. Have the client perform occupation-based, tabletop activities that require numerous mental shifts and variations within the task (eg, tasks involving shifting from color to the written word or the substitution of visual instructions for verbal instructions).

2. If the client is physically perseverating, as for example, while putting his shirt on, physically guide the client to the next step in the process.

Utilizing an Adaptive Approach

1. During occupation-based activities, ask the client to perform, for example, a kitchen task that includes hot and cold meal preparation and functional categorization. Observe whether the client can shift and organize his behavior within the overall activity. Provide cuing when necessary to compensate for the impaired mental flexibility to increase the client's independence.

2. Utilize external aids such as written or audiotape instructions for relevant areas of function to compensate for the deficit.

3. Provide breaks between activities to allow time for the client to mentally shift to the next activity.[116]

4. Teach the client and his or her family about the deficit and how it will affect his or her daily life.

Utilizing a Dynamic Interactional Approach

1. Apply concepts from a DIA by altering task demands (surface characteristics) and type and amount of feedback for mental shifting between stimulis depending on the client's performance. Provide occupation-based activities that require mental flexibility/shifting in a variety of context or settings.

2. Identify which cognitive domains are affected by the client's mental inflexibility. For example, the client's mental inflexibility may be an underlying cause for his or her decreased categorization or problem solving. This information can be extrapolated from the interpretation of the results from dynamic assessment tools such as the TCA, previously described.

3. Identify which task characteristics and environmental factors facilitate performance, and provide treatment in a variety of contexts or settings. As the client improves, progress the client by altering additional task characteristics. For example, if the client is able to shift from one step of preparing a cup of coffee to another without environmental distractions, progress the client to performing the task with graded environmental distractions. This would be done if the DIA pointed to environmental distractions as the cause of a decrease in the client's attentional shifting. The following is an example of changing environmental factors. During DIA (such as the TCA), it may have been revealed that the client was able to mentally shift only between two groups of objects or could only shift his or her behavior if there was a physical component to the activity. In cases such as these, altering the task characteristics would be indicated. Activities would be initiated that required shifting from one task to another in multi-contexts and progressed to two shift requirements, then three, etc. The same principle would be utilized for the client who required a physical component to shift his or her behavior. Treatment would begin with activities that had a physical component and progress to more abstract activities.

Abstraction

Abstraction, or concept formation, is one of the most crucial cognitive functions that an individual performs. Abstract thinking is the ability to conceptualize and make inferences from information.[15] It is fundamental to thinking and communication.[20] Concept formation and abstraction require the individual to be able to identify features that are common to a group of objects and discover rules that relate these conceptual features. In other words, abstract thinking requires categorization abilities. In addition, the individual must be able to "...relate information to a hierarchal order, determine the relevance of the information according to a particular situation, sequence information, and solve problems."[116]

Impaired abstraction is a commonly occurring deficit exhibited by the ABI client. Clients with poor abstraction have limited imagination and stick to people, objects, and events that catch their eye at once.[104] These clients fail to form concepts or generalize from individual events, fail to plan ahead, are unable to go beyond the immediate stimulus situation, and have difficulty explaining their ideas.[20,117] The client is unable to analyze the relationship between objects and their properties.[93] They view information in a concrete or factual fashion and often appear rigid in their approach.[5,15] The client's ability to understand a concept is dependent on how clearly and concretely it is presented.[20]

Some researchers consider memory deficits as a partial cause of this concrete thinking.[94,99] Severe anterograde amnesia in cases of brain injury is associated with subtle or severe problems with abstraction and decreased "mental flexibility," which in turn, results in the client's inability to learn and integrate new information for future conceptualization.[99] Theoretically, clients with poor abstraction are unable to perceive similarities and differences or to identify the important features in objects and events because they are unable to keep these objects and events in mind.[94] Owing to a memory deficit, they are unable to make comparisons or are unable to retain the comparisons they have already made.

EVALUATION OF ABSTRACTION

Test 1 – Concept Formation and Abstraction[90]

Concept formation involves the ability to define objects, compare and differentiate, establish logical relationships, and categorize. The following sample questions illustrate the evaluation of each of these components of concept formation and abstraction.

Definition-Abstraction

The client is asked to define a specific word (eg, chair, apple).

Scoring

Nonstandardized
The therapist notes how the client makes use of abstract categories.

Comparison-Differentiation

The client is asked to relate a pair of ideas through the following:

1. *Common ground* (eg, refrigerator and stove, dresser and sofa).

2. *Differences* (eg, the difference between a fox and a dog or a bed and a chair).

Scoring

Nonstandardized
The therapist notes whether the client is able to identify similarities and differences between the paired ideas presented.

Logical Relationships

The client is asked to relate a word to a given series, (eg, a dog is a _____, a knife is a _____).

Scoring

Nonstandardized
The therapist notes the client's ability to establish logical relationships through completion of the series presented.

Opposites

The client is asked to supply the opposite of the word the therapist gives him (eg, high-low, tall-short).

Scoring

Nonstandardized
The therapist notes the client's ability to supply the opposite.

Categories

The client is asked to identify the word that does not belong in a series of words the therapist provides (eg, father, mother, brother, sister, friend).

Scoring

Nonstandardized
The therapist notes the client's ability to identify the word that does not belong in the series.

Validity

To improve validity, rule out decreased attention, memory, and aphasia (especially comprehension) as causes of poor performance.

Table 10-5

Applying for a Job Checklist

Locating Available Jobs

1. Purchase newspaper ☐
2. Purchase trade journals ☐
3. Network with friends and colleagues ☐
4. Review ads for appropriate possible job ☐
5. Develop a question list for initial phone contact ☐
6. Contact chosen potential employers to find out if the job is still available, and use your question list for the initial phone contact ☐

TREATMENT OF ABSTRACTION

Utilizing an Adaptive Approach

1. If the client is unable to abstract, teach the client how to make greater use of his or her concrete thinking skills in problem solving.[93]

2. Provide information in a factual manner, and avoid using abstract concepts whenever possible.[15]

3. Parente and Herrmann outline the following strategy to assist the client to compensate for decreased abstract thinking.[20]

    a) Break down the concept into smaller pieces, and give concrete and clear examples to illustrate the concept.

    b) Have the client identify the relevant dimensions of the concept.

    c) Have the client ask others to explain what they mean. Then, the client should provide his or her own examples of what he or she thinks the other person means and ask if he or she is correct.

4. Identify which concepts or rules are lacking in the client's understanding, which affect his daily occupations, and address those—for example, the need for a daily hygiene program, dress code to go out on a date, or applying for a job. The therapist, for instance, could generate with the client a checklist for applying for a job with items such as how to locate available jobs, how to set up an interview, develop a resume, etc. Table 10-5 shows a checklist for one of the components in applying for a job (ie, locating available jobs).

Generalization and Transfer

Although the terms generalization and transfer are often used interchangeably and both involve the use of skills in contexts or environments other than those of their original use, they are actually two separate concepts.[63] Transfer of learning involves training skills applicable in specific situations.[99] It relates the effect of training specific skills and the extent to which these abilities facilitate or limit new learning.[20,73] Modern theories of transfer of learning focus on the concept of the "problem space" or similarity of cognitive processing demands common to two tasks.[73] It is believed positive transfer will occur when the client uses the same knowledge in a similar way in successive tasks. It is also assumed that positive transfer occurs only as long as the same training is used in the same way across a sequence of tasks. Hypothetically, two types of learning can transfer: declarative (the client's existing storehouse of knowledge) and procedural (a specific skill that may apply in only one situation).[73]

As previously described in Chapter 1 (page 16), the DIA is concerned with information processing and the transfer of learning. Toglia describes how the characteristics of an activity can influence the client's ability to transfer new learning.[64] This includes both the surface and conceptual characteristics of a given task. Transfer of learning is easiest, for example, if two activities share physical characteristics or look the same.[64] As the physical characteristics of an activity become more divergent, transfer becomes more difficult. Toglia conceptualizes transfer of learning as a horizontal continuum that emphasizes "sideways learning" and "...represents activities or situations that remain at a similar level of complexity but gradually differ in physical or superficial similarity."[64]

The continuum spans from near transfer to very far transfer and is described by Toglia as follows[63,64]:

> *Near transfer*—Only one or two task characteristics are changed.
>
> *Intermediate transfer*—Three to six characteristics are changed; new task shares same physical characteristics of the original task but are less readily identified
>
> *Far transfer*—Conceptually similar to the original task but completely different or shares only one surface characteristic
>
> *Very far transfer*—Generalization or the spontaneous application of what has been learned in treatment to everyday functioning

Generalization, as just described in Toglia's very far transfer category, involves the ability to use a newly learned strategy in a novel situation. The therapist can increase the amount of generalization by varying the task elements while simultaneously keeping the organization relatively constant.[73] The client will, therefore, begin to understand how the same organizational technique can apply in a variety of settings. Successful generalization provides the client with the adaptability to perform correctly across a variety of environments and tasks as well as the ability to perform tasks without need for further instructions.[99] However, although generalization of learning evolves from the client, "...at the same time, the activity and environmental demands may be changed so that strategies are practiced within the information processing capabilities of the person."[64]

In summary, the surface characteristics of a given task will dictate the amount of transfer of learning that is required. The adaptive approach with direct treatment in ADLs, for example, requires only near transfer. Transfer of learning from restorative cognitive and perceptual tasks will have more than three to six surface characteristics, which differ from functional tasks and would, therefore, require intermediate transfer. Transfer will also be more successful if the training and transfer problems both require the same type of processing.[118] Some theorize that in addition to surface characteristics of a task affecting transfer, the way in which the client learns to organize the task is a predictor of how much transfer will occur. It is recommended, therefore, that the therapist show the client how the organization applies in a variety of different settings. If the client does not understand how a given strategy or organization applies to everyday life, then transfer will be minimal. As Fuhrer and Keith state, "...the extent to which skills learned in the clinical setting can be transferred to other environments such as home, community, school, or work is another crucial question in rehabilitation."[119]

EVALUATION OF GENERALIZATION AND TRANSFER

The client's ability to transfer new learning can change through the course of treatment due to spontaneous neurological recovery and, therefore, needs to be evaluated on an ongoing basis.[120] In addition, because transfer of learning depends on the use of previously acquired information, it is inherently dependent on the client's memory capacity.[118]

Test 1 – Modification of Activities of Daily Living[120]

Description

Modify ADL treatment from one day to the next at the beginning of treatment. For example, modify the surface characteristics during dressing training. One day, place all clothes out in an organized manner, and the next, place them on the bed in a haphazard manner. Watch for the client's response.

Scoring

If the client is unable to handle change in one or two surface characteristics, this indicates difficulty with near transfer.[120] An inability to handle a change of three to six surface characteristics indicates difficulty with intermediate transfer. If the client is confused or has difficulty, then he or she may be functioning at an association learning level. If the client can perform the task, then he or she is showing a capacity for representational learning.[120]

Dynamic Assessment

Description

DIA is not one specific test, but rather a qualitative, process-oriented evaluation. The components of the evaluation are an awareness assessment, strategy investigation and task grading, and response to cuing.

Scoring

The strategies the client utilizes in a given task are identified (through observation and probing questions). Cues and tasks are altered if the client has difficulty. The therapist identifies how many task characteristics can be changed before performance breaks down. The client's ability for near, intermediate, and far transfer are evaluated. The types of cuing and task alteration that facilitate client performance are also recorded. Strategy use is evaluated and recorded in a variety of environments (multicontext).

TREATMENT OF GENERALIZATION AND TRANSFER

*Utilizing a Restorative Approach**

1. Strategies can be taught to the client; however, that does not guarantee he or she will use them. The therapist must provide opportunities and different situations where the client may apply them.

2. Generalization requires that the client recognize that the new situation is similar to an old one.[63]

3. Research has shown "…strategies learned in therapy will generalize to the real world to the extent that the client learns mental organizations that transfer intact…"[73]

The restorative approach should only be used if the client has demonstrated at least near transfer ability.

4. If the goal is a transferable skill (eg, to use when the client returns to work) create a simulated work environment and visit the client's employer. Assure the client that he or she has the necessary skills by performing the targeted job tasks.

5. The skills required to perform complex tasks do not transfer well; successful performance requires practice under conditions that closely match the intended context. Use near transfer tasks for complex skills.

6. Parente and Herrmann outline the following helpful treatment guidelines[20]:

   a) Train mental sets that are useful in a variety of different situations.

   b) Train specific skills that transfer.

   c) Focus on relevant tasks. The client should perceive they are relevant to his or her goals.

   d) Vary the training examples.

   e) Provide overlearning and verification.

   f) Avoid reorganization (ie, train the client with systems/tasks he or she will eventually be using). For example, do not work on cooking skills with a microwave if he or she will only be using a cooktop.

Utilizing an Adaptive Approach

1. Identify the client's potential placements and plan treatment so that the context does not require the client to reorganize or unlearn anything. For example, placement of hygiene and dressing items should be consistent every day. The client's kitchen and job site station should also remain consistent. Provide environmental adaptations and cuing through written instructions to compensate for client's impaired generalization ability.

2. Utilize external aids (eg, audiotaped instructions and signs) to assist clients in daily occupational performance tasks.

3. Educate the client and his or her family as to the generalization and/or transfer deficit and the need for consistent routines and environmental set-up.

Utilizing a Dynamic Interactional Approach

1. Target the processing strategies or behaviors you want to teach the client in a variety of different tasks.

2. Begin with near transfer tasks, and use the same strategies in tasks that gradually differ in surface characteristics.[63,64]

3. Provide multicontext training, and teach the client the variety of conditions to which the strategy can be applied.[63,64]

4. Increase task complexity when the client has demonstrated that he or she can use the strategy effectively in a variety of different situations.[63,64]

SECTION III

OCCUPATION-BASED EVALUATIONS OF EXECUTIVE FUNCTION

Test 1 – The Kitchen Task Assessment[121]

Description

This assessment tests the client's ability to complete the task of making cooked pudding from a commercial package. Please refer to Table 10-6 for details of the administration of the kitchen task assessment (KTA). The therapist provides the necessary assistance to the client for successful task completion.

Scoring

Performance is scored on the following areas: initiation, organization, performance of all steps, sequencing, judgment and safety, and task completion. The level of support required from the therapist is scored: 0 (independently competent), 1 (required verbal cue), 2 (required physical assists), and 3 (totally incapable). Please refer to Table 10-7 for scoring guidelines.

Validity and reliability measures were generated in a study of Alzheimer's clients.

Validity

Results of factor analysis indicated that all factor loadings exceeded 0.88.

Construct validity was established through highly significant correlations with several neuropsychological tests (ie, Token Test Short Version, Trail Making Part A, and the Crossing Off Test).

Reliability

Inter-rater reliability: Pearson correlation for the total score was 0.853 (p = < 0.0001). The range was 0.632 for safety to 1.0 for initiation. The coefficient alpha (measures the internal consistency of the test) ranged from 0.5 to 0.963. The high reliability coefficients support the structure of the test.

Test 2 – Woodrow Wilson Executive Function Route Finding Task[35]

Description

The Woodrow Wilson Executive Function Route Finding Task (EFRFT) consists of an open ended route finding task. Ratings address task understanding, information seeking, retaining directions, error detection, error correction, and on-task behavior. Please refer to Table 10-8 for detailed information on assessment scoring and interpretation guidelines. The assessment also contains guidelines or rules for cuing, which are summarized in Table 10-9.

Validity

The EFRFT correlated with perceptual organization (p < 0.01), verbal comprehension (p < 0.01), and the short-term Category Test (p < 0.05).

Reliability

Inter-rater reliability with Pearson Correlation r = 0.94 (p < 0.001)

Table 10-6

Administration Procedure for the Kitchen Task Assessment

Pretest Set-Up

1. Place to the left on the counter:

   2 or 3 flavors of pudding mix (the kind that requires cooking, not instant)

   a 1-1½ quart saucepan with a heat-resistant handle

   a wooden spoon

   a rubber scraper

   a 2 cup glass measuring cup

   4 small dishes (paper cups will do)

2. Have a quart of milk in the refrigerator.

3. Print the instructions in large letters on a piece of paper and mount the instructions where the person can read them. Use the same instructions that are on the box, except add "pour into cups."

4. Have hand soap and paper towels near the sink.

Before You Begin the Assessment

Determine the individual's ability to respond to verbal or physical assistance or both by instructing him or her to wash his or her hands. If the person can not do this, either with or without assistance, the test should not be administered, as the person will not be able to follow cues and will be unsuccessful.

Instructions

Tell the person:

- To mix a box of pudding and pour the mixture into four dishes
- That the milk is in the refrigerator
- How the stove works and what burner to use
- That the instructions are on the box and on the wall
- To begin when ready
- You will cue only after you have determined he or she cannot perform without help (wait 5 seconds) UNLESS safety is an issue.

Reprinted from reference 121: Baum C, Edwards D. Cognitive performance in senile dementia of the Alzheimer's type: the kitchen task assessment. Am J Occup Ther. 1994;47(5):435-436. Reprinted with permission from Republication Licensing Service (RLS) Copyright Clearance Center, Inc.

Observations During Validity/Reliability Study

The clients generally needed not to be told what to do but to think for themselves about what needed to be done.[35]

Test 3 – Behavioral Assessment of Dysexecutive Syndrome[122]*

Although the behavioral assessment of dysexecutive syndrome (BADS) is sometimes administered by a neuropsychologist, a description is included here because it is a test battery that is aimed at predicting everyday problems arising from problems with executive function.

Description

This test battery includes the Rule Shift Cards Test (measures the ability to shift from one rule to another and keep track of the color of the previous card and the current rule), Action Program

---

This BADS is distributed by Harcourt Assessment, 19500 Bulverde Road, San Antonio, TX 78259, 1-800-211-8378.

Table 10-7

Scoring Guide for the Kitchen Task Assessment

Initiation   Did he or she begin the task after being told to begin? If not, did he or she begin when reminded (verbal), or did you have to open the box and hand it to him or her (physical)?

Organization   Was he or she able to get the milk from the refrigerator and use the tools appropriately? Some may use the tools or equipment incorrectly; for example, some try to cook in the measuring cup. Did the person respond to verbal help, or did he or she require physical assistance?

Performance of all steps   Did he or she perform all the major steps—measuring, stirring, pouring—alone? Did you have to assist him or her—for example, to light the stove? Was it verbal or physical assistance?

Sequencing   Was he or she able to do the tasks in a functional sequence? During sequencing, it is essential not to overdo. Some people stir the mixture initially in the cup. This is permissible if he or she has the right amount of milk and all of the mix from the box. Some people pour the hot mixture into the measuring cup before filling the serving dishes. This, too, is permissible. A problem arises when the person does not perform the tasks necessary to proceed with the activity (ie, pour milk or powder into the dishes or turn on the stove before starting).

Judgment   Evaluation is based on how the person manages the stove and the hot pudding. Because of the possibility of injury, the examiner must be alert to the subject's needs. Give physical assistance if the person is in danger.

Completion   Evaluation is based on whether the person knows he or she is finished. Some will continue the process and do chores such as scraping the pan after it is empty or moving the dishes around on the counter. He or she may put the dishes in the sink but is not required to clean up. Saying that you will wash the dishes is not considered a verbal cue; however, you must wait until he or she puts the pudding in the dishes before you offer to clean up.

Reprinted from reference 121: Baum C, Edwards D. Cognitive performance in senile dementia of the Alzheimer's type: the kitchen task assessment. Am J Occup Ther. *1994;47(5):436. Reprinted with permission from Republication Licensing Service (RLS) Copyright Clearance Center, Inc.*

Test (measures action plan development and problem solving of a novel practical task), Key Search Test (measures planning, self-monitoring, abstraction), Temporal Judgment Test (measures temporal sense), Zoo Map Test (measures planning, self-monitoring), Modified Six Elements Test (organization), and Dysexecutive Questionnaire (examines emotional and personality changes, motivational changes, behavior changes, and cognitive changes).

Validity

Validity measures are presented in the manual for the BADS.

Reliability

Measures of inter-rater and test-retest reliability are contained in the manual for the BADS.

Test 4 – The Arnadottir OT, Activities of Daily Living Neurobehavioral Evaluation (A-One) Instrument[123]

Description

Test format includes the primary ADLs with items that address neurobehavioral deficits. It is composed of two parts. Part 1 is the Functional Independence Scale and Neurobehavioral Impairment Scale, which consists of the Neurobehavioral Specific Impairment Subscale and the Neurobehavioral Pervasive Impairment Scale. Table 10-10 contains a sample (dressing) of the Neurobehavioral Specific Impairment Subscale. Part II is used to convert the results of Part I to reveal information pertaining to central nervous system (CNS) dysfunction.

Table 10-8

Woodrow Wilson Rehabilitation Center, Executive Function Route-Finding Task

Name: _____   Date of Evaluation: _____ / _____ / _____
Examiner: _____   Disability code: _____

Instructions

"I am going to give you an exercise, which involves your finding an unfamiliar office, _____.
How you do this is up to you. I will go with you but cannot answer questions about how to find the office. I want you to do this exercise as quickly and efficiently as possible. Before you begin, I would like you to tell me what I have asked you to do."

I. Task understanding

1. Failure to grasp nature of task despite several elaborations.
2. Faulty understanding of important element(s) requiring specific or explanatory cuing and elaboration (eg, "How am I supposed to know where it is?").
3. Distorts peripheral detail requiring slight clarification or a nonspecific cue (eg, "Can you tell me where it is?").
4. Shows a clear grasp or asks for clarification appropriately (eg, "Can I get someone to take me there?"). Initiates the task spontaneously.

II. Information-seeking

1. Aimless wandering.
2. Follows a hunch without gathering information first (unless shows prior knowledge of destination) or exhaustive door-to-door search.
3. Gathers information before commencing search, but without appraisal of information source.
4. Shows judgment in use of information sources (eg, selects staff over clients, clarifies confusing directions, and verifies information with another person).

III. Retaining directions (functional memory)

1. Continual forgetting of directions or name of destination and failure to use suggested means of compensating (eg, note taking) unless cued repeatedly.
2. Needs repeated non-specific cuing or provision of concrete strategy to compensate for memory deficits.
3. Forgets detail(s) but compensates after non-specific cue (eg, "How might you keep yourself from forgetting the destination?").
4. Paraphrasing or clarification sufficient for remembering, or spontaneous compensation (eg, note taking).

IV. Error detection (self-monitoring)

1. Continued errors without self-detection even after repeated examiner cues.
2. Some spontaneous awareness of errors but more instances of cuing required.
3. Some cuing required but more instances of spontaneous error detection shown.
4. Verifies correctness independently when appropriate; may exploit incidental information (eg, signs) to prevent errors.

V. Error correction (troubleshooting)

1. Helpless or perseverative behavior.
2. Inefficient strategy (eg, returns to original information source).
3. Seeks help immediately once aware of error.
4. Reasons efficiently (eg, looks for signs; considers where may have erred in following directions to self-correct).

VI. On-task behavior

1. Must be held to task in ongoing fashion (eg, distractible, stimulus-bound).
2. Digression from task requiring cues to redirect attention to task.
3. Incidental behaviors (eg, small talk) interfere with efficiency.
4. Any incidental behaviors (eg, waving to a friend) do not hinder performance observably.

(continued)

Table 10-8 *(continued)*
Woodrow Wilson Rehabilitation Center, Executive Function Route-Finding Task

Potential Contributing Problems

Emotional
_____ Indifference, lack of effort
_____ Poor frustration tolerance
_____ Self-criticism, depression
_____ Defensiveness
_____ Thought disturbance
_____ Other _____

Communication
_____ Speech reception
_____ Expressive speech
_____ Reading ability
_____ Other _____

Motor
_____ Manual limitations
_____ Ambulation difficulties
_____ Other _____

Interpersonal
_____ Self-consciousness/shyness
_____ Social skills
_____ Requesting information
_____ Flirting
_____ Interrupting
_____ Other _____

Perceptual
_____ Visual acuity
_____ Auditory acuity
_____ Right-left confusion
_____ Other _____

Evaluation of Overall Independence

	Client's rating	Examiner's rating	Overall
Extensive cuing required	_____	_____	_____
Appreciable cuing needed (specific cues or several nonspecific cues)	_____	_____	_____
Occasional nonspecific cuing required	_____	_____	_____
Independent of cuing	_____	_____	_____

Scoring summary

Tasking understanding	1	2	3	4
Information seeking	1	2	3	4
Retaining directions	1	2	3	4
Error detection	1	2	3	4
Error correction	1	2	3	4

Overall average _____

Table 10-9

Rules for Cuing During the Executive Function Route-Finding Task

1. When to cue:

   a) A nonspecific cue is given when the client deviates from the path approaching the goal (not necessarily most direct) and passes up a subsequent opportunity for correction (eg, sign, staff person, office doorway that might lead to information, path leading towards goal).

   b) A specific cue is given following a nonspecific cue after the client fails to attempt correction or passes another opportunity for correction in doing so.

2. Nature of cues:

   a) A nonspecific cue alerts the client to monitor performance (ie, "Tell me what you need to do now"), which is essentially a means to assist the client to be aware of the process of executive functioning.

   b) A specific cue provides information on how to execute the task by providing the client directive guidance in carrying out aspects of the task.

Reprinted with permission from John Wiley and Sons Ltd, reference 36: Boyd TM, Sautter SW. Route-finding: a measure of everyday executive functioning in the head-injured adult. App Cogn Psychol. 1993;7:175.

Table 10-10

Dressing Section of the Specific Neurobehavioral Impairment Scale

Name _____   Date _____

Activities of Daily Living Functions   *Neurobehavioral Impairment Score*

Dressing	Present	Absent	Comment
Motor apraxia			
1. Has difficulties related to motor planning. May grab a shirt or a sock, but has trouble adjusting the grasp according to needs.	☐	☐	
2. Difficulties with buttons or fastenings because of clumsy hand movements: R/L side?	☐	☐	
Ideational apraxia			
1. Does not know what to do with shirt, pants, or socks.	☐	☐	
2. Misuses clothes. Starts to put leg into armhole or arm into leg hole.	☐	☐	
(a) Other apraxia:	☐	☐	
Unilateral body neglect			
1. Does not dress the affected body side.	☐	☐	
2. Does not pull down shirt all the way on the affected side, or shirt gets stuck on the affected shoulder without the person trying to correct it or realizing what is wrong.	☐	☐	
Somatagnosia			
1. Starts putting legs into armholes or arms into legholes.	☐	☐	
(b) Other body-scheme disorders:	☐	☐	

(continued)

Table 10-10 *(continued)*

Dressing Section of the Specific Neurobehavioral Impairment Scale

Activities of Daily Living Functions	*Neurobehavioral Impairment Score*		
Dressing	**Present**	**Absent**	**Comment**
Spatial-relation disorders			
1. Unable to find armholes, legholes, or bottom of shirt.	☐	☐	
2. Pull sleeve in the wrong direction.	☐	☐	
3. Unable to differentiate front from back or inside from outside of clothes.	☐	☐	
4. Aims correctly at armholes but misses it without noticing.	☐	☐	
5. Matches buttons and buttonholes incorrectly.	☐	☐	
6. Puts hand into sleeve through distal instead of proximal opening.	☐	☐	
7. Legholes end up inside of pants at the top opening without the person realizing it or being able to correct it.	☐	☐	
8. Puts arm through neckhole.	☐	☐	
9. Unable to learn to tie lace one-handed when other hand is paralyzed. This may be the reason for refusing to try the method.	☐	☐	
10. Attempts to turn shirt front to back with the shirt on by pulling at the bottom of the shirt, not realizing that the shirt will not turn while arms are in the sleeves. Similarly, may try to turn pants front to back after placing one leg into leghole, by pulling at the waist opening.	☐	☐	
11. Places foot in the wrong leghole.	☐	☐	
Unilateral spatial neglect			
1. Does not pay attention to clothes	☐	☐	
(c) Other spatial-relations problems:	☐	☐	
Perseveration			
1. Repeats movements or acts and cannot stop them once initiated. Attempts, for example, to put on shirt without any progress. May pull the front edge of a long sleeve up arm way past the wrist.	☐	☐	
2. Attempts to button many buttonholes onto the same button.	☐	☐	
3. Attempts to put the same arm into both sleeves.	☐	☐	
4. Persists motorically in looking for the hole of a sock on the toe side, although the hole cannot be found there.	☐	☐	
(d) Other perserveration problems:	☐	☐	
Organization and Sequencing			
1. Has difficulty sequencing the steps of the activity. Will, for example, dress the unaffected arm before the affected one, then run into trouble dressing the affected arm.	☐	☐	
2. Does not include all steps of the activity. Does not, for example, complete the fastenings (buttons, zippers, laces) as required by the nature of the activity.	☐	☐	
3. Will stop the activity after each step and will have to be "programmed" by the therapist to continue.	☐	☐	
4. Will put on the shoes before putting on the trousers.	☐	☐	
(e) Other organization problems:	☐	☐	

Reprinted with permission from Elsevier Publishing, reference 123: Arnadottir G. The Brain and Behavior: Assessing Cortical Dysfunction Through Activities of Daily Living. *St. Louis, Mo: CV Mosby; 1990.:234-236.*

Scoring

The Functional Independence Scale focuses on the traditional functional level of independence. The Neurobehavioral Scale Measures the number and type of neurobehavioral deficits that interfere with function. Both are scored with a four-point scale with scoring criteria for each functional task.

Validity

Content validity was established through extensive literature review and expert opinion within the field.

Reliability

The average Kappa coefficients for the degree of agreement between raters was 0.84, $p < 0.01$ (three items $p < 0.05$).

Additional normative validity, reliability, and normative studies have been performed and are summarized in: *The Brain and Behavior: Assessing Cortical Dysfunction Through Activities of Daily Living.*[123]

Test 5 – Daily Living Questionnaire[64]

Description

The Daily Living Questionnaire (DLQ) was designed to assess difficulties that persons with subtle cognitive impairments may experience in everyday life. A revised version, DLQ-2, asks the person to rate the degree of cognitive difficulty or mental effort experienced with different activities. Part I of the revised scale is divided into subscales that correspond to the organization of the ICF (cognitive symptoms or impairments, activity limitation, and participation restrictions).

The DLQ-2 provides a comprehensive self-report of the person's level of function that can be used as a foundation for treatment planning and goal setting. It may also be helpful in identifying early changes in cognitive function, tracking functional changes, and measuring the effectiveness of treatment in persons with subtle cognitive impairments.

Reliability

Pilot data indicates high internal consistency-reliability for the separate subscales: Activity Limitation = 0.92; Participation Restrictions = 0.88; Cognitive symptoms (impairments) = 0.92. The DLQ-2 also asks persons to review the questionnaire and identify the five most important activities or concerns. The second part of the DLQ-2 includes seven questions about role performance and satisfaction with everyday functioning. The DLQ has been formally piloted on persons who have Lupus and who have mild cognitive impairment (MCI) and is currently under further development.

References

1. Anderson V, Levin HS, Jacobs R. Executive functions after frontal lobe injury: a developmental perspective. In: Stuss D, Knight R, eds. *Principles of Frontal Lobe Function*. New York, NY: Oxford University Press; 2002.
2. Constantinidou F, Thomas RD, Best P. Principles of cognitive rehabilitation: an integrative approach. In: Ashley MJ, ed. *Traumatic Brain Injury: Rehabilitative Treatment and Case Management*. 2nd ed. Boca Raton, Fla: CRC Press; 2004.
3. Josman N, Jarus T. Construct-related validity of the Toglia Category Assessment and the Deductive Reasoning test with children who are typically developing. *Am Occup Ther*. 2001;55(5):524-530.
4. Raskin SA. Executive functions. In: Raskin SA, Mateer CA, eds. *Neuropsychological Management of Mild Traumatic Brain Injury*. New York, NY: Oxford University Press; 2000.
5. Golisz, Toglia J. Perception and Cognition. In: Crepeau E, Cohn ES, Schell BAB, eds. *Willard and Spackman's Occupational Therapy*. Philadelphia, Pa: Lippincott, Williams and Wilkins; 2003.

6. Evans J. Rehabilitation of the dysexecutive syndrome. In: Suchoff I, Ciuffreda K, Kappor N, eds. *Visual and Vestibular Consequences of Acquired Brain Injury.* Santa Ana, Calif: Optometric Extension Program Inc; 2001.

7. Manly T, Hawkins K, Evans J, et al. Rehabilitation of executive function: facilitation of effective goal management on complex tasks using periodic auditory alerts. *Neuropsychologia.* 2002;40:271-281.

8. Braver T. The role of prefrontal cortex in normal and disordered cognitive control: a cognitive neuroscience perspective. In: Stuss D, Knight R, eds. *Principles of Frontal Lobe Function.* New York, NY: Oxford University Press; 2002.

9. Elliott R. Executive functions and their disorders. *Br Med Bull.* 2003;65:49-59.

10. Levine B, Stuss DT, Milberg WP, et al. The effects of focal and diffuse brain damage on strategy application: evidence from focal lesions, traumatic brain injury and normal aging. *J Int Neuropsychol Soc.* 1998;4(3):247-264.

11. Shimamura AP. Memory retrieval and executive control processes. In: Stuss D, Knight R, eds. *Principles of Frontal Lobe Function.* New York, NY: Oxford University Press; 2002.

12. Dritschel BH, Kogan L, Burton A, et al. Everyday planning difficulties following traumatic brain injury: a role for autobiographical memory. *Brain Inj.* 1998;12(10):875-886.

13. Ylvisaker M, Szekeres SF. Metacognitive and executive impairment in head-injured children and adults. *Top Lang Disord.* 1989;9(2):34-49.

14. Evans J. Rehabilitation of executive deficits. In: Wilson BA, ed. *Neuropsychological Rehabilitation.* Lisse, The Netherlands: Sweets and Zeitlinger; 2003.

15. Hibbard MR, et al. The neuropsychological evaluation: a pathway to understanding the sequelae of brain injury. In: Suchoff I, Ciuffreda K, Kappor N, eds. *Visual and Vestibular Consequences of Acquired Brain Injury.* Santa Ana, Calif: Optometric Extension Program, Inc; 2001.

16. Pohjasvaara T, Leskela M, Vataja R, et al. Post-stroke depression, executive dysfunction and functional outcome. *Eur J Neurol.* 2002;9(3):269-275.

17. Stablum F, Umilta C, Mogentale C, Carlan M, Guerrini C. Rehabilitation of executive deficits in closed head injury and anterior communicating artery aneurysm patients. *Psychol Res.* 2000;63(3-4):265-278.

18. Giles G. Lack of insight following severe brain injury. In: Giles G, Clark-Wilson J, eds. *Rehabilitation of the Severely Brain-Injured Adult.* 2nd ed. Cheltenham: Stanley Thornes Publ; 1999.

19. Katz N, Hartman-Maeir A. Metacognition: the relationships of awareness and executive functions to occupational performance. In: Katz N, ed. *Cognition and Occupation In Rehabilitation.* Bethesda, Md: American Occupational Therapy Association Press; 1998.

20. Parente R, Herrmann DJ. *Retraining Cognition: Techniques and Applications.* 2nd ed. Austin, Tex: Pro Ed; 2003.

21. Goel V, Grafman J, Tajik J, Gana S, Danto D. A study of the performance of patients with frontal lobe lesions in a financial planning task. *Brain.* 1997;120(Pt 10):1805-1822.

22. Case R. The role of the frontal lobes in the regulation of cognitive development. *Brain Cogn.* 1992;20:51-73.

23. Grafman J. Plans, actions, and mental sets: managerial knowledge units in the frontal lobes. In: Perecman E, ed. *Integrating Theory and Practice in Clinical Neuropsychology.* Hillsdale, NJ: Lawrence Erlbaum Assoc; 1989.

24. Grafman J, Litvan I. Importance of deficits in executive functions. *Lancet.* 1999;354:1921-1923.

25. McDonald BC, Flashman LA, Saykin AJ. Executive dysfunction following traumatic brain injury: neural substrates and treatment strategies. *Neurorehabilitation.* 2000;17(4):333-344.

26. Feinstein A. Mood and motivation in rehabilitation. In: Stuss D, Knight R, eds. *Cognitive Rehabilitation.* New York, NY: Cambridge University Press; 1999.

27. Moscovitch M, Winocur G. The frontal cortex and working with memory. In: Stuss D, Knight R, ed. *Principles of Frontal Lobe Function.* New York, NY: Oxford University Press; 2002.

28. Stuss T, Alexander MP. Executive functions and the frontal lobes: a conceptual view. *Psychol Res.* 2000;63:289-298.

29. Stuss DT, Alexander MP, Palumbo CL, et al. Organizational strategies of patients with unilateral or bilateral frontal lobe injury in word list learning tasks. *Neuropsychology.* 1994;8:355-373.

30. Hanks A, Rapport LJ, Millis SR, Deshpande SA. Measures of executive functioning as predictors of functional ability and social integration in a rehabilitation sample. *Arch Phys Med Rehab.* 1999;80(9):1030-1037.

31. Goverover Y, Hinojosa J. Categorization and deductive reasoning: predictors of instrumental activities of daily living performance in adults with brain injury. *Am J Occup Ther.* 2002;56(3):509-515.

32. Mazaux J, Masson F, Levin HS, et al. Long-term neuropsychological outcome and loss of social autonomy after traumatic brain injury. *Arch Phys Med Rehabil.* 1997;78(12):1316-1320.

33. Duran L, Fisher A. Evaluation and intervention with executive functions impairment. In: Unsworth C, ed. *Cognitive and Perceptual Dysfunction: A Clinical Reasoning Approach to Evaluation and Intervention.* Philadelphia, Pa: FA Davis; 1999.

34. Burgess P, Veitch E, de Lacy Costello A, Shallice T. The cognitive and neuroanatomical correlates of multitasking. *Neuropsychologia.* 2000;38(6):848-863.
35. Boyd TM, Sautter SW. Route-finding: a measure of everyday executive functioning in the head-injured adult. *App Cogn Psychol.* 1993;7:171-181.
36. Bieman-Copland S, Dywan J. Achieving rehabilitative gains in anosognosia after TBI. *Brain Cogn.* 2000;44:1-18.
37. Fischer S, Gauggel S, Trexler LE. Awareness of activity limitations, goal setting and rehabilitation outcome in patients with brain injuries. *Brain Inj.* 2004;18(6):547-562.
38. Sherer M, Boake C, Levin E, et al. Characteristics of impaired awareness after traumatic brain injury. *J Int Neuropsychol Soc.* 1998;4(4):380-387.
39. Levine B, Robertson IH, Clare L, et al. Rehabilitation of executive functioning: an experimental-clinical validation of goal management training. *J Int Neuropsychol Soc.* 2000;6(3):299-312.
40. Mateer C. The rehabilitation of executive disorders. In: Stuss D, Knight R, eds. *Cognitive Neurorehabilitation.* New York, NY: Cambridge University Press; 1999.
41. Liu KP, Chan CC, Lee TM, Li LS, Hui-Chan CW. Self-regulatory learning and generalization for people with brain injury. *Brain Inj.* 2002;16(9):817-824.
42. Abreu BC, Seale G, Scheibel RS, et al. Levels of self-awareness after acute brain injury: how patients' and rehabilitation specialists' perceptions compare. *Arch Phys Med Rehabil.* 2001;82(1):49-56.
43. Prigatano G. Motivation and awareness in cognitive neurorehabilitation. In: Stuss DT, Robertson IH, eds. *Cognitive Neurorehabilitation.* New York, NY: Cambridge University Press; 1999.
44. Barco P, Grosson B. Bolesta MM, Werts D, Stout R. Training awareness and compensation in postacute head injury rehabilitation. In: Kreutzer JS, Wehman PH, eds. *Cognitive Rehabilitation For Persons with Traumatic Brain Injury: A Functional Approach.* Baltimore, Md: Paul H. Brooks Publishing; 1991.
45. Knight R. Prefrontal cortex: the present and the future. In: Stuss D, Knight R. *Principles of Frontal Lobe Function.* New York, NY: Oxford University Press; 2002.
46. Prigatano G, Klonoff PS. A clinician's rating scale for evaluating impaired self-awareness and denial of disability after brain injury. *Clin Neuropsychol.* 1998;12(1):56-67.
47. Burgess P, Shallice T. Response suppression: initiation and strategy use following frontal lobe lesions. *Neuropsychologia.* 1999;34(4):263-273.
48. Anderson SW, Tranel D. Awareness of disease states following cerebral infarction, dementia, and head trauma: standardized assessment. *Clin Neuropsychol.* 1989;3(4):327-339.
49. Doehring DG, Reitan RM, Klove H. Changes in patterns of intelligence test performance associated with homonymous visual field defects. *J Nerv Ment Dis.* 1961;132:227-233.
50. Prigatano G, Altman IM, O'Brien KP. Behavioral limitations that traumatic-brain-injured patients tend to underestimate. *Clin Neuropsychol.* 1990;4(2):163-176.
51. Prigatano G. Disturbances of self-awareness of deficit after traumatic brain injury. In: Prigatano GP, Schacter DL, eds. *Awareness of Deficit After Brain Injury.* New York, NY: Oxford University Press; 1991.
52. Godfrey HP, Partridge FM, Knight RG, Bishara S. Course of insight disorder and emotional dysfunction following closed head injury: a controlled cross-sectional follow-up study. *J Clin Exp Neuropsychol.* 1993;15(4):503-515.
53. McGlynn SM. Behavioral approaches to neuropsychological rehabilitation. *Psychol Bull.* 1990;108(3):420-4410.
54. Parente R. Executive skills training. In: Parente R, Herrmann D, eds. *Retraining Cognition: Techniques and Applications.* Gaithersburg, Md: Aspen Publications; 1996.
55. Gasquoine PG, Gibbons TA. Lack of awareness of impairment in institutionalized, severely and chronically disabled survivors of traumatic brain injury: a preliminary investigation. *J Head Trauma Rehab.* 1994;9(4):16-24.
56. Ayres AJ. *Southern California Sensory Integration Tests.* Los Angeles, Calif: Western Psychological Services; 1972.
57. Fleming JM, Strong J, Ashton R. Self-awareness of deficits in adults with traumatic brain injury: how best to measure? *Brain Inj.* 1996;10(1):1-15.
58. Sherer M, Boake C, Silver BV, et al. Assessing awareness of deficits following acquired brain injury: the awareness questionnaire. *J Int Neuropsychol Soc.* 1995;1:163.
59. Sherer M, Bergloff P, High WM, et al. Contribution of impaired self-awareness to predicting employment outcome after traumatic brain injury. *J Int Neuropsychol Soc.* 1997;3:75.
60. Sherer M, Boake C, Clement V, et al. Awareness of deficits after traumatic brain injury: comparison of patient, family, and clinician ratings. *J Int Neuropsychol Soc.* 1996;2:17.
61. Prigatano G. *Neuropsychological Rehabilitation After Brain Injury.* Baltimore, Md: Johns Hopkins University Press; 1986.
62. Toglia J. Personal Communication; 2005.

63. Toglia J. A dynamic interactional approach to cognitive rehabilitation. In: Katz N, ed. *Cognition and Occupation Across The Life Span.* Bethesda, Md: American Occupational Therapy Association Press; 1998.

64. Toglia J. A dynamic interactional approach to cognitive rehabilitation. In: Katz N, ed. *Cognition and Occupation Across The Life Span.* Bethesda, Md: American Occupational Therapy Association Press; 2005.

65. Berkeland R, Flynn, N. Therapy as learning. In: Christiansen C, Baum C, eds. *Occupational Therapy: Performance, Participation, and Well-Being.* Thorofare, NJ: SLACK Incorporated; 2005.

66. Namerow NS. Cognitive and behavioral aspects of brain-injury rehabilitation. *Neurologic Rehabil.* 1987;5(4):569-583.

67. Bruce M. Cognitive rehabilitation: intelligence, insight, and knowledge. In: Royee CB, ed. *AOTA Self Study Series: Cognitive Rehabilitation.* American Occupational Therapy Association Press; 1994.

68. Fetherlin JM, Kurland L. Self-instruction: a compensatory strategy to increase functional independence with brain-injured adults. *Occup Ther Pract.* 1989;1(1):75-78.

69. Manchester D, Wood RL. Applying cognitive therapy in neurobehavioral rehabilitation. In: Wood RL, McMillan TM, eds. *Neurobehavioral Disability and Social Handicap Following Traumatic Brain Injury.* Philadelphia, Pa: Psychology Press; 2001.

70. Chittum WB, Johnson K, Chittum JM, et al. Road to awareness: an individualized training package for increasing knowledge and comprehension of personal deficits in persons with acquired brain injury. *Brain Inj.* 1996;10(10):763-776.

71. Lezak M. *Neuropsychological Assessment.* New York, NY: Oxford University Press; 1983.

72. Duchek J. Cognitive dimensions of performance. In: Christiansen C, Baum C, eds. *Occupational Therapy: Overcoming Human Performance Deficits.* Thorofare, NJ: SLACK Incorporated; 1991.

73. Parente R. Effect of monetary incentives on performance after traumatic brain injury. *Neuro Rehabil.* 1994;4(3):198-203.

74. Evans JJ, Emslie H, Wilson BA. External cuing systems in the rehabilitation of executive impairments of action. *J Intern Neuropsychol Soc.* 1998;4(4):399-408.

75. Baker SC, Rogers RD, Owen AM, et al. Neural systems engaged by planning : a PET study of the Tower of London Test. *Neuropsychologia.* 1996;34(6):515-526.

76. Harrington DO. *The Visual Fields.* 4th ed. St. Louis, Mo: CV Mosby; 1976.

77. Craine JF. The retraining of frontal lobe dysfunction. In: Trexler LE, ed. *Cognitive Rehabilitation Conceptualization and Intervention.* New York, NY: Plenum Press; 1982.

78. Burgess P. Strategy application disorder: the role of the frontal lobes in human multitasking. *Psychol Res.* 2000;63(3-4):279-288.

79. Duncun J. Disorganization of behavior after frontal lobe damage. *Cogn Neuropsychol.* 1986;3(3):271-290.

80. Cohen RF, Mapou RL. Neuropsychological assessment for treatment planning: a hypothesis-testing approach. *J Head Trauma Rehabil.* 1988;3(1):12-23.

81. Grafman J, Kampen D, Rosenberg J, Salazar AM, Boller F. The progressive breakdown of number processing and calculation ability: a case study. *Cortex.* 1989;25:121-133.

82. Dehaene S, Changeux JPA. Hierarchal neuronal network for planning behavior. *Proc Natl Acad Sci U S A.* 1997;94:13293-13298.

83. Goel V, Grafman J. Role of the right prefrontal cortex in ill structured planning. *Cogn Psychol.* 2000;17(5):415-436.

84. Cicerone KD, Wood J. Planning disorder after closed head injury: a case study. *Arch Phys Med Rehabil.* 1987;68:111-113.

85. Benedict RHB. The effectiveness of cognitive remediation strategies for victims of traumatic head injury: a review of the literature. *Clin Psych Rev.* 1989;9:605-626.

86. Shallice T, Burgess P. Deficits in strategy application following frontal lobe damage in man. *Brain.* 1991;114:727-741.

87. Wilson BA. Compensating for cognitive deficits following brain injury. *Neuropsychol Rev.* 2000;10(4):233-243.

88. Anderson S, Manzel K. Matrix reasoning as an index of fluid intelligence following frontal lobe damage. *J Int Neuropsychol Soc.* 2001;7:234-235.

89. Bourne LE, Dominowski RL, Loftus EF. *Cognitive Processes.* Englewood Cliffs, NJ: Prentice-Hall; 1979.

90. Christenson AL. *Luria's Neuropsychological Investigation.* New York, NY: Spectrum Publications; 1975.

91. Dimitrov J, Grafman J, Hollnagel C. The effects of frontal lobe damage on everyday problem solving. *Cortex.* 1996;32:357-366.

92. Patterson KE, Baddeley AD. When face recognition fails. *J Exp Psychol Hum Learn Mem.* 1977;3:406-417.

93. Goldstein FC, Levin H. Disorders of reasoning and problem solving ability. In: Meir MJ, Benton AL, Diller L, eds. *Neuropsychological Rehabilitation.* New York, NY: Guilford University Press; 1987.

94. Meltzer M. Poor memory: a case report. *J Clin Psychol.* 1983;39(1):3-10.

95. Rabbit P. Changes in problem solving ability in old age. In: Birren J, Schaie K, eds. *Handbook of Psychology of Aging.* New York, NY: Van Nostrand Reinhold Co; 1977.

96. Hoyer W, Rebok G, Svold S. Effects of varying irrelevant information on adult age differences in problem solving. *J Gerontol.* 1979;34(4):553-560.

97. Schonfield D. Translations in gerontology—from lab to life: utilizing information. *Am Psychol.* 1974;29:796-901.

98. Adamovich BLB. Cognition, language, attention and information processing following closed head injury. In: Kreutzer JS, Wehman PH, eds. *Cognitive Rehabilitation For Persons with Traumatic Brain Injury: A Functional Approach.* Baltimore, Md: Paul H Books Pub; 1991.

99. Ben-Yishay Y, Diller L. Cognitive remediation in traumatic brain injury: update and issues. *Arch Phys Med Rehabil.* 1993;74:204-213.

100. Waltz JA, Knowlton BJ, Holyoak KJ, et al. A system for relational reasoning in human prefrontal cortex. *Psychol Sci.* 1999;10:119-125.

101. Parsons LM, Osherson D. New evidence for distinct right and left brain systems for deductive versus probabilistic reasoning. *Cereb Cortex.* 2001;11:954-965.

102. Bolger J. Cognitive retraining: a developmental approach. *Clin Neuropsychol.* 1982;4:55-70.

103. Okkema K. *Cognition and Perception in the Stroke Patient.* Gaithersburg, Md: Aspen Publishers; 1993.

104. von Crameon D, von Cramon D, Mai N. The influence of a cognitive remediation programme on associated behavioural disturbances in patients with frontal lobe dysfunction. In: von Steinbuchel N, von Cramon D, Poppel E, eds. *Neuropyschological Rehabilitation.* Berlin, Springer-Verlag; 1992.

105. Dougherty PM, Radomski MV. *A Dynamic Assessment Approach for Adults with Brain Injury: The Cognitive Rehabilitation Workbook.* Gaithersburg, Md: Aspen Publishers; 1993.

106. Berardi-Coletta B, Buyer LS, Dominowski RL, Rellinger ER. Metacognition and problem solving: a process oriented approach. *J Exp Psych Learn Mem Cogn.* 1995;21(1):205-223.

107. Goldberg E, Podell K. Adaptive decision making, ecological validity, and the frontal lobes. *J Clin Exp Psychol.* 2000;22:56-68.

108. Bechara A, Tranel D, Damasio H. Characterization of the decision-making deficit of patients with ventromedial prefrontal cortex lesions. *Brain.* 2000;123(Pt 11):2189-2202.

109. Bechara A, Damasio H, Damasio AR. Emotion, decision making and the orbitofrontal cortex. *Cereb Cortex.* 2000;10(3):295-307.

110. Ashley M. Evaluation of traumatic brain injury following acute rehabilitation. In: Ashley M, ed. *Traumatic Brain Injury Rehabilitative Treatment and Case Management.* Boca Raton, Fla: CRC Press; 2004.

111. Josman N. Reliability and validity of the Toglia Category Assessment Test. *Can J Occup Ther.* 1999;66:33-42.

112. Goldberg E, Bougakov D. Novel approaches to the diagnosis and treatment of frontal lobe dysfunction. In: Christenson A, Uzzel BP, eds. *International Handbook of Neuropsychological Rehabilitation.* New York, NY: Plenum Publishers; 2000.

116. Malec J. Training the brain-injured client in behavioral self-management skills. In: Edelstein BA, Couture ET, eds. *Behavioral Assessment and Rehabilitation of the Traumatically Brain-Damaged.* New York, NY: Plenum Press; 1984.

114. Parker RS. *Traumatic Brain Injury and Neuropsychological Impairment.* New York, NY: Springer Verlag; 1990.

115. Averbach S, Katz N. Cognitive rehabilitation: a retraining model for clients with neurological disabilities. In: Katz N, ed. *Cognition and Occupation Across the Live Span.* Bethesda, Md: American Occupational Therapy Association Press; 2005.

116. Shiffman LM. Cerebrovascular accident. In: Early MB, ed. *Physical Dysfunction Practice Skills for the Occupational Therapy Assistant.* St. Louis, Mo: Mosby Year-Book; 1998.

117. Goldstein G. Comprehensive neuropsychological assessment batteries. In: Goldstein G, Hersen M, eds. *Handbook of Psychological Assessment.* New York, NY: Pergamon Press; 1984.

118. Brown SC, Craik FIM. Encoding and retrieval of information. In: Tulving E, Craik FIM, eds. *The Oxford Handbook of Memory.* New York, NY: Oxford University Press; 2000.

119. Fuhrer MJ, Keith RA. Facilitating patient learning during medical rehabilitation: a research agenda. *Am J Phys Med Rehabil.* 1998;77:557-561.

120. Neistadt ME. Assessing learning capabilities during cognitive and perceptual evaluations for adults with traumatic brain injury. *Occup Ther Health Care.* 1995;9(1):3-16.

121. Baum C, Edwards D. Cognitive performance in senile dementia of the Alzheimer's type: the kitchen task assessment. *Am J Occup Ther.* 1994;47(5):431-436.

122. Wilson B, Alderman N, Burgess PW, et al. *Behavioral Assessment of the Dysexecutive Syndrome.* London: Harcourt Assessment; 1996.

123. Arnadottir G. *The Brain and Behavior: Assessing Cortical Dysfunction Through Activities of Daily Living.* St. Louis, Mo: CV Mosby; 1990.

Resources

Alexander M, Stuss P. Disorders of frontal lobe functioning. *Semin Neurol.* 2000;20(4):427-437.

Alexander M. Disorders of language after frontal lobe injury: evidence for the neural mechanisms of assembling language In: Stuss D, Knight R, eds. *Principles of Frontal Lobe Function.* New York, NY: Oxford University Press; 2002.

Arenberg D, Robertson-Tchabo E. Learning and aging. In: Brirren J, Schaie K, eds. *Handbook of the Psychology of Aging.* New York, NY: Van Nostrand Reinhold Co; 1997.

Baddeley A. The central executive: a concept and some misconceptions. *J Int Neuropsychol Soc.* 1998;4:523-526.

Ben-Yishay Y. *Working Approaches to Remediation of Cognitive Deficits in Brain-damaged Persons.* Rehabilitation Monograph 62. New York, NY: University Medical Center; 1981.

Bransford JD, Sherwood, R, Vye N, Rieser J. Teaching, thinking and problem solving. *Am Psychologist.* 1986;42(10):1078-1089.

Burgess P, Alderman N, Evans J, et al. The ecological validity of tests of executive function. *J Intern Neuropsychol Soc.* 1998;4(6):547-558.

Cook EA, Thigpen R. Identification and management of cognitive perceptual deficits in the rehabilitation patient. *Rehab Nurs.* 1993;18(5):3110-3113.

Dagher A, Owen AM, Boecker H, Brooks DJ. Mapping the network for planning: a correlational PET activation study with the Tower of London task. *Brain.* 1999;122(Pt 10):1973-1987.

Evans J. *Rehabilitation of the Dysexecutive Syndrome.* Philadelphia, Pa: Taylor and Francis, Inc; 2001.

Fuster J. Physiology of executive functions: the perceptual action cycle. In: Stuss D, Knight R, eds. *Principles of Frontal Lobe Function.* New York, NY: Oxford University Press; 2002.

Grafman J. The structured event complex and the human prefrontal cortex. In: Stuss D, Knight R, eds. *Principles of Frontal Lobe Function.* New York, NY: Oxford University Press; 2002.

Hansen CS. Traumatic brain injury. In: van Deusen J, ed. *Body Image and Perceptual Dysfunction in Adults.* Philadelphia, Pa: WB Saunders; 1993.

Kafer KL, Hunter M. On testing the face validity of planning/problem-solving tasks in a normal population. *J Intern Neuropsychol Soc.* 1997;3:108-119.

Kreutzer JS, Marwitz JH, Seel R, Serio CD. Validation of a neurobehavioral functioning inventory for adults with traumatic brain injury. *Arch Phys Med Rehab.* 1996;77:116-124.

Levine B, Dawson D, Boutet I, Schwartz ML, Stuss DT. Assessment of strategic self-regulation in traumatic brain injury: its relationship to injury severity and psychosocial outcome. *Neuropsychology.* 2000;14:491-500.

Levine SP, Horstmann HM, Kirsch NL. Performance considerations for people with cognitive impairment in accessing assistive technologies. *J Head Trauma Rehabil.* 1992;7(3):46-58.

Metcalfe J. Insight and metacognition. In: Mazzoni G, Nelson T, eds. *Metacognition and Cognitive Neuropsychology.* Mahwah, NJ: Lawrence Erlbaum Assoc; 1998.

Nieber E, Koch C. Computational architectures for attention. In: Parasuraman R, ed. *The Attentive Brain.* Cambridge, Mass: MIT Press; 1998.

Oddy M, McMillan TM. Future directions: brain injury services in 2010. In: Wood RL, McMillan TM, eds. *Neurobehavioral Disability and Social Handicap Following Traumatic Brain Injury.* Philadelphia, Pa: Taylor and Francis, Inc; 2001.

Partiot A, Grafman J, Sadato N, et al. Brain activation during the generation of non-emotional and emotional plans. *Neuroreport.* 1995;6(10):1269-1272.

Schacter DL, Prigatano GP. Forms of unawareness. In: Prigatano GP, Schacter DL, eds. *Awareness of Deficit After Injury.* New York, NY: Oxford University Press; 1991.

Schraw G, Dunkle ME, Bendixen LD. Cognitive processes in well-defined and ill-defined problem solving. *App Cogn Psych.* 1995;9:523-538.

Squire LR, Knowlton BJ. Learning about categories in the absence of memory. *Psychology.* 1995;92:14270-12474.

Stuss DT. Biological and psychological development of executive functions. *Brain Cogn.* 1992;20:8-23.

Tanaka J, Taylor M. Object categories and expertise: is the basic level in the eye of the beholder? *Cogn Psychol.* 1991;23:457-482.

Ullman M. Disorder of body image after stroke. *Am J Nurs.* 1964;64:89-91.

Vazzetti D. Capacity, content, control: a model for analyzing the cognitive demands of activity. *Occup Ther Pract.* 1989;1(1):9-17.

Woolcock WW. Generalization strategies. In: Wehman P, Kreutzer JS, eds. *Vocational Rehabilitation for Persons with Traumatic Head Injury.* Rockville, Md: Aspen Publishers; 1990.

Zola SM. Memory, amnesia, and the issue of recovered memory: neurobiological aspects. *Clin Psychol Rev.* 1998;(8):915-932.

CHAPTER 11

ACALCULIA

Acalculia

The ability to perform calculations is crucial to many areas of occupational performance. The skill is used for tasks such as reading price tags, paying bills, counting out money for a purchase, addressing letters, measuring for a recipe, or writing checks.[1,2] Apart from language, calculations are perhaps the only culturally determined semantic system that the majority of the population is expected to acquire and master.[3] Our "number sense" is useful for survival and helps us make sense of a world of discrete objects that form sets and whose combinations follow the rules of arithmetic.[4]

An individual's internal representation of numerical quantities develops rapidly in the first year of life.[4] This ability underlies our ability, later in life, to learn symbols for numbers and perform simple calculations.[4,5] Our adult numerical skills not only include these simple calculations but also include the ability to translate among Arabic numerals, written number names, and spoken number names.[6] Dehaene outlines the following number processing skills of the normal adult[4]:

1. *Read, write, produce, or comprehend numerals in both Arabic and verbal forms*

2. *Convert numbers in these formats to internal quantities and vice-versa*

3. *Compute single-digit addition, subtraction, multiplication, and division operations*

4. *Coordinate several such elementary operations to solve a complex, multidigit arithmetic problem*

In order to understand and interpret any problems the client may have with calculations, it is important to understand the theoretical underlying mechanisms required for successful performance. This successful performance depends on different types of knowledge, including arithmetic facts (ie, 4 x 5 = 20), knowledge of procedures (ie, use of carrying over), and conceptual knowledge (ie, understanding the principles underlying the facts and the procedures).[7]

It is generally assumed that the cognitive numerical processing mechanisms include numeral comprehension, numeral production, and cognitive processes specific to arithmetic.[8,9] They include components of comprehension of operation symbols (eg, =) and words (eg, plus), retrieval of arithmetic facts, and execution of calculation procedures.[9,10] The number processing system is generally distinguished from the calculation system. The number processing system includes the number comprehension and number production subsystems.[10] The calculation system, on the other hand, includes the comprehension of operation symbols, the retrieval of arithmetic facts, and the execution of arithmetic procedures.[9-11] Within each of these subsystems, a further distinction is made between components for processing Arabic numbers (ie, numbers in digit form such as 362) and components for processing verbal numbers.[2]

The number comprehension subsystem translates Arabic or verbal number inputs into internal semantic representation for use in subsequent cognitive processing.[2] Within the Arabic and verbal number comprehension components, a distinction is made between lexical and syntactic processing. Lexical processing is the comprehension of the individual elements in a number. For example, the digit 3 or the word three. Syntactic processing involves the analysis of the relations among elements. This skill refers to word order or the ability to produce an internal representation of the number as a whole.[2]

As previously described, number production components serve to translate internal semantic representations of numbers into sequences of digit or word representations for output.[2,11] Performing calculations requires the three elements of cognitive processes for number comprehension and production and cognitive processes that are specific to calculation procedures. These processes include comprehension of operation symbols or words, retrieval of number facts, and execution of the procedures themselves. Retrieval of number facts is central to almost any form of arithmetic problem solving.[11]

The number processing and calculation system model is summarized in Figure 11-1 and Figure 11-2. Although the number processing and calculation system model is generally accepted, some theorists believe it to be somewhat oversimplified.[12] These theorists describe an alternative theory of encoding complex. They hypothesize that excitatory and inhibitory associative processes contribute collectively to the performance of numerical tasks. Rather than assuming that brain damage would selectively impair comprehension, calculation, or production, this model suggests that partial dysfunction might by associated with selective damage to inhibitory processes.[12] A nonmodular system, in which multiple numerical codes activate one another in the course of numeral processing and arithmetic tasks, is envisioned.[9] These numerical codes are assumed to be interconnected in an associative network.

McClosky presents a model of number processing for which "…all transcoding, including reading aloud both Arabic numerals and written number names, occurs via a single route."[9] Still others propose a multiroute model, which includes both semantic and nonsemantic routes. These theorists hypothesize that the activation of one of the two routes will inhibit the function of the other route.[4] Others hypothesize that internal representations of numbers are not abstract but rather are format specific.[6] According to this model, "…number transcoding and calculations are based on a series of modality-specific codes (eg, verbal, visual, and visuospatial) that can be directly interconnected without the mediation of an abstract code."[6] Dehaene and Cohen support this concept by proposing a "Triple-Code Model," which includes the three main representations of numbers as follows: visual Arabic code, an analogical quantity or magnitude code, and a verbal code.[13]

Hittman-Delazer et al describe three components of the arithmetic system.[5] These components are 1) arithmetic facts, which are thought to be stored in a specific semantic network system from where they can be retrieved as "labels" without a calculation process, 2) arithmetic procedures, defined as sequences of steps necessary to perform multi-digit operations, and 3) a recognition system for arithmetic signs.[5] Other theorists add a fourth component of conceptual knowledge. This involves the understanding and use of arithmetic principles.

Dyscalculia Battery: Number-Processing Section

	Item	Correct Response
Magnitude Comparison Tasks		
Arabic Numbers	108 150	Point to "150"
Spoken verbal numbers	☐ "fifty" ☐ "fifteen"	Point to square representing "fifty"
Written verbal numbers	eleven thousand eighteen three hundred eighty-five	Point to "eleven thousand eighteen"
Transcoding Tasks		
Arabic to spoken verbal numbers	190	"one hundred ninety"
Spoken verbal to written verbal numbers	"nineteen"	nineteen
Spoken verbal to Arabic numbers	"four thousand fifty-seven"	4,057
Arabic to written verbal numbers	5	five
Written verbal to spoken verbal numbers	ninety-two	"ninety-two"
Written verbal to Arabic numbers	three thousand twenty-four	3,024

Figure 11-1. Examples of test items from the number-processing section of the dyscalculia test battery.[2] (Reprinted with permission from Macaruso P, Harley W, McCloskey M. Assessment of acquired dyscalculia. In: Margolin DM, ed. *Cognitive Neuropsychology in Clinical Practice.* New York, NY: Oxford University Press; 1992:4055.)

Recent neuroimaging studies have lent support to the concept of multiple network involvement in numerical processing abilities. Both cortical and subcortical networks have been found to underlie the ability to understand, produce and mentally manipulate numbers in various formats.[14] Research has shown even extremely simple calculations, such as 5 − 2, involve multiple brain areas.[4] One functional magnetic resonance imaging (fMRI) study indicated brain regions including parietal, frontal, and anterior cingulate areas were activated during number processing.[15] A study by Ruechert et al also revealed that activation during calculations involved the coordinated effort of several different cortical areas.[16] Another fMRI study of eight college students demonstrated that the parietal areas as well as the prefrontal cortex and possibly the thalamus are all activated during numerical processing.[17] A study conducted by Chochon et al confirmed the involvement of the left and right parietal areas in calculations but state they may not be functionally equivalent.[15] In addition, this study demonstrated that there exists partially distinct cerebral networks or circuits that underlie distinct arithmetic operations.[15] A study conducted by Dehaene et al supports the notion of distinct networks when their study results pointed to partially distinct networks for multiplication and number comparisons.[18]

Indeed, deficits in acalculia have been reported as the result of numerous brain regions.[1] It can occur with a number of other deficits such as aphasia or as part of Gerstmann's syndrome[13,19] or as a primary deficit involving any or all four arithmetic operations.[10] Denburg and Tranel have described three general categories of acalculia, which are summarized in Table 11-1.

Dyscalculia Battery: Calculation Section

	Item	*Correct Response*
Operation Symbol and Word Comprehension Tasks		
Operation symbol comprehension	subtraction 6 + 2 6 X 2 6 − 2	point to 6 − 2
Operation word comprehension	addition "nine times six"	"No"
Written Arithmetic Tasks		
Addition	752 +978	752 +978 1730
Subtraction	86 −37	86 −37 49
Multiplication	30 x84	30 x84 120 +2400 2520
Oral Arithmetic Tasks		
Addition	"five plus eight"	"thirteen"
Subtraction	"seventeen minus nine"	"eight"
Multiplication	"six times three"	"eighteen"

Figure 11-2. Examples of test items from the calculation section of the dyscalculia test battery.[2] (Reprinted with permission from Macaruso P, Harley W, McCloskey M. Assessment of acquired dyscalculia. In: Margolin DM, ed. *Cognitive Neuropsychology in Clinical Practice.* New York, NY: Oxford University Press; 1992:4055.)

Table 11-1

General Categories of Acalculia

Type	*Description*	*Lesion Site*
Acalculia with alexia and agraphia for numbers	Calculation deficits occur as a result of impaired reading or writing of numbers	Primarily left hemisphere (especially parietal)
Acalculia of the spatial type	Impaired spatial organization of numbers, related to visual neglect, misalignment of numbers, and number inversions	Primarily right hemisphere lesions
Anarithmetia (primary acalculia)	Acalculia that does not conform to the previous two categories	Primarily left hemisphere lesions, but can occur following right hemisphere lesions

Adapted from reference 1: Denburg N, Tranel D. Acalculia and disturbances of the body schema. In: Heilmann, Valenstein E, eds. Clinical Neuropsychology. 4th ed. New York, NY: Oxford University Press; 2003.

Even two seemingly similar operations such as subtraction and multiplication can be dissociated (ie, the client is able to perform one operation but not the other).[6] Some studies, in fact, have found that subtraction appears to be better preserved than multiplication and addition.[20] One study has also described a client who exhibited acalculia for addition, subtraction, and division, but had intact multiplication.[10] This client also had intact ability to distinguish math signs. These results point to the possibility of different processing systems responsible for each of the basic arithmetic operations. Another study of clients with major left hemisphere lesions showed their inability to name, add, subtract, or multiply digits accompanied with an intact ability to state which of two numbers is larger.[6]

Tohgi et al support these findings in a description of a client with a left frontal lobe infarct.[21] The client was able to add and subtract numbers but could not multiply or divide.[21] The deficit was attributed to a difficulty in retrieving facts from the multiplication table and the calculation procedures themselves.

Corbett et al describe still another clinical picture related to acalculia.[22] A 60-year-old male with a subcortical infarct had difficulties in numerical syntax, a loss of ability to manipulate math concepts, and impaired working memory.[22] This study is one of several that have demonstrated that localization for number processing and calculations is not limited to cortical structures.[23]

Sokol et al describe a client with ABI with impaired retrieval of arithmetic facts but intact abilities in execution of calculation procedures.[24] These authors point to two separate functionally distinct components in the cognitive calculation system.

Rosselli and Ardila studied 41 clients with left hemisphere damage and 21 clients with right hemisphere damage.[25] All groups presented difficulties with calculations tasks. Left hemisphere clients showed a significantly higher number of errors in reading numbers and arithmetic signs, counting backwards, and performing successive operations. These clients, however, showed a better comprehension of written numbers. Lucchelli and DeRenzi also describe a client with good comprehension of operation symbols but impaired retrieval of math facts and execution of calculation procedures.[26]

Takayama et al describe clients who could read, repeat, and accurately verbalize numbers; had normal counting ability; understood the basic processes of calculation, and showed little difficulty in the retrieval of table values.[27] Their errors were made in the process where a number of steps were carried out simultaneously. These steps included retrieval of the number fact or table value, appropriate spatial alignment of the digits, appropriate procedural access, and retention and use of any integers remaining from the previous product.[27] These authors concluded that a working memory deficit could have a strong effect on multi-digit arithmetic problems and that the left parietal lobe may be a specialized area for working memory for calculation.[27]

Delazer and Benke describe a 56-year-old female with a left parietal tumor who demonstrated that arithmetic facts could be represented at a superficial level without really understanding the operation she performed.[20] A client studied by Hittman-Delazer et al demonstrated the opposite.[5] Despite this client's inability to perform arithmetic fact problems such as $2 + 3$, he was able to process algebraic expressions and had an excellent understanding of complex arithmetic text problems. He understood arithmetic principles and applied them in a variety of tasks. The client's clinical picture lead these authors to hypothesize that conceptual knowledge (in addition to arithmetic fact knowledge and arithmetic procedures) is a functionally independent component of the calculation system.[5]

The previously described theoretical models, neuroimaging, and clinical research studies indicate that acalculia can be manifest in a number of different ways. Calculation ability is likely mediated by several cognitive processes including, language, memory, visual spatial, and attentional abilities.[1,7,20] In addition, conceptual knowledge or abstraction is considered to be an important part of the calculation or number processing system.[5] Semenza et al associate a calculations deficit with either a deficit in the knowledge or memory of the procedure or a monitoring deficit.[7] They build on this concept by outlining the characteristics of the client's performance that would

Table 11-2

Characteristics of a Failure of Arithmetic Procedures and Possible Associated Underlying Cause

Deficit of Knowledge/ Memory of the Procedure	Monitoring Deficit
Consistent and systematic errors occurring as a result of a faulty strategy	Inconsistent and unsystematic errors reflecting no strategies
No breakdown in performance as the operation proceeds	Breakdown in performance as the operation proceeds, starting would be typically correct
No problem in knowing when an operation or subsets of the operation are completed	Difficulty in ending operation or parts of operations
Modification of performance with training	No effect of training
Possible awareness about the specific difficulty	A general lack of awareness about the quality of performance

Adapted from reference 7: Semenza C, Miceli L, Girelli L. A deficit for arithmetical procedures: lack of knowledge or lack of monitoring? Cortex. 1997;33(3):483-498.

indicate the type of calculation deficit. These characteristics and associated deficits are summarized in Table 11-2.

Acalculia can have broad implications relating to the client's occupational performance and, therefore, warrants a complete evaluation. Assessment of calculation skills should be varied and include written and oral calculation, comprehension and use of operations, and tasks involving the spatial components of arithmetic.[1] The assessment should parse out a true primary calculation deficit versus one that is secondary to deficits in areas such as language, attention, memory, or executive skills.[1] It is also important initially to find out, perhaps through family interviews, the client's premorbid calculation abilities.

EVALUATION OF ACALCULIA

Test 1 – Clinical Observations

Description

Observe the client during occupation-based activities involving number processing abilities (ie, measuring during kitchen tasks, calculating money during a purchase on a community outing, balancing his or her checkbook, etc).

Test 2 – Dyscalculia Battery[2]

Description

This test battery has items representing both the number processing system and calculations system. Within each of these major sections are items covering all the component skills. Please refer to Figure 11-1 and Figure 11-2 for examples of test items.

Test 3 – Functional Calculations Evaluation

Description

An evaluation can be developed that contains test items for recognition of numbers, simple mathematical operations, and complex mathematical operations, including concepts associated with these operations.[28,29] Test items that are functionally oriented should be incorporated into the evaluation (eg, coin recognition, calculating change, check writing, or budgeting).

Scoring

Nonstandardized
The clinician measures the client's level of performance on each category of tasks described.

Validity

To improve validity, rule out poor visual attentiveness and oculomotor skills, decreased attention, problem solving, mental inflexibility, and aphasia as causes of poor performance.

TREATMENT FOR ACALCULIA

Utilizing a Restorative Approach

(Note: The therapist should frequently monitor the client's progress using this approach for acalculia, as no evidence-based research using the approach was located by the author.)

1. Identify which aspect or aspects of the number processing or calculations system are impaired. Ask the client to perform repetitive related tasks, beginning with one-step operations and progressing to multiple-step operations as the client improves.

2. Utilize computer retraining with software that has been designed for the specific restoration of number processing and calculations skills.

Utilizing an Adaptive Approach

1. Identify how the client's acalculia is affecting function, and provide environmental adaptations as needed—as, for example, the use of a calculator. Ideally, the calculator should either be solar powered or have a long life battery.[30] Training should include calculator use in activities of daily living (ADLs) or instrumental activities of daily living (IADLs) such as use in a restaurant or grocery store during a community outing.

2. If the client is unable to balance his or her checkbook, use an electronic checkbook, which combines calculator and checkbook balancing features.[30] The RadioShack checkbook calculator (Fort Worth, Tex) is simple to use and can keep accurate records of a checking account as well as two charge accounts at the same time.[30]

3. If the client is unable to use a telephone, then a telephone with memory can assist.

4. Alter the mode of presentation of material as needed based on the evaluation. For example, if the evaluation showed the client could not read Arabic numbers, then write out in words important numbers such as phone numbers or addresses. If the client can comprehend numbers when presented visually but not auditorily, then use only the visual mode.

References

1. Denburg N, Tranel D. Acalculia and disturbances of the body schema. In: Heilmann, Valenstein E, eds. *Clinical Neuropsychology.* 4th ed. New York, NY: Oxford University Press; 2003.
2. Macaruso P, Harley W, McCloskey M. Assessment of acquired dyscalculia. In: Margolin DM, ed. *Cognitive Neuropsychology in Clinical Practice.* New York, NY: Oxford University Press; 1992:4055.
3. Spiers PA. Acalculia revised: current issues. In: Deloche G, Seren X, eds. *Mathematical Disabilities: A Cognitive Neuropsychological Perspective.* Hillsdale, NJ: Lawrence Erlbaum Assoc; 1987.
4. Dehaene S. Cerebral basis of number counting and calculation. In: Gazzaniga, Michael S, ed. *The New Cognitive Neuroscience.* 2nd ed. Cambridge, Mass: MIT Press; 2000.

5. Hittman-Delazer M, Sailer U, Benke T. Impaired arithmetic facts but intact conceptual knowledge—a single-case study of dyscalculia. *Cortex.* 1995;31(1):139-147.

6. Cipolotti L, Butterworth B. Toward a multiroute model of number processing: impaired number transcoding with preserved calculations skills. *J Exp Psychol.* 1995;124(4):375-390.

7. Semenza C, Miceli L, Girelli L. A deficit for arithmetical procedures: lack of knowledge or lack of monitoring? *Cortex.* 1997;33(3):483-498.

8. Basso A, Burgio F, Caporali A. Acalculia, aphasia and spatial disorders in left and right brain-damaged patients. *Cortex.* 2000;36(2):265-280.

9. McCloskey M. Cognitive mechanisms in numerical processing: evidence from acquired dyscalculia. *Cognition.* 1992;44:107-157.

10. Lample Y, Eshel Y, Gilad R, Sarova-Pinhas I. Selective acalculia with sparing of the subtraction process in a patient with left parietotemporal hemorrhage. *Neurology.* 1994;44(9):1759-1761.

11. McCloskey M, Harley W, Sokol SM. Models of arithmetic fact retrieval: and evaluation in light of findings from normal and brain-damaged subjects. *J Exp P Psych Learning Mem Cogn.* 1991;17(3):377-397.

12. Clark JM, Campbell JID. Integrated versus modular theories of number skills and acalculia. *Brain Cogn.* 1991;17:204-3-239.

13. Dehaene S, Cohen L. Cerebral pathways of calculation: double dissociation between rote verbal and quantitative knowledge of arithmetic. *Cortex.* 1997;33(2):210-250.

14. Delazer M, Girelli L, Semenza C, Denes G. Numerical skills and aphasia. *J Int Neuropsychol Soc.* 1999;5(3):213-221.

15. Chochon F, Cohen L, van de Moortele PF, Dehaene S. Differential contributions of the left and right inferior parietal lobules to number processing. *J Cogn Neurosci.* 1999;11(6):617-630.

16. Ruechert L, Lange N, Partiot A, et al. Visualizing cortical activation during mental calculation with functional MRI. *Neuroimage.* 1996;3(2):97-103.

17. Rickard TC, Romero SG, Basso G, et al. The calculating brain: an fMRI study. *Neuropsychologia.* 2000;38(3):325-335.

18. Dehaene S, Tzourio N, Frak V, et al. Cerebral activations during number multiplication and comparison: a PET study. *Neurolpsychologia.* 1996;34(11):1097-1106.

19. Grafman J, Kampen D, Rosenberg J, Salazar AM, Boller F. The progressive breakdown of number processing and calculation ability: a case study. *Cortex.* 1989;25:121-133.

20. Delazer M, Benke T. Arithmetic facts without meaning. *Cortex.* 1997;33(4):697-710.

21. Tohgi H, Saitoh K, Takahashi S, et al. Agraphia and acalculia after a left prefrontal (F1, F2) infarction. *J Neurol Neurosurg Psychiatry.* 1995;58:629-632.

22. Corbett AJ, McCusker EA, Davidson OR. Acalculia following a dominant-hemisphere subcortical infarct. *Arch Neurol.* 1986;43(9):964-966.

23. Kahn HJ, Whitaker HA. Acalculia: an historical review of localization. *Brain Cogn.* 1991;17:102-1151.

24. Sokol SM, McCloskey M, Cohen NJ, Aliminosa D. Cognitive representations and processes in arithmetic: inferences from the performance of brain-damaged subjects. *J Exp Psych Learning Mem Cogn.* 1991;17(3):355-376.

25. Rosselli M, Ardila A. Calculation deficits in patients with right and left hemisphere damage. *Neuropsychologla.* 1989;27(5):607-617.

26. Lucchelli F, DeRenzi E. Primary dyscalculia after a medical frontal lesion of the left hemisphere. *J Neurol Neurosurg Psychiatry.* 1993;56:304-307.

27. Takayama Y, Sugishita M, Akiguchi I, Kimura J. Isolated acalculia due to left parietal lesion. *Arch Neurol.* 1994;1:2860-291.

28. Lezak M. *Neuropsychological Assessment.* New York, NY: Oxford University Press; 1983.

29. Luria AR. *Higher Cortical Functions in Man.* 2nd ed. New York, NY: Basic Books Inc; 1980.

30. Parente R, Herrmann D. External aids to cognition. In: Parente R, Herrmann D, eds. *Retraining Cognition: Techniques and Applications.* 2nd ed. Austin, Tex: PRO-ED Inc; 2003.

Resources

Benson DF. Disorders of visual gnosis. In: Brown JW, ed. *Neuropsychology of Visual Perception.* Hillsdale, NJ: Lawrence Erbaum Assoc; 1989.

Wheatley C. Evaluation of cognitive dysfunction. In: Early MB, ed. *Physical Dysfunction: Practice Skills for the Occupational Therapy Assistant.* St. Louis, Mo: Mosby; 1998.

CHAPTER 12

FACTORS THAT INFLUENCE THE CLIENT'S VISION, PERCEPTION, AND COGNITION

Many areas of skill have an influence on the client's vision, perception, or cognition. For example, aphasia, sensory loss, and visual and perceptual deficits can all complicate or interfere with the client's cognitive abilities. As previously described, in addition to these internal factors, the external environment can have an affect on performance. Detailed information about these areas has been presented elsewhere in this book. In addition to these areas, factors such as age, motivation, depression, fatigue, behavior, and secondary medical conditions can influence the client's cognitive, perceptual, and visual skills. These additional factors are subsequently described.

The Relationship of Age to Visual, Perceptual, and Cognitive Evaluation and Treatment

The incidence of cerebral vascular accident (CVA) escalates rapidly with advancing age, from 3.3 per 100,000 persons under 35 to 1800 or more in those 85 years old or older.[1] One study reports that of 578 clients who had sustained CVAs, 76.5% were between the ages of 60 and 99 years.[2] Despite research and clinical evidence that the majority of the clients who sustain a CVA are elderly, functional neurological changes that occur as the result of normal aging are rarely taken into account during visual, perceptual, and cognitive evaluation and treatment. The following section will acquaint the reader with the major changes related to the normal aging process that may affect visual, perceptual, and cognitive functioning.

SENSORY LOSS

Sensory loss, involving any of the primary senses, as well as proprioceptive and vestibular function loss are common in the elderly.[3-7] The age-related changes in all of the client's sensory systems can lead to distorted representations of the external world, which in turn, can lead to declines in cognitive performance.[7] The age-related sensory changes subsequently described should be treated with a view of how they affect the client's overall cognitive function. The therapist should

Table 12-1

Changes in the Visual System Associated with Age

Structural Component	Age-Related Change	Functional Implications
Cornea	Appearance change	Loss of luster, limited amount of fluid bathing the cornea
	Accumulation of lipids	Increased astigmatism with increased blurred vision (independent of near or farsightedness)
Iris	Decreased permeability	May contribute to glaucoma
Ciliary Muscle	Atrophy of muscle	Decreased mobility of the lens which causes decreased muscle effectiveness
Pupil	Decreased pupil size	Restricted amount of light reaching retina; difficulty in seeing dark objects or objects in dim light
	Decreased pupillary reflex	Decreased dark adaptation and recovery from glare
Lens	Lens growth	Decreased accommodative ability
	Decreased refractive index of lenses	Uneven refracture properties, which can result in double vision in one eye
	Yellowing	Reduces amount of light reaching retina and changes light composition; alters color vision
Vitreous	Contracts	May separate from retina (the retina itself may also detach)

encourage the client to use technological aids, such as a hearing aid or glasses, to maximize occupational performance through improved environmental sense and interaction.[4]

VISION

Visual acuity and adaptability decline with age.[3,6,8-11] Decreased depth perception and peripheral vision may also occur.[6,12] Changes occur in the cornea, pupil, iris, lens, vitreous, and ciliary muscles of the eyes.[8,12-14] Common age-related conditions that will affect vision include macular degeneration, glaucoma, cataracts, and arteriosclerosis. Macular degeneration results in a loss of central vision, which can start to manifest around age 70 and becomes more significant through the 80s and 90s.[5] The condition occurs from fluid that leaks from the deeper layers of the retina.[15] This leak causes pressure that pushes the retina up and detaches it from the nourishing layer.[15] Glaucoma results from increased intraocular pressure that affects the flow of blood and nutrients to the optic disk.[15] This condition, if severe enough, can cause field loss and eventually complete blindness.[15] Cataracts are the result of a loss of transparency of the crystalline lens and result in an impairment of the overall clarity of vision.[15] Arteriosclerosis can cause a hardening of the retinal arteries, which will ultimately affect vision.

Table 12-1 summarizes changes in the visual system associated with age.

AUDITION

Hearing loss caused by aging is always bilateral and usually symmetrical.[16] Age-related changes might include decreased inner ear function, thickening of the tympanic membrane, loss of elasticity of the ossicular chain, and atrophy of the cochlear organ or Corti.[12,16] As a result of the structural changes of the auditory system, any or all of the following functional changes might occur:

1. High frequency loss
2. All frequency loss
3. Neural problems that result in decreased speech comprehension and discrimination
4. Problems in determining the source of a sound
5. Distortion of environmental sound
6. Difficulty hearing in the presence of background noise
7. Impaired intellectual functioning

REMAINING SENSORY SYSTEMS

Research has indicated that in at least a portion of the elderly population, there is a reduced sensitivity to taste, smell, touch, vibration, temperature, kinesthesia, and pain.[8,17] Proprioceptive and vestibular loss are also common. The effect of vestibular loss on vision, perception, and cognition is covered in Chapter 3.

AUTONOMIC NERVOUS SYSTEM

Age-related changes in the hypothalamus have been observed and seem to result in decreased maintenance of homeostasis.[18,19] Age-related changes occur in the metabolism and regulatory mechanisms of an organism. Aging is characterized by a progressive decrease in the intensity of adaptive processes.[20] It is believed that with aging, autonomic nervous system changes take place throughout all aspects of the system. These changes lead to shifts in the reflectory regulation of inner organs, a decrease in the organism's adaptive capacities, a decrease in the reliability of homeostatic regulatory mechanisms, easier disruption of regulatory mechanisms, and the development of disorders in old age.[19]

PERCEPTION

In view of the close relationship between vision and perception, it can be expected that age-related visual changes will influence perceptual abilities in the elderly. For example, the decreased accommodative power and poor lens transmissiveness previously described can, in turn, affect distance vision, sensitivity to glare, and depth and color perception.[13] Losses in acuity and distance perception, visual closure, or part-whole perception may also be deficient.[13] The elderly client may exhibit decreased visual discrimination, figure-ground, visual memory, and spatial relations.[21] The quality of stereopsis depends on brightness and contrast. Therefore, any age-related process that reduces retinal illumination would impair binocular depth perception.[13] Decreased pattern recognition and poor attentional processing during visual search have also been documented.[22-24]

In addition to distance, depth, and color perception, the elderly client's visual fields may be altered. This age-related change involves the retina and the nervous system in general. Age-related circulatory changes can cause a metabolic change in the retina, which in turn, is reflected by changes in the size of the visual field.[13]

COGNITION

Research has indicated that decreased brain weight and volume and a decrease in the cells of the cerebral cortex occur with age.[25,26] Research has shown with advancing age, there is a progressive deterioration of the frontal and medial temporal lobe regions of the brain.[27] Since the cerebral cortex is intricately involved with higher intellectual functioning, cognitive and behavioral changes might be expected with age. Nearly all aspects of human performance are guided by cognition.[28] Although there is no universal effect of aging on learning, age-related changes in memory, processing ability, attention, and executive functions such as problem solving, mental flexibility, or abstraction are well documented.[27,29-33]

The documentation of decreased memory of one type or another in the elderly is abundant.[34-43] Age-related deficits in overall cognitive performance appear less evident when performance tasks do not require retrieval or processing of information.[33] Some authors believe that age-related memory loss is primarily a storage and retrieval problem. This retrieval deficit is present in the elderly for both episodic and semantic memory and is especially apparent in tasks that require a large degree of self-initiated activity.[27,37,39,44] This retrieval deficit begins when an individual is in his or her 40s and 50s and increases significantly beyond the age of 70.[39] Others believe that nonverbal memory is a particular problem for the elderly and that they will benefit from the use of verbal cues to improve their performance.[43,45] Craik, Byrd, and Swanson believe age-related deficits in memory appear to be related to cognitive tasks that require a greater amount of effort for processing than automatic processing.[46] Age-related memory loss has also been attributed to the inefficient use of learning strategies.[34,47] For example, the elderly do not use repetition, visual imagery, verbal mediation, association encoding, mnemonics, or organization strategies as often or as effectively as younger individuals.[34,47,48] Inefficient use of all or any of these strategies means that the retrieval cues are minimal.[34] Retrieval deficits in the elderly in association with new information do not appear to generalize to very old memory. In addition, recent research has indicated that any changes with aging in either the capacity or duration of iconic memory are slight if they exist at all.[22] No major changes in echoic memory were noted.[22] Older adults seem to have more problems with remembering contextual or source information and especially have difficulty when information is new and not conceptually well organized.[39] Implicit memory, as well as general knowledge of the world, vocabulary, and well-learned skills are generally not as affected by age.[39]

Decreased spatial memory has also been documented in the elderly.[38] Age differences in face recognition memory are also apparent by the fifth decade.[49] This difference becomes especially pronounced by the seventh decade.[49] Additional age-related deficits include a decreased ability to acquire knowledge about a novel environment and decreased bilateral coordination.[46]

A generalized slowing of cognitive processes and reaction time in the elderly has also been documented.[3,29,31,44,50] This decreased processing ability has been associated with an inability to perform postural or balance activities while doing a cognitive task.[31,51,52] It may also affect memory or abstraction and tasks that require holding and processing multiple items in memory.[3] The elderly client can display diminished ability for abstract and complex conceptualization and poor mental flexibility.[8,47] These deficits, along with decreased memory, can cause difficulty in adapting to new situations, solving novel problems, and changing from one mental set to another.[8,47] There is, indeed, documentation of poor problem solving ability among the elderly.[8,30,34,53,54]

IMPLICATIONS FOR EVALUATION

Some of the age-related deficits described in this section may or may not be present in a given individual. It is vital for the therapist to obtain a clear picture of the premorbid status of the elderly client with acquired brain injury (ABI) prior to visual, perceptual, or cognitive evaluation and treatment. Vision should be evaluated prior to testing, and measures that involve small visual stimuli should be avoided if possible. Responses that require fine color discrimination, especially in the blue spectrum, may be invalid.[55] One should use color contrasts, increased amount of light, and clean prescription glasses when indicated. Determine the client's hearing acuity. Evaluate the effects of modifying your voice, identify the best position to sit or stand to reinforce what is said, and make sure that the client's hearing aid is clean.[12] Consult vision and hearing experts when there is a question.

Always remember that for the elderly, testing is often a threatening experience. The fear of testing may in fact limit their risk taking and inhibit their response. Consider the environment when testing; the elderly are more easily distracted by irrelevant stimuli than younger individuals.[56]

Finally, consider fatigue in testing.[34,36] Mental fatigue at any age can cause various sensory and perceptual changes, slowed and disorganized performance, and perhaps short-term memory impairment.[49] Evaluate the client at different times of day as he or she may be disoriented in the morning or fatigued in the afternoon.[57]

IMPLICATIONS IN TREATMENT

The areas to consider for evaluation are also applicable to treatment. In addition, the therapist should limit redundant and extraneous information and treat in a nondistracting environment.[34,36] Repetition and practice are indicated because the elderly (along with the young) can benefit from this.[2] For example, research has shown that the elderly, like the young, have the capability of improving their skill in divided attention through practice.[58] Intensive and extensive mnemonics training can also help the elderly.[59] Formal training in mnemonics has increased the learning proficiency of some elderly adults.[59] The extent of benefit, however, depends on the extent of training.

Allow sufficient time for the client to respond, and utilize cues that will most benefit the client (eg, verbal, visual, touch, or movement) in addition to practice and cuing. The elderly client who has sustained a CVA can benefit from controlled sensory stimulation and sensory integrative techniques.[60] Training activities that target psychosocial skills and foster self-efficacy beliefs (belief about one's ability to perform) can help the elderly client's cognitive ability.[27] Home-based activities or services appear to be particularly important for the elderly client.[57] This not only can increase client awareness but requires less transfer of learning.

Sleep Disorders

Clients who have sustained an ABI are at risk for various types of sleep disorders that, often times, remain undiagnosed.[61-65] These disorders may be the result of pre-existing conditions secondary to a comorbid psychiatric condition such as depression or the ABI itself, and can contribute to decreased independence in activities of daily living (ADLs) and overall functional outcome.[61,62,66,67] Common disorders can include sleep apnea, periodic limb movement disorder (PLMD), and hypersomnolence (excessive daytime sleepiness).[61,66] These disorders can affect attention, concentration, complex problem solving, and memory.[61,62,65] They can affect the client's memory, perception, and overall judgment.[68]

Motivation

The client's motivation to participate in the treatment process will ultimately affect functional outcome.[69] Decreased motivation subsequent to ABI is a common occurrence and can have a physical or psychological cause. Brain injury affecting the mesolimbic/mesocortical circuitry, for example, has been associated with poor client motivation.[70] Research has indicated that for these clients, medication can help.[70]

Various psychological factors can affect client motivation. Depression, for example, can cause the client to believe he or she cannot enjoy anything and, therefore, does not have the impulse to try.[71] The time, energy, frustration, and pain experienced during therapy can also affect a client's motivation.[71] His or her belief in recovery, therapist competence, and ability to relate the relevance of therapeutic activities to his or her life will also determine level of motivation. The client's previous interests, accomplishments, and activities that were meaningful, therefore, are important to incorporate into the therapeutic process. Therapeutic activities should have relevance and goals, or activities should reflect the client's cognitive abilities. As Rosenfeld states, therapeutic activities should facilitate strong occupational engagement.[71] These activities will help motivate the client with ABI.

Depression

Depression is one of the major emotional disorders often present subsequent to an ABI.[3,67,72-77] One study indicated a poststroke depression rate of 20% to 25%,[78] while another indicated more than half of 106 acute CVA clients suffered from depression.[79] Anxiety and depression for prolonged periods have also been observed in the adult traumatic brain injury (TBI) client.[74,80] One study of clients with TBI indicated depression and anxiety tend to persist and may worsen over time, even at long-term follow up if left untreated.[81] Documented post-TBI anxiety symptoms include free-floating anxiety, fearfulness, intense worry, generalized uneasiness, social withdrawal, interpersonal sensitivity, and anxiety dreams.[67] Symptoms of post-ABI depression can include perseverative thoughts, poor initiation, slowed reaction times, and poor ability to predict the quality of activity performance.[82] Depression in the aphasic client may be overlooked due to his or her inability to express feelings of distress.[72]

The occupational therapist can screen for depressive symptoms during the initial evaluation as well as through medical records review and ongoing observation for behavioral changes during the rehabilitative process. Rosenfeld recommends that a referral should be made if five of the following symptoms are present for more than several weeks[71]:

1. *Disrupted sleep patterns*—Frequent interruptions, early awakening
2. *Loss of interest*—In previously valued activities, relationships
3. *Guilt*—Feeling self-worthlessness, unrealistic self-blame
4. *Decreased energy*—Decreased vitality
5. *Impaired concentration*—Significant decrease
6. *Change in appetite*—Anorexia and weight loss or overeating and weight gain
7. *Impaired psychomotor*—Agitation or retardation
8. *Suicidal*—Ideas, impulses, plans, actions

It is well documented that post-ABI depression can affect the client's cognitive abilities,[3,27,82,83] as well as the client's ultimate functional outcome.[71,84-87] The cause of post-ABI depression, however, remains unclear. Some believe the persistent dependency in ADLs along with the social isolation common to the client with ABI contribute to depression.[61,66] Others look to neuroimaging and pharmacological advances to identify neuroanatomic and neurochemical associations of depression.[71] Still others advocate that post-ABI depression is the result of both psychological and organic difficulties.[67] Rao and Lyketsos build on this concept in their belief that transient post-ABI depression is caused by disrupted brain physiology, while prolonged depression is associated with a psychological base related to physical and cognitive impairment.[67]

No matter what the purported underlying cause of post-ABI depression, the therapist should consider the symptoms in the evaluation and treatment of vision, perception, and cognition as well as overall functional abilities. The therapist should strongly support yet challenge the depressed client as well as listen empathetically and address his or her concerns.[71]

Behavior and Personality Changes

Personality changes and/or behavioral problems often occur subsequent to an ABI. The client may exhibit challenging, disruptive, or aggressive behaviors, which will have a major impact on rehabilitation.[88,89] He or she may be confused, agitated, or noncompliant.[80] Clients who have sustained injury to the orbitofrontal area may display a behavioral dyscontrol disorder.[67,90] Symptoms could include impulsiveness, lability, reduced anger control, aggressiveness, sexual acting out, perseveration, and generally poor social judgment.[89] Inappropriate behavior could range from tactless remarks that are offensive to inappropriate advances.[91] On rare occurrences, the client with ABI may develop a manic disorder or an affective bipolar disorder.[72,80]

Most clinicians believe the etiology of psychiatric problems after an ABI are related to postinjury changes, premorbid personality, psychosocial, and environmental factors.[67] Premorbid occurrences of alcoholism or psychiatric illness as well as factors such as marital problems or financial instability can all be risk factors for psychiatric problems after ABI.[67] Generalized treatment can include pharmacotherapy, psychotherapy, and family education and support. General guidelines for treatment of the client with a behavioral problem can include the following[75]:

1. Allow rest time.
2. Keep the environment simple.
3. Give feedback and set goals.
4. Be calm and redirect to task.
5. Provide choices.
6. Keep instructions simple.
7. Decrease the chance of failure.
8. Vary treatment activities.
9. Overplan the treatment session.
10. Analyze the tasks you are asking the client to perform.

Management of the client with behavioral problems requires a consistent approach and effort from all members of the treatment team. Techniques being used with the individual client should also be taught to the family or caregiver. Many behavior management approaches can be utilized, and the reader is encouraged to refer to techniques described in previous chapters as well as to the references to seek out additional detailed information.

Additional Factors Affecting Performance

As previously described in the section on aging, many other sequelae of ABI can affect the client's visual, perceptual, and/or cognitive skills. These can range from language impairment such as aphasia to sensory memory loss.[66,82,92] Tactile inattention, proprioception, and stereognosis, for example, may all affect the outcome of cognitive treatment.[92]

Medications can affect the client's cognitive function.[3,57] Oftentimes, the client will be taking several medications, which can decrease his or her cognitive reserve and result in lethargy or confusion.[3,57] The therapist, therefore, should review what medications the client is taking as well as the potential side effects and interactions.

Research has indicated that many chronic diseases can cause decreased cognitive performance.[3,27,44,93,94] These can include chronic hypo or hyper forms of thyroid function, hypertension, hyperlipidemia, and diabetes.[3,27,93-96] If the client suffers from any of these conditions, the therapist should consult with the client's family or caregiver pertaining to the client's premorbid cognitive abilities.

References

1. Robins M, Baum H. Incidence, part II. *Stroke.* 1981;12(2):45-58.
2. Moskowitz E, Lightbody E, Freitag NS. Long-term follow-up of the post stroke patient. *Arch Phys Med Rehab.* 1972;53:167-172.
3. Fillit H, Butler RN, O'Connell AW, et al. Achieving and maintaining cognitive vitality with aging. *Mayo Clin Proc.* 2002;77(7):681-696.
4. Fisher DL. Cognitive aging and adaptive technologies. In: Stern PC, Carstensen LL, eds. *The Aging Mind: Opportunities in Cognitive Research.* Washington, DC: National Academy Press; 2000.
5. LaGrossa J. The plague that threatens the greatest generation. *Advance for Occupational Therapy Practitioners.* June 28, 2004.
6. Peralta A. Older adults and multidiagnosis patients. In: Early MB, ed. *Physical Dysfunction: Practice Skills for the Occupational Assistant.* St. Louis, Mo: CV Mosby; 1998.
7. Schneider B. Sensation, cognition, and levels of processing in aging. In: Naveh-Benjamin M, Moscovitch M, Roediger HL III, eds. *Perspectives on Human Memory and Cognitive Aging.* Ann Arbor, Mich: Psychology Press; 2001.
8. Filskov S, Boll T. *Handbook of Clinical Neuropsychology.* New York, NY: John Wiley & Son, Inc; 1981.
9. Hirvela H, Koskela P, Laatikainen L. Visual acuity and contrast sensitivity in the elderly. *Acta Opthalmol Scand.* 1995;73(2):111-115.
10. Hoyer WJ, Rybash JM. Age and visual field differences in computing visual-spatial relations. Psych Aging. 1992;7(3):339-342.
11. Vaughan WJ, Smitz P, Fatt I. The human lens—a model system for the study of agong. In: Ordy JM, Bizzee KR, eds. *Aging. Vol 10. Sensory System and Communication in the Elderly.* New York, NY: Raven Press; 1979.
12. Carter R, Buseck S, Shields E. *Aging: Sensory Losses.* New York, NY: American Journal of Nursing Co; 1980. (Study guide and videotape).
13. Fozard J, Wolf E, Bell B, McFarland R, Podolsky S. Visual perception and communication. In: Birren J, Schaie K, eds. *Handbook of Psychology of Aging.* New York, NY: Van Nostrand Reinhold Co; 1977.
14. Podolsky S, Schachar R. Clinical manifestations of diabetic retinopathy and other diseases of the eye in the elderly. In: Ordy JM, Bizzee KR, eds. *Aging. Vol 10. Sensory Systems and Communications in the Elderly.* New York, NY: Raven Press; 1979.
15. Aloisio L. Visual dysfunction. In: Gillen G, Burkhardt A, eds. *Stroke Rehabilitation: A Function-Based Approach.* St. Louis, Mo: Mosby Inc; 2004.
16. Pickett JM, Bergman M, Levitt H. Aging and speech understanding. In: Ordy JM, Bizzee KR, eds. *Aging. Vol 10. Sensory Systems and Communication in the Elderly.* New York, NY: Raven Press; 1979.
17. Jackson OL. Brain function, aging, and dementia. In: Umphred DA, ed. *Neurological Rehabilitation.* 2nd ed. St. Louis, Mo: CV Mosby; 1990.
18. Diamond MC. The aging brain: some enlightening and optimistic results. *Am Sci.* 1978;66:66-71.

19. Frolkis V. Aging of the autonomic nervous system. In: Birren J, Schaie K, eds. *Handbook of the Psychology of Aging.* New York, NY: Van Nostrand Reinhold Co; 1977.
20. Drachman D, Leavitt J. Memory impairment in the aged: storage vs retrieval deficit. *J Exp Psychol.* 1972;93(2):302-308.
21. Su C, Chien T, Cheng K, Lin T. Performance of older adults with and without cerebrovascular accident on the test of visual perceptual skills. *Am J Occup Ther.* 1995;49(6):491-499.
22. Kausler DH. *Learning and Memory in Normal Aging.* San Diego, Calif: Academic Press; 1994.
23. Madden DJ. Adult age differences in the time course of visual attention. *J Gerontol.* 1990;45:9-16.
24. Russo R, Parkin AJ. Age differences in implicit memory, more apparent than real. *Memory Cogn.* 1993;21:72-80.
25. Bondareff W. The neural basis of aging. In: Birren J, Schaie K, eds. *Handbook of the Psychology of Aging.* New York, NY: Van Nostrand Reinhold Co; 1977.
26. Brody H, Vijayashankar N. Anatomical changes in the nervous system. In: Finch CE, Hayfbeck L, eds. *Handbook of the Biology of Aging.* New York, NY: Van Nostrand Reinhold Co; 1977.
27. Dawson D, Winocur G, Moscovitch M. The psychosocial environment and cognitive rehabilitation in the elderly. In: Stuss DT, Winocur G, Robertson IH, eds. *Cognitive Neurorehabilitation.* New York, NY: Cambridge University Press; 1999.
28. Duchek J. Cognitive dimensions of performance. In: Christiansen C, Baum C, eds. *Occupational Therapy: Overcoming Human Performance Deficits.* Thorofare, NJ: SLACK Incorporated; 1991.
29. Charness N, Bosman E. Compensation through environmental modification. In: Dixon R, Backman L. *Compensating for Psychological Deficits and Declines.* Wahmah, NY: Lawrence Erlbaum Associates; 1995.
30. Levine B, Stuss DT, Milberg WP, et al. The effects of focal and diffuse brain damage on strategy application: evidence from focal lesions, traumatic brain injury and normal aging. *J Neuropsychol Soc.* 1998;4(3):247-264.
31. Rankin JK, Woollacott MH, Shumway-Cook A, Brown LA. Cognitive influence on postural stability: a neuromuscular analysis in young and older adults. *J Gerontol.* 2000;55(3):M112-M119.
32. Salthouse TA. What and when of cognitive aging. *Am Psychol Soc.* 2004;13:140-144.
33. Woodruff-Pak DS, Hanson C. Plasticity and compensation in brain memory systems in aging. In: Dixon RA, Backman L, eds. *Compensating For Psychological Deficits and Declines.* Mahwah, NJ: Lawrence Erlbaum Assoc; 1995.
34. Arenberg D, Robertson-Tchabo E. Learning and aging. In: Birren J, Schaie K, eds. *Handbook of the Psychology of Aging.* New York, NY: Van Nostrand Reinhold Co; 1977:421-449.
35. Baum B, Hall K. Relationship between constructional praxis and dressing in the head injured adult. *Am J Occup Ther.* 1981;35(7):438-442.
36. Birren J, Renner V. Research on the psychology of aging: principles and experimentation. In: Birren JE, Schaie KW, eds. *Handbook of the Psychology of Aging.* New York, NY: Van Nostand Reinhold Co; 1977.
37. Craik F, Grady C. Aging, memory and frontal lobe functioning. In: Stuss D, Knight R, eds. *Principles of Frontal Lobe Function.* New York, NY: Oxford University Press; 2002.
38. Denneg NW, Dew JR, Kihlstrom JF. An adult developmental study of the encoding of spatial location. *Exp Aging Res.* 1992;18:25-32.
39. Glitsky EL, Glitsky ML. Memory rehabilitation in the elderly. In: Stuss DT, Winocur G, Robertson IH, eds. *Cognitive Neurorehabilitation.* New York, NY: Cambridge University Press; 1999.
40. Kahan RL, Zarit SH, Hilbert NM, Neiderehe G. Memory complaints and impairment in the aged. *Arch Gen Psychiat.* 1975;32;1569-1573.
41. Kolb B, Wishaw I. *Fundamentals of Human Neuropsychology.* New York, NY: NH Freeman and Co; 1990.
42. Riege W, Inman V. Age differences in nonverbal memory tasks. *J Gerontol.* 1979;36(1):51-58.
43. Riege WH, Klane LT, Metter EJ, Hanson WR. Decision speed and bias after unilateral stroke. *Cortex.* 1982;18:345-355.
44. Wilson RS, Bennett DA, Swartzendruber A. Age-related change in cognitive function. In: Nussbaum PD, ed. *Handbook of Neuropsychology and Aging.* New York, NY: Plenum Press; 1997.
45. Kramer N, Farbik L. Assessment of intellectual changes in the elderly. In: Raskin A, Jarbik L, eds. *Psychiatric Symptoms and Cognitive Loss in the Elderly.* New York, NY: Hemisphere Pub; 1979.
46. Craik F, Byrd M, Swanson JL. Patterns of memory loss in three elderly samples. *Psychol Aging.* 1987;2:79-86.
47. Lezak M. *Neuropsychological Assessment.* New York, NY: Oxford University Press; 1983.
48. Brown J. *Aphasia, Apraxia and Agnosia, Clinical and Theoretical Aspects.* Springfield, Ill: Charles C Thomas Pub; 1972.
49. Crook TH, Larrabee GJ. Changes in facial recognition memory across the adult lifespan. *J Gerontol Psychol Sci.* 1992;47:138-141.
50. Salthouse TA. Aging and measures of processing speed. *Biol Psych.* 2000;54:35-54.

51. Brauer SG, Woollacott M, Shumway-Cook A. The interacting effects of cognitive demand and recovery of postural stability in balance-impaired elderly persons. *J Gerontol.* 2001;56(8):489-496.

52. Lajoie Y, Teasdale N, Bard C, Fleury M. Upright standing and gait: are there changes in attentional requirements related to normal aging? *Exp Aging Res.* 1996;22(2):185-189.

53. Delaney RC, Ravdin LD. The neuropsychology of stroke. In: Nussbaum PD, ed. *Handbook of Neuropsychology and Aging.* New York, NY: Plenum Press; 1997.

54. Young M. Problem-solving performance in two age groups. *J Gerontol.* 1966;21:505-509.

55. Bracy O. Computer-based cognitive rehabilitation. *Cognit Rehab.* 1983;1(1):7-8.

56. Crook T. Psychometric assessment in the elderly. In: Raskin A, Javick L, eds. *Psychiatric Symptoms and Cognitive Loss in the Elderly.* New York, NY: Hemisphere Publishing Co; 1979:207-220.

57. Raskin SA. Cognitive remediation of mild traumatic brain injury in an older age group. In: Raskin SA, Mateer CA, eds. *Neuropsychological Management of Traumatic Brain Injury.* New York, NY: Oxford University Press; 2000.

58. Barron A, Mattila WR. Response slowing of older adults: effects of time limit contingencies on single and dual task performances. *Psychol Aging.* 1989;4:66-72.

59. Verhaegen P, Marcoen A, Grossenms L. Improving memory performance in the aged through mnemonic training: a meta-analytic study. *Psychol Aging.* 1992;7:242-251.

60. Ordy JM, Brizzee KR. Sensory coding: sensation perception, information processing, and sensory motor integration from maturity to old age. In: Ordy JM, Bizzee KR, eds. *Aging. Vol 10. Sensory Systems and Communication in the Elderly.* New York, NY: Raven Press; 1979.

61. Ashley MJ, Ashley SM. Discharge planning in traumatic brain injury rehabilitation. In: Ashley MJ, ed. *Traumatic Brain Injury: Rehabilitative Treatment and Case Management.* 2nd ed. Boca Raton, Fla: CRC Press; 2004.

62. Castriotta RJ, Lai JM. Sleep disorders associated with traumatic brain injury. *Arch Phys Med Rehabil.* 2001;82(10):1403-1406.

63. Findley LJ, Barth JT, Powers DC, et al. Cognitive impairment in patients with obstructive sleep apnea and associated hypoxemia. *Chest.* 1986;90(5):686-690.

64. LaChappelle DL, Finlayson MA. An evaluation of subjective and objective measures of fatigue in patients with brain injury and healthy controls. *Brain Inj.* 1998;12:649-659.

65. Masel BE, Scheibel RS, Kimbark T, Kuna ST. Excessive daytime sleepiness in adults with brain injuries. *Arch Phys Med Rehabil.* 2001;82(11):1403-1406.

66. Dobkin BH. Rehabilitation and recovery of the patient with stroke. In: Mohr JP, Choi D, Grotta J, Wolf P, eds. *Stroke: Pathophysiology, Diagnosis, and Management.* 4th ed. Philadelphia, Pa: Churchill Livingstone; 2004.

67. Rao V, Lyketsos CG. Psychiatric aspects of traumatic brain injury. *Psychiatr Clin North Am.* 2002;25(1):43-69.

68. Teasdale J. Selective effects of emotion on information-processing. In: Baddeley A, Weiskrantz L, eds. *Attention: Selection, Awareness, and Control.* Oxford: Clarendon Press; 1993.

69. Macciocchi SN, Eaton B. Decision and attribution bias in neurorehabilitation. *Arch Phys Med Rehabil.* 1995;76(6):521-524.

70. Powell JH, al-Adawi S, Morgan J, Greenwood RJ. Motivational deficits after brain injury: effects of bromocriptine in 11 patients. *J Neurol Neurosurg Psychiatry.* 1996;60(4):416-421.

71. Rosenfeld MS. Motivating elders with depression in SNFs. *OT Practice.* 2004;9(11):21-28.

72. Feinstein A. Mood and motivation in rehabilitation. In: Stuss DT, Winocur G, Robertson IH, eds. *Cognitive Neurorehabilitation.* New York, NY: Cambridge University Press; 1999.

73. McKinlay WW, Watkiss AJ. Cognitive and behavioral effects of brain injury. In: Rosenthal M, Griffith ER, Kreutzer JS, eds. *Rehabilitation of the Adult and Child with Traumatic Brain Injury.* 3rd ed. Philadelphia, Pa: FA Davis; 1983.

74. Morton MV, Wehman P. Psychosocial and emotional sequelae of individuals with traumatic brain injury: a literature review and recommendations. *Brain Inj.* 1995;9:81-92.

75. Persel CS, Persel CH. The use of applied behavior analysis in traumatic brain injury rehabilitation. In: Ashley MJ, ed. *Traumatic Brain Injury: Rehabilitative Treatment and Case Management.* 2nd ed. Boca Raton, Fla: CRC Press; 2004.

76. Ramasubbu R, Robinson RG, Flint AJ, et al. Functional impairment associated with acute poststroke depression: the Stroke Data Bank Study. *J Neuropsychiatry Clin Neurosci.* 1998;10(1):26-33.

77. Steffens DC, Helms MJ, Ranga Rama Krishnan K, Burke GL. Cerebrovascular disease and depression symptoms in the Cardiovascular Health Study. *Stroke.* 1999;30(10):2159-2166.

78. Gainotti G. Assessment and treatment of emotional disorders. In: Halligan P, Kischka U, Marshall JC, eds. *Handbook of Clinical Neuropsychology.* New York, NY: Oxford University Press; 2003.

79. Kauhanen M, Korpelainen JT, Hiltunen P, et al. Poststroke depression correlates with cognitive impairment and neurological deficits. *Stroke.* 1999;30(9):1875-1880.

80. Cummings JL. Neuropsychiatric manifestations of right hemisphere lesions. *Brain Language.* 1997;57:22-37.

81. Perino C, Rago R, Cicolin A, et al. Mood and behavioural disorders following traumatic brain injury: a clinical evaluation and pharmacological management. *Brain Inj.* 2001;15(2):139-148.

82. Golisz, Toglia J. Perception and cognition. In: Crepeau E, Cohn ES, Schell BAB, eds. *Willard and Spackman's Occupational Therapy.* Philadelphia, Pa: Lippincott, Williams and Wilkins; 2003.

83. Satz P, Forney DL, Zaucha K, et al. Depression, cognition, and functional correlates of recovery outcome after traumatic brain injury. *Brain Inj.* 1998;12(7):537-553.

84. Bacher Y, Korner-Bitensky N, Mayo N, Becker R, Coopersmith H. A longitudinal study of depression among stroke patients participating in a rehabilitation program. *Can J Rehabil.* 1990;4:27–37.

85. Burton LA, Volpe BT. Depression after head injury: do physical and cognitive sequelae have similar impact? *J Neurol Rehabil.* 1992;8:63-67.

86. Herrmann N, Black SE, Lawrence J, Szekely C, Szalai JP. The Sunnybrook Stroke Study: a prospective study of depressive symptoms and functional outcome. *Stroke.* 1998;29(3):618-624.

87. Rosenthal M, Christensen BK, Ross TP. Depression following traumatic brain injury. *Arch Phys Med Rehabil.* 1998;79(1):90-103.

88. Mateer CA, Raskin S. Cognitive rehabilitation. In: Rosenthal M, Griffith ER, Kreutzer JS, eds. *Rehabilitation of the Adult and Child with Traumatic Brain Injury.* 3rd ed. Philadelphia, Pa: FA Davis; 1983.

89. Ylvisaker M, Jacobs HE, Feeney T. Positive supports for people who experience behavioral and cognitive disability after brain injury: a review. *J Head Trauma Rehabil.* 2003;18(1):7-32.

90. Mysiw JW, Sandel EM. The agitated brain injured patient. Part 2: pathophysiology and treatment. *Arch Phys Med Rehabil.* 1997;78:213-220.

91. Wood R, McMillan TM. *Neurobehavioral Disability and Social Handicap Following Traumatic Brain Injury.* Philadelphia, Pa: Psychology Press; 2001.

92. Lincoln N. Outcome Measurement in Cognitive Rehabilitation. In: Stuss DT, Winocur G, Robertson IH, eds. *Cognitive Neurorehabilitation.* New York, NY: Cambridge University Press; 1999.

93. Arvanitakis Z, Wilson RS, Bienias JL, et al. Diabetes mellitus and risk of Alzheimer disease and decline in cognitive function. *Arch Neurol.* 2004;61:661-666.

94. Madden DJ, Blumenthal JA. Interaction of hypertension and age in visual selective attention performance. *Health Psychol.* 1998;17:76-83.

95. Elias MF, Robbins MA, Elias PK, Streeten DH. A longitudinal study of blood pressure in relation to performance on the Wechsler Adult Intelligence Scale. *Health Psychol.* 1998;17(6):486-493.

96. Gregg EW, Yaffe K, Cauley JA, et al. Is diabetes associated with cognitive impairment and cognitive decline among older women? Study of Osteoporotic Fractures Research Group. *Arch Intern Med.* 2000;160(2):174-180.

Resources

Arenberg D. A longitudinal study of problem solving in adults. *J Gerontol.* 1974;29:656-658.

Burvill P, Johnson G, Jamrozik K, et al. Prevalence of depression after stroke: the Perth Community Stroke Study. *Br J Psychiatry.* 1995;166(3):320-327.

Cabeza R, Grady CL, Nyberg L, et al. Age-related differences in neural activity during memory encoding and retrieval: a positron emission tomography study. *J Neurosci.* 1997;17(1):391-400.

Guilleminault C, Yuen KM, Gulevich MG, et al. Hypersomnia after head-neck trauma: a medicolegal dilemma. *Neurology.* 2000;54(3):653-659.

House A, Dennis M, Mogridge L, et al. Mood disorders in the year after the first stroke. *Br J Psychiatry.* 1991;158:83-92.

Nilsson LG, Soderlund H. Aging, cognition, and health. In: Naveh-Benjamin M, Moscovitch M, Roediger HL III, eds. *Perspectives on Human Memory and Cognitive Aging.* Ann Arbor, Mich: Psychology Press; 2001.

Paradiso S, Chemerinski E, Yazici KM, et al. Frontal lobe syndrome reassessed: comparison of patients with lateral or medial frontal brain damage. *J Neurol Neurosurg Psychiatry.* 1999;67(5):664-667.

Parikh RM, Robinson RG, Lipsey JR, et al. The impact of poststroke depression on recovery in activities of daily living. *Arch Neurol.* 1990;47(7):785-789.

Spikman J, Timmerman ME, Zomeren van AH, Deelman BG. Recovery versus retest effects in attention after closed head injury. *J Clin Exp Neuropsychol.* 1999;21(5):585-605.

Stuss DT, Winocur G, Robertson IH, eds. *Cognitive Neurorehabilitation.* New York, NY: Cambridge University Press; 1999.

CHAPTER 13

The Use of Computers and Computerized Technology in Visual, Perceptual, and Cognitive Retraining

Computers

The application of computer technology to health care has increased rapidly in recent years. Its use in rehabilitation has become established in the United States, Canada, Great Britain, Australia, and other developed countries.[1] Probably the most recent use of computers in health care has been in direct client treatment. Such use can range from prevocational applications, to environmental control, to visual, perceptual, or cognitive retraining.[2-5] Computer programs have been designed and used to assess reaction time, visual scanning, attention, speed of information processing, memory, and problem solving.[4,6-9] The concept of using the computer as an adaptive or prosthetic device has also gained popularity.[10-12] As computers become more portable, and powerful, their use with people with disabilities continues to expand.[13] It is only natural that occupational therapists have shown an increased interest in computers and technology as a whole.[14]

Computer advocates believe computers to be the ultimate in flexibility and readily modifiable.[15] In addition, it is believed computer use saves therapists time, provides an objective measure of performance, and provides immediate feedback to the client.[16] Computer programs can control stimulus exposure time and level of difficulty, which can be systematically altered to meet the client's individual needs.[16] Small and affordable computers and general availability of hard or fixed discs have expanded the potential for computer use in visual, perceptual, or cognitive retraining.[15] In addition to these advances in hardware, new software is available that can modify keyboard use and that is specifically designed for the restoration of cognitive deficits.[2,15,17,18]

Despite its apparent advantages and increased use, the effectiveness of computer use in visual, perceptual, and cognitive retraining remains controversial. Microcomputer-based assessment and treatment of visual processing has been examined in a number of empirical studies.[1,19,20] Robertson et al report improvement of visual scanning with verbal cuing using computer mediated tasks.[19] These gains also generalized to a degree to reading and dialing a telephone. These same authors also report improvement in other visuospatial skills after computer training.

Computer retraining has also been effective with the restoration of visual neglect.[8,19] Some authors caution, however, that although there have been indications that computers can assist in the rehabilitation of visual neglect, there is no conclusive evidence that computerized therapy is better than a noncomputerized approach.[1,19]

Computer-based cognitive retraining has focused primarily on the areas of attention and memory.[21] In a study of 40 brain-injured clients who received computer-assisted cognitive retraining, significant gains in memory, problem solving, and attention were reported.[9] Marks et al report brain injury clients who received computer memory retraining improved their memory test performance and that these gains were maintained over time.[22] There was no indication, however, that these gains generalized to other tasks. Glisky reports that traumatic brain injury (TBI) clients with memory and learning deficits were able to learn considerable amounts of new knowledge and skills (though at a slower rate than normal) that are relevant to activities of daily living (ADLs).[7] These goals were accomplished primarily by computer retaining. Training involved the vanishing cues method for which the client was provided with as many initial letters of a target word as needed in order to produce the answer. The computer gradually withdraws the letters across learning trials until the client is able to answer without cues. He goes on to state that although these goals could be accomplished by other means, the clients in his study tended to like using the computer over other external aids. However, Batchelor et al question these results when reporting the results of their study of 47 TBI clients.[16] These authors compared performance of those clients who received computer cognitive retraining with those who received traditional treatment. Their study failed to support the hypothesis that computer training is more effective than traditional treatment in improving memory, attention, information processing, and higher cortical functions. In addition, they point out that those studies claiming that computer retraining is better are primarily anecdotal in nature or single case studies.

Increased attentional abilities have also been reported with computer retraining.[20,21] Research has supported the use of the computer as an enhancement to traditional rehabilitation techniques for rehabilitation of attentional deficits. In fact, it is felt that although more research is indicated in order to clarify the mechanisms involved, the research to date suggests that the remediation of attentional skills may be one of the more promising areas of computerized cognitive rehabilitation.[1]

As of yet, computer-assisted cognitive rehabilitation (CACR) as a restorative tool remains unproven. CACR as an adaptive or compensatory approach, however, has shown great promise.[23] One study showed significantly more effective performance on a cooking task with computer generated cuing than without it.[10,11] Another study described a microcomputer organizer that was effective in compensating for the client's decreased memory by increasing functional performance.[24] It is becoming accepted that the microcomputer can be helpful as a memory prosthesis to assist in storage and retrieval of ADL information.[1] Kim et al also describe the successful use by a 22-year-old TBI client of a microcomputer as a memory aid.[25] Although computer cognitive restoration with the goal of deficit reduction remains controversial, research suggests its use as a cognitive prosthesis is an effective intervention.[12]

Computerized Technology

COGNITIVE PROSTHETICS

Lynch describes cognitive prosthetics as any computer-based system that has been designed for a specific client to accomplish one or more designated tasks related to functional activities.[23] These prosthetics can range from speechware to smart houses.[26,27] The everyday use of cognitive prosthetics has a wide range of applications. Wilson provides the following examples[27]:

1. *Use of the telephone*

    a) Photographs of 10 people important in the client's network are pasted on to the telephone buttons. Each button is programmed to dial the number of the person in the photograph.

    b) A video-phone link is provided between the client's home and the care center or main helper.

    c) A big red 'Help' button is provided to automatically call the day center or a relative.

2. *Entrance and exits*

    a) A floodlight is installed by the front door that lights up when someone approaches.

    b) A movement detector can be connected to a verbal message that indicates someone is approaching.

    c) An infrared key is provided for opening doors.

    d) Environmental control systems may be installed to open and close doors from a distance.

3. *Temperature control*

    a) A fitted control system for showers and baths can ensure that water is neither too hot nor too cold.

    b) A central control can be used to regulate the temperature of rooms.

4. *Alarm systems*

    a) Alarms can be fitted to sound when the cooker or other electric appliances are left on and unused for a certain length of time.

    b) An alarm system can sound when the person leaves the house in order to prevent wandering.

    c) In case of fire or any other emergency, an alarm rings in an alarm or care center. A voice message is relayed to the client telling him or her to leave the house because of the emergency.

Cognitive prosthetics can either be portable or nonportable and simple or complex. Nonportable devices can include electric timers that run off electricity (ie, alarm clock or device that turns lights or the sprinkler system on).[28] Portable devices can include memo watches or personal data assistants (PDAs).[28,29] Memo watches can store the date and time of appointments accompanied by a directive presented on the screen of the watch. Some memo watches can download or upload files on a computer.[28]

PERSONAL DATA ASSISTANTS

PDAs can vary in weight and size, and if a client has motor impairments, a family member can enter input for the client.[28] In some geographical areas, a wireless card can be attached to the PDA for internet access. All PDAs provide a written directive on a screen when a signal is presented.[28] Some PDAs contain a physical keyboard, and one study of clients with TBI indicated that these clients preferred the keyboard PDAs and used them more than those without the keyboard.[30]

PDAs can be used as a prosthetic for prospective memory as well as for storing phone numbers, addresses, directions, etc. A study of 12 TBI clients indicated that PDAs were useful in a high proportion of clients for assisting with memory-dependent functions.[29] PDAs can store and produce a variety of information relevant to the client's individual daily life.[31] If a client has prosopagnosia, pictures of friends or relatives can be stored and labeled and then retrieved before the client attends a family or social gathering. In addition to the picture and label, additional personal information can be stored and retrieved to further assist the client.

Kim et al outline the following areas to consider before using a PDA as an external aid for the client: 1) computer design, 2) client characteristics (ie, average or above average intelligence, retained or mildly impaired reasoning, insight into deficits, adequate initiation, and decreased functional memory), and 3) cost.[25] Some clients will not be interested in working or learning on the computer or any computerized device.[32] Clients who have previous computer knowledge, who will be using the computer at home or at work, and enjoy the computer are the best candidates.[32] In addition to these considerations, the client should be trained daily in the use of the device for at least 1 to 2 weeks.[28]

ELECTRONIC AIDS TO DAILY LIVING

Electronic aids of daily living (EADLs) were previously termed environmental controls. As Lange and Smith state, the change in name reflects an emphasis on how the specific technology assists occupational performance rather than focusing on the technology itself.[33] EADLs can now assist the client with visual, perceptual, and/or cognitive impairments. Lange and Smith provide the following examples of EADLs that can assist these clients[33]:

> *Microwaves that automatically cook any type of food to appropriate doneness, sensors that monitor water temperature to prevent scalding, controls to select water temperature and pressure for individual faucets, refrigerators that scan bar codes on food items passed in front of a sensor, compile a shopping list and send the list via the internet for at-home delivery.*

These authors also project future EADLs that could include auditory scanning for use with the client with visual impairments.[33]

Smart houses are also now being designed and used with dementia clients and could conceivably be adapted for the client with acquired brain injury (ABI). These smart houses use new computer technology and video cameras to monitor and control the living environment.[27]

ACCESS AND MODIFICATION TO COMPUTERIZED TECHNOLOGY

Today's technology can provide many input devices for use by the client with ABI. ABI clients may require and use a mouse, an inverted trackball, an oversized joystick, a light pen, or a touch screen.[34] The keyboard may be modified with large contrasting stickers on the keys for the client with decreased acuity.[35] The font size and style may be enlarged for the client with decreased figure ground, or an antiglare monitor can be used for the client with sensitivity to light.[35] Clients with cognitive problems can utilize the help key to facilitate understanding and proper use.

These are just a few of the modifications available to increase computer access. The use of a computer or computerized technology as a prosthetic or compensatory device by the client with ABI will only be successful if it is customized to the individual client's needs and abilities.[26] It is encouraging that new products specifically designed for individuals with cognitive disabilities are now reaching the market.[13] In addition, the use of digital versatile disk (DVD) recorders in the home opens up a new field of video-based training or instruction in a less expensive and more flexible manner than previously possible.[23] Computer software is also now focusing more on commonly impaired functional tasks such as driving or everyday math skills.[23] As Anson states, "…as access techniques are slowly being refined, computer programmers are beginning to consider accessibility in their design."[36]

Two resources for information on cognitive technology devices follow[13]:

1. *Partnership for People With Disabilities: Consortium for Handheld Technology*

   Information website of Virginia Commonwealth University's Consortium for Handheld Technology, which conducts research on assistive technology for cognition: http://www.vcu.edu/partnership/pda

2. *National Brain Injury Association website*

   www.biausa.org/page/AT

Before leaving the topic of computer use in visual, perceptual, and cognitive retraining, it is important to address the need for a conceptual framework for its application. Aptly stated by Dunn, the vast array of software being utilized underscores the need for an integrative conceptual framework to guide computer cognitive rehabilitation efforts and allow for the categorization of software in terms of specific cognitive functions.[1] As with any approach, there needs to be a theoretical model or models to guide technology use in rehabilitation and related empirical research that evaluates these efforts.

Several authors recently have attempted to answer this need for a conceptual framework for technology use. Levin outlines six areas of computer use and relates them back to behavioral theory[37]:

1. *Computer as a learning lab*—Client receives training in the use of disc drive, mouse, etc. Client practices logic and organizational skills within the practical context of applying computer technology.

2. *Information acquisition*—Enables experts in particular professional disciplines to create computer-assisted resources that imitate their own decision making processes and professional judgment

3. *Computer as orthotic device*—Simplifies otherwise complex tasks (eg, memory prompts, checklists)

4. *Simulations*—(ie, video games), allows practice of complex skills in a protected environment

5. *Drill and practice*—Discrete tasks are presented one at a time.

6. *Computer-assisted multitasking*—This approach is based on behavioral theory. The emphasis is on creating ways to help the therapist control environmental contingencies for specific training objectives and goals.

Levin views behavior, including self-managed behavior, as based on or selected by the environment rather than internal cognitive sources.[37] His computer work is based on this assumption. The therapist arranges training in a hierarchy based on observations of client interaction with the external environment.

Dunn utilizes this concept of the importance of human-environment interactions in his computer work.[1] Dunn conceptualizes a human-machine systems model whereby technology is conceptualized as a highly complex mechanized part of the environment.[1] An interaction between the individual and the computer, or any technology, is a process of input, output, and feedback. This human-machine systems model contains two important concepts outlined as follows[1]:

1. *Machine-assisted approach*—Involves temporary use of technology to reduce impairments that lead to disability—for example, training related to attentional deficits.

2. *Machine-dependent approach*—Involves relatively permanent application of technology to accommodate impairment—for example, a speech synthesizer.

In other words, the machine-assisted approach is a restorative approach and the machine-dependent is an adaptive approach.

Computers and computerized technology are fundamental tools used by the individual in contemporary society. The occupational therapist can no longer view CACR as a specialty area of expertise.[38] In addition to its use as an intervention, whether restorative or adaptive, incorporation of the computer as an occupation-based activity is now likely. As with any intervention, attention is focused on the activity and input method, which are modified to meet physical as well as visual, perceptual, or cognitive goals.[38] The occupational therapist should have and apply a foundation of knowledge and skills in this area.[13] As with any area, the therapist should stay current with the ongoing changes in technology and how they relate to practice. In the not-so-distant future, for example, there will exist the ability for neuron to computer interface, which may allow computers to function as memory aids for brain cells. There are now technologies that can create the right chemical environment to coax neuronal regrowth to damaged areas. In addition, the appropriateness of application and efficacy of all new technological developments need to be evaluated.[27] The effective use of rehabilitation technology requires not just the hardware and software, but the "orgware" or human system for appropriate use.[1] In utilizing the computer, the person-environment fit must be considered. Future research should contain efficacy studies based on a sound conceptual framework with good controls. Only then can practice be refined.

References

1. Dunn KW. Information technology and brain injury rehabilitation. In: Finlayon MAJ, Garner SH, eds. *Brain Injury Rehabilitation: Clinical Considerations.* Baltimore, Md: Williams and Wilkins; 1994.
2. Bracy O. Computer-based cognitive rehabilitation. *Cogn Rehabil.* 1983;1(1):7-8.
3. Hansen CS. Traumatic brain injury. In: Van Deusen J, ed. *Body Image and Perceptual Dysfunction in Adults.* Philadelphia, Pa: WB Saunders; 1993.
4. Milner D. Use of microcomputers in the treatment of patients with physical disabilities. *Phys Disab Center Sect Newsletter.* 1984;7(2):1.
5. Weber MP. About this issue. *Phys Disab Spec Inter Sect Newsletter.* 1984;2(2):1.
6. Adamovich BLB. Cognition, language, attention and information processing following closed head injury. In: Kreutzer JS, Wehman PH, eds. *Cognitive Rehabilitation For Persons with Traumatic Brain Injury: A Functional Approach.* Baltimore, Md: Paul H Brooks Publishing Co; 1991.
7. Glisky EL. Computer-assisted instruction for patients with traumatic brain injury: teaching of domain-specific knowledge. *J Head Trauma Rehabil.* 1992;7(3):1-12.
8. Robertson SL, Jones LA. Tactile sensory impairments and prehensile function in subjects with left hemisphere cerebral lesions. *Arch Phys Med Rehabil.* 1994;75:1108-1117.
9. Ruff RM, Baserr CA, Johnston JW, Marshal LF, Klauber SK, Klauber MR, Minteer M. Neuropsychological rehabilitation: an experimental study with head injured patients. *J Head Trauma Rehabil.* 1989;4(3):20-36.
10. Kirsch NL, Levine SP, Lajiness-O'Neill R, Schnyder M. Computer-assisted interactive task guidance: facilitating the performance of a simulated vocational task. *J Head Trauma Rehabil.* 1992;7(3):13-25.
11. Kirsh NL, Levine SP, Fallon-Krueger M, Jaros LA. The microcomputer as an "orthotic" device for patients with cognitive deficits. *J Head Trauma Rehabil.* 1987;2(4):77-86.
12. Lynch WJ. Software update. *J Head Trauma Rehabil.* 1994;9(2):105-108.
13. Gentry T. A brain in the palm of your hand: assistive technology for cognition. *OT Practice.* 2005;10(19):10-12.
14. Smith RO. The role of occupational therapy in a developmental technology model. *Am J Occup Ther.* 2000;54:339-340.
15. Gianutsos R. The computer in cognitive rehabilitation; it's not just a tool anymore. *J Head Trauma Rehabil.* 1992;7(3):26-35.

16. Batchelor J, Shores EA, Marosszeky JE, Sandanam J. Lovarini M. Focus on clinical research: cognitive rehabilitation of severely closed-head injured patients using computer-assisted and noncomputerized treatment techniques. *J Head Trauma Rehabil.* 1988;3(3):78-85.

17. Lynch WJ. The use of electronic games in cognitive rehabilitation. In: Trexler LE, ed. *Cognitive Rehabilitation—Conceptualization and Intervention.* New York, NY: Plenum Press; 1982.

18. Parente R. Cognitive rehabilitation and the use of computers. Paper presented to Baltimore Adult Communications Disorders Interest Group.

19. Robertson I, Gray J, Mckenzie S. Microcomputer-based cognitive rehabilitation of visual neglect: three multiple baseline single case studies. *Brain Inj.* 1988;2(2):151-163.

20. Sohlberg MM, Mateer CA. *Introduction to Cognitive Rehabilitation: Theory and Practice.* New York, NY: Guilford Press; 1989.

21. Thomas-Stonell N, Johnson P, Schuller R, Jutai J. Evaluation of a computer-based program for remediation of cognitive-communication skills. *J Head Trauma Rehabil.* 1994;9(4):25-37.

22. Marks C, Parente R, Anderson J. Retention of gains in outpatient cognitive rehabilitation therapy. *Cogn Rehabil.* 1986;4(3):20-23.

23. Lynch WJ. Historical review of computer-assisted cognitive retraining. *J Head Trauma Rehabil.* 2002;17(5):446-457.

24. Giles G, Shore M. The effectiveness of an electronic memory aid for a memory-impaired adult of normal intelligence. *Am J Occup Ther.* 1989;43(6):409-411.

25. Kim HJ, Burke DT, Dowds MM, George J. Utility of a microcomputer as an external memory aid for a memory-impaired head injury patient during in-patient rehabilitation. *Brain Inj.* 1999;13(2):147-150.

26. Chute DL, Bliss ME. ProsthesisWare: concepts and caveats for microcomputer-based aids to everyday living. *Exp Aging Res.* 1994;20:229-238.

27. Wilson BA. Memory rehabilitation in brain injured people. In: Stuss DT, Winocur G, Robertson IH, eds. *Cognitive Neurorehabilitation.* New York, NY: Cambridge University Press; 1999.

28. Herrmann D, Brubaker B, Yoder C, Sheets V, Tito A. Devices that remind. In: Durso FT, Nickerson RS, Schvaneveldt RW, et al, eds. *Handbook of Applied Cognition.* New York, NY: John Wiley & Sons; 1999.

29. Kim HJ, Burke DT, Dowds MM Jr, Boone KA, Park GJ. Electronic memory aids for outpatient brain injury: follow-up findings. *Brain Inj.* 2000;14(2):187-196.

30. Wright P, Rogers N, Hall C, et al. Comparison of pocket-computer memory aids for people with brain injury. *Brain Inj.* 2001;15(9);787-800.

31. Wilson BA. Memory rehabilitation: compensating for memory problems. In: Dixon R, Backman L, eds. *Compensating for Psychological Deficits and Declines.* Mahwah, NY: Lawrence Erlbaum Associates; 1995.

32. Aloisio L. Visual dysfunction. In: Gillen G, Burkhardt A, eds. *Stroke Rehabilitation: A Function-Based Approach.* St. Louis, Mo: Mosby Inc; 2004.

33. Lange ML, Smith R. The future of electronic aids to daily living. *Am J Occup Ther.* 2002;56:107-109.

34. Pedretti L, et al. Treatment of disturbances in tactile sensation, perception, cognition, and vision. In: Early MB, ed. *Physical Dysfunction: Practice Skills for the Occupational Therapy Assistant.* St. Louis, Mo: Mosby Inc; 1998.

35. Bain BK. Assistive technology in occupational therapy. In: Crepeau E, Cohn ES, Schell BAB, eds. *Willard and Spackman's Occupational Therapy.* Philadelphia, Pa: Lippincott, Williams and Wilkins; 2003.

36. Anson D. The future of computer access. *Am J Occup Ther.* 2001;55:106-108.

37. Levin W. Computer applications in cognitive rehabilitation. In: Kreutzer JS, Wehman PH, eds. *Cognitive Rehabilitation for Persons With Traumatic Brain Injury: A Functional Approach.* Baltimore, Md: Paul H. Brooks Co; 1991.

38. Phillips B, et al. Computer: tools to engage and participate in occupation. *OTAC.* September 2004: 13-23.

Resources

Bergman MM. Computer-enhanced self-sufficiency: part 1. Creation and implementation of a text writer for an individual with traumatic brain injury. *Neuropsychology.* 1991;5(1):17-23.

Kasten E, Sabel BA. Visual field enlargement after computer training in brain-damaged patients with homonymous deficits: an open pilot trial. *Restorative Neurol Neurosci.* 1995;8:113-127.

Niemann H, Ruff RM, Baser CA. Computer-assisted attention retraining in head-injured individuals: a controlled efficacy study of an outpatient program. *J Consult Clin Psychol.* 1990;58(6):811-817.

Parente FJ, Anderson JK. Techniques for improving cognitive rehabilitation: teaching organization and encoding skills. *Cognit Rehabil.* 1983;1:20-22.

COMMON STATISTICAL TERMS AND ANALYSES USED IN CLINICAL RESEARCH STUDIES

Analysis of covariance (ANCOVA) – Used when the research design cannot provide adequate control; statistical control is achieved by measuring one or more confounding variables in addition to the dependent variable (ie, the ANOVA accounts for the confounding factors in the analysis).

Analysis of variance (ANOVA) – Specifically designed to compare more than two means.

Analysis of variance of regression – The observed relationship between x and y did not occur by chance.

Chi square – Can be used for data analysis and descriptive purposes; useful in establishing group equivalence following random assignment; can confirm the validity of the randomization process. (Should not be used as an alternative to more precise tests [such as t test or analysis of variance] when data can be measured on a continuous scale. It is sensitive to sample size).

Coefficient of determination – Measure of proportion indicating the accuracy of prediction based on x.

Coefficient of variation – To account for the relationship between the mean and standard deviation; the variability across distributions is compared using this statistic.

Coefficient of variation (CV) – Measure of variability that can be used to describe data measured on the interval or ratio scale.

Correlation coefficients – Used to quantitatively describe the strength and direction of a relationship between two variables.

Cronbach alpha – Most common statistical index used for internal consistency; can be used for yes/no scales or scales with more than two response choices.

Discriminant analysis – Form of regression; technique for distinguishing two or more groups based on a set of characteristics that are predictors of group membership.

Factor analysis – Examines the structure within a large number of variables, in an attempt to explain the nature of their inter-relationships.

Intraclass correlation coefficient (ICC) – Can be used to assess reliability among two or more ratings; does not require the same number of raters for each subject; useful index in a variety of analysis situations .

Kappa statistic – Chance corrected measure of agreement (ie, also looks at the proportion of agreements expected by chance).

Linear regression – Examines two variables that are linearly related or correlated (x = independent variable, y = dependent variable).

Meta-analysis – A special case of secondary analysis, which is a statistical method of combining the results of a series of independent, previously published studies carried out for the same general purpose.

Multivariate analysis of variance (MANOVA) – Used to account for the relationship among several dependent variables when comparing groups; can be applied to all types of experimental designs.

Paired t-test – Used in studies where subjects are used as there own controls.

Pearson product-moment coefficient of correlation – Appropriate for use when x and y are continuous variables with underlying normal distributions on the interval or ratio scales.

Procedures for multiple comparison test – (For example, comparing multiple treatments for one problem) – Newman-Keuls Test, Scheffe's comparison, Bonferroni T-test.

Spearman rank correlation coefficient – Nonparametric analogue to the Pearson r, to be used with ordinal data.

Standard error of measurement – The standard deviation of the measurement errors reflects the reliability of the response.

Standardized scores – Scores that are expressed in terms of standard deviations

T-test – Used for evaluating the comparisons between two means; should not be used when comparing more than two means.

Resource

Portney L, Watkins M. *Foundations of Clinical Research: Applications to Practice*. 2nd ed. Upper Saddle River, NJ: Prentice Hall Health; 2000.

APPENDIX B

EVALUATION INDEX

GLOSSARY OF TERMS

Anosognosia – Client fails to recognize the presence or severity of his or her paralysis.

Abstract learning – Highest level of learning for which the individual can gain and store knowledge of rules that have been abstracted independently from the spatial and temporal contexts.

Abstract thinking – Ability to conceptualize and make inferences from information.

Acalculia – Inability to perform calculations.

Accommodation – Process by which the refractive power of the eye changes to ensure for a clear retinal image.

Adaptation – One makes changes in or adapts the environment of the client to compensate for his or her deficits.

Adaptive approach – Promotes adaptation of and to the environment to capitalize on the client's abilities; provides training in actual occupational behavior and assumes certain functions cannot be recovered or restored completely.

Agnosia – Inability to recognize familiar objects.

Alternating attention (attentional flexibility) – Alternating back and forth between mental tasks, (eg, chopping vegetables while periodically checking food on the stove).

Ambient vision – Initially organizes and stabilizes the visual field; peripheral vision.

Amblyopia – Loss of acuity in one eye.

Anterograde disorientation – Inability to learn new environments with an ability to find their way in older ones (have known for at least 6 months).

Apperceptive visual agnosia – Inability to recognize, copy, match, or discriminate visual stimuli and cannot even recognize simple shapes.

Apraxia – Inability to perform certain skilled purposeful movements in the absence of loss of motor power, sensation, and coordination.

Arteriosclerosis – Hardening of the arterial walls.

Association learning – Learning that occurs when an individual makes an association between two events.

Associative visual agnosia – Ability to describe the features and shape of an object with an inability to recognize it.

Astigmatism – Vision is blurred both at near and distance; eye is oval shape rather than spherical.

Attention – An active process that helps to determine which sensations and experiences are alerting and relevant to the individual; means by which one can orient in order to receive incoming information.

Auditory agnosia – Inability to recognize differences in sounds, including both word and nonword sounds.

Automatic processing – Subcortical processing.

Autotopagnosia – Disturbance of body scheme.

Benchmarking – Compares outcomes from practice conditions with evaluation and treatment methods associated with a research study.

Body scheme – The representation of the spatial relations among the parts of the body.

Bottom-up assessment – Specific assessments that are designed to measure component skills such as attention or constructional praxis.

Brain plasticity – The brain's adaptive capacity to change.

Cataracts – Result of loss of transparency of the lens resulting in reduced visual acuity.

Categorization – Assignment of objects, people, or events into groups based on commonalities.

Client-centered practice – Therapist is engaged by the client to help him or her reach identified goals; client and therapist develop a collaborative relationship with the therapist creating an environment that facilitates change; the client holds the most important information regarding his or her needs.

Client and Family education – Transfer of specific knowledge to the client and family that relates to the client's needs and priorities.

Clinical observation – Direct observation of occupational performance generally of motor, visual, perceptual, and cognitive factors that appear to impede client performance.

Clinical reasoning – Thinking and decision making process the therapist utilizes to plan, direct, perform, and reflect on client care.

Color agnosia – Inability to recognize colors such that the client cannot pick out a color or name the color on command.

Compensation – Response to loss or deficiency that can involve changing an activity and\or the environment to meet the client's capabilities; can be external (provided by outside sources) or situational (a technique used by the client so he or she does not depend on others).

Concentration – The ability to do mental work while attending; the process of active encoding in working memory.

Conditional reasoning – Examines and tries to understand how the client's capabilities affect occupational performance.

Consolidation – Integration of new memories with the individual's existing cognitive linguistic framework.

Constraint induced therapy (CIT) – Functionally based intervention designed to improve motor control in individuals with upper extremity hemiplegia; consists of two main components: 1) constraining the movement of the affected upper extremity and 2) intensive, repetitive, and targeted training of the paretic arm.

Construct validity – Measures how much test scores conform to previous theoretical relationships.

Constructional apraxia – The impairment in producing designs in two or three dimensions, copying, drawing, or construction either on command or spontaneously, which cannot be attributed to perceptual impairments, ideomotor apraxia, organizational impairments, or primary motor or sensory impairment.

Content validity – How well the test represents the total universe of the content of the skill being measured.

Contrast sensitivity – Low contrast acuity.

Controlled processing – Used when new information is being considered.

Convergence – Increase in the angle of the visual axes.

Convergent thinking – Thinking process used in recognizing and analyzing relevant and missing information.

Criterion validity – Measures how much a particular test agrees with another established accurate measure of a given trait.

Decision making – Form of problem solving for which the problem is to choose from several options to make a decision.

Declarative memory – Enables conscious recollection of past facts and events.

Deductive reasoning – Process of drawing conclusions about a given situation based on certain principles in a systematic manner.

Depth perception – The ability to judge depth and distances.

Diplopia – Double vision.

Divergence – Decrease in the angle of the visual axes.

Divided attention – Ability to do several things at once; requires the ability to allocate attentional resources, switch between tasks that cannot be done simultaneously, and timesharing of processing resources.

Dressing apraxia – The inability to dress oneself because of a disorder in body scheme and\or spatial relations.

Dynamic assessment – Assesses the individual's latent capacity, and aims to measure his or her potential to learn; assumes cognitive abilities are modifiable and changes and learning take place through task experience; attempts to modify performance through examiner assistance.

Dynamic interactional theory (DIT) – Assumes cognition is an ongoing outcome of the interaction among the individual, the task, and the environment; client performance is analyzed by evaluating the underlying processing strategies and conditions that change performance as well as the client's potential for learning; processing strategies and self-awareness are fundamental aspects of cognition that interact dynamically with external factors (task and environment) and internal factors (individual's structural capacity).

Ecology of Human Performance Model – Assumes it is impossible to understand an individual without understanding his or her context.

Egocentric – Concerned with the individual.

Egocentric disorientation – Topographical disorientation that is secondary to visual disorientation.

Emmetropia – Absence of refractive error.

Encoding – Begins with selective attention and is the means by which information is transformed in working memory so that it can be stored efficiently in long-term memory.

Episodic memory – Knowledge of a previously experienced event along with the awareness or understanding that the event occurred in the individual's past.

Errorless learning – Clients are cued as they learn a new skill to prevent them from making any errors; if an error is made, it is corrected immediately; cuing is reduced as the client becomes more competent.

Esotropia – Eyes turn in.

Ethical reasoning – Considers not what can be done but what should be done.

Executive function – Variety of skills that govern the majority of cognitive processing and come into play during nonroutine activities.

Explicit memory – Consists of information that can be consciously declared to have been learned or experienced.

Exotropia – Eyes turn out.

Field of fixation – Area within which central fixation can be accomplished by moving the eyes but not the head.

Figure ground perception – The ability to distinguish the foreground from the background.

Functional magnetic resonance imaging (fMRI) – A form of magnetic resonance imaging that registers blood flow to functioning areas of the brain

Focal vision – Provides attention to important features of an object for perception and discrimination.

Focused attention – The ability to respond to different kinds of stimulation; implies a body posture and orientation appropriate to receiving sensory information and taking motor action; the mind is free of extraneous thoughts, and an effort is made to keep sensory channels open.

Form discrimination – The ability to distinguish different types of forms.

Frame of reference – Mechanism that links theory to practice.

Functional approach – Top-down approach that works directly with actual occupations to maximize the client's independence; can be domain specific and\or involve specific adaptations or compensations.

Functional reorganization – Type of brain plasticity that involves reweighting of functional interactions within an existing network of brain regions.

Generalization – The ability to use a newly learned strategy in a novel situation.

Glaucoma – Intraocular pressure too high to maintain the normal physiology of the eye; commonly damages the optic nerve that will result in visual field loss and, if left uncontrolled, can lead to total blindness.

Haptic system – Nonvisual means one can use to recognize an object; contains both cutaneous and kinesthetic receptors.

Heading disorientation – Inability to generate directional information from landmarks that are recognizable; inability to perceive and remember the spatial relationships among landmarks in their environment.

Hyperopia – Farsightedness; vision is blurred at near but not at a distance.

Hypertropia – One eye turns up.

Hypophoria – Eye turns down.

Ideational apraxia – Inability to carry out a sequence of motor acts that is caused by a disruption of the conception rather than the execution of the motor act.

Ideomotor apraxia – Inability to imitate gestures or perform a purposeful task on command even though the client fully understands the idea or concept of the task

Implicit memory – Does not require conscious awareness of a prior experience to remember.

Incentive learning – The understanding that the use of a particular strategy in everyday life will result in getting something in return.

Inductive reasoning – Formulation of a solution based on details that lead to a standard conclusion.

Initiation – Starting a task or activity.

Interactive reasoning – Occurs during the therapeutic process, and tries to understand the client's needs, interests, and values in order to understand the disability from the client's perspective.

Internal consistency – Measures whether all parts of the evaluation are highly intercorrelated so that the skill being measured is being measured by all items.

Inter-rater reliability – Examines whether two or more raters can independently assign similar ratings to the individual performing the evaluation.

Intransitive movements – Movements that convey ideas or feelings.

Intra-rater reliability – Measures variation that occurs with one rater as a result of multiple administrations of the same evaluation.

Lagophthalmos – Defective closure of the lid.

Landmark agnosia – Inability to use prominent, relevant landmarks, or environmental features for the purpose of orientation.

Learned nonuse – Clients stop using affected extremity because it is too frustrating.

Limb kinetic apraxia – Difficulty in making fine, precise movements with the limb contralateral to a central nervous system (CNS) lesion.

Long-term memory – Holds an unlimited amount of information in a permanent state for hours or years.

Macular degeneration – Results in a central blind spot or scotoma and significant central vision loss.

Memory – The process by which an individual encodes, stores, and retrieves information; perception that has been stored at an earlier time that can then be brought forward.

Mental flexibility – The ability to initiate, stop, and switch actions depending on feedback from the environment related to those actions.

Midline shift – Information to the right of the client's midline is well attended and to the left of midline is poorly attended.

Model of human occupation (MOHO) –Incorporates a systems view of the individual; assumes behavior is both dynamic and context driven and occupation is essential for self-organization; views the individual as composed of the three elements of volition, habituation, and performance capacity.

Myopia – Nearsightedness; vision is blurred at a distance but not at near.

Near point of convergence – Nearest point on which the eyes can converge.

Neural plasticity – Creation of new brain circuits either by forming new connections among remaining neurons or by generating new neurons.

Neurodevelopmental treatment (NDT) – Comprehensive management approach to motor recovery as it relates to activities of daily living (ADLs); includes concepts drawn from motor learning, organization of movement, environmental influence on movement, and cognitive processing as it relates to movement performance and analysis.

Nondeclarative memory – Information that is learned or acquired during the development of skill learning.

Norms – Statistics that have been generated from a well-defined group that has been evaluated using a test in a standardized manner.

Nystagmus – Involuntary rhythmic oscillation of one or both eyes.

Occupational Adaptation Model (OA) – Deals with human adaptation and occupation; the adaptation process develops from an interaction between the person and occupational environment in response to occupational challenges that occur within the context of performing occupational roles.

Ocular dysmetria – Difficulty controlling the range of voluntary movement of the eyes.

Optokinetic reflex – Activated during sustained movement and takes over the function of the vestibular ocular reflex (VOR).

Oral apraxia – Difficulty in forming and organizing intelligible words although the musculature required to do so remains intact.

Orientation – Recognition of one's self with regard to time, place, and person within one's personal environment.

Oscillopsia – Sensation that the world is moving.

Pattern recognition – Ability to identify shape, contour, general, and specific features of an object.

Person-Environment-Occupation (PEO) Model – Focuses on the dynamic nature of occupational performance and the interaction of the three elements of the person, environment, and occupation.

Positron emission tomography (PET) scan – Imaging technique useful in showing how a tissue or organ is functioning; can show the blood flow through the brain

Planning – The attainment of a goal through a series of intermediate steps which do not necessarily lead directly toward that goal.

Pragmatic reasoning – Reasoning based on practice contexts such as organizational culture, resources, length of stay, reimbursement issues, therapist's personal context, etc.

Problem solving – Integration of several cognitive skills that are used to take down barriers towards a goal.

Procedural reasoning – Diagnostic reasoning; strategies used to determine what the client's problems might be and how to address those problems.

Prosopagnosia –Inability to identify a known individual by his or her face.

Prospective memory – Remembering to complete an activity or carry out a task at a time in the future.

Ptosis – Drooping of the upper eyelid.

Qualitative assessment – Provides non-numerical data that can highlight problems and provide in-depth information about those problems; important characteristics of the client's performance are described, and the therapist observes the process of how a client performs a task or activity.

Quantitative assessment – Static assessment that provides quantitative measurements of developed abilities; concerned with the products of learning rather than the learning process itself.

Refraction – Evaluation of the optical system of the eye.

Refractive error – Deviation from emmetropia.

Reliability – Consistency and accuracy.

Representational learning – An internal representation of events is formed, which includes how events are organized and retrieved.

Restorative approach – Rehabilitation focused on the impairment underlying the client's disability; examines foundational factors that are contributing to the client's limitations; aims at promoting or enhancing brain recovery or reorganization.

Retinopathy – Pathology related to the retina.

Retrieval – Process of recovering previously encoded information.

Saccadic eye movements – Sequenced rapid eye movements that change the line of sight; jump eye movements.

Scotoma – Blind spot in the field of vision.

Selective attention – Activating and inhibiting responses selectively; involves discrimination of stimulus information and differentiating responses; helps goal directed behavior, and is critical for perception; assures that an individual does not perceive a superposition of all stimuli present at a given time in our visual field by suppressing the nonattended stimuli such that only one stimulus is processed at a given time in higher cortical areas (unilateral neglect is an illustration of a disruption of the selective attentional network).

Self-awareness – Knowledge of one's cognitive abilities.

Self-monitoring – Individual's ability to evaluate and regulate the quality and quantity of his or her behavior.

Semantic memory – Involves general facts or knowledge about the world.

Sensory memory – First phase of an individual's information processing; very short-term, modality specific memory that is either transferred for further analysis or it degenerates.

Simultagnosia – Inability to recognize a compound visual array.

Smooth pursuit eye movements – Those movements that keep an image steady on the retina; visual scanning.

Spatial relations – The ability to perceive the position of two or more objects in relation to the self and to each other.

Standardized test – Test that has been administered to a large sample of the population the examiner wants to test so that he or she knows how the average person in this population scores on the test; generates norms.

Stereopsis – Three-dimensional vision.

Strabismus – Misalignment of the eyes.

Sustained attention – Vigilance; maintaining attention for a long time; the ability to self-sustain mindful conscious processing of stimuli whose repetitive, nonarousing qualities would otherwise cause habituation and distraction to other stimuli; ensures that goals are maintained over time; associated with right hemisphere specialization.

Tactile agnosia – Inability to recognize objects through touch although tactile, thermal, and proprioceptive functions are still intact.

Test-retest reliability – Measures the test's stability over time; test is given to an individual several times.

Top-down assessments – Examines the client's performance in a particular occupational performance task as a way to understand possible underlying causes of poor performance.

Topographagnosia – Impairment in the interpretation of maps, house plans, etc.

Topographical disorientation – The inability to follow a familiar route or a new route once it has become familiar.

Validity – Refers to how well a test measures what it purports to measure.

Vergence – Change in the relative position of the visual axes.

Vergence system – Aligns the eye to maintain binocular fixation and binocular vision.

Vestibular ocular reflex (VOR) – Along with vestibular controlled eye movements and visually controlled eye movements, maintains a stable gaze; activated in the labyrinth; stabilizes gaze by producing an eye movement of equal velocity and opposite direction to the head movement.

Vigilance – The ability to sustain attention over a period of time. Thirty seconds is considered a vigilant period in a mental status examination; a control process that coordinates functional components of attention (alertness, arousal, and selectivity) to direct attention to significant feature of the environment.

Visual acuity – Resolution power of the eye.

Visual agnosia – Inability to recognize visual stimuli despite adequate primary visual function such as acuity, oculomotor function, and visual fields.

Visual cognition – Highest level of visual skills integration within the nervous system; serves as the basis for academic activities; ability to mentally manipulate and integrate visual information to solve problems, plan, etc.

Visual extinction – Inability or severe limitation in perceiving two objects displayed at once with an ability to process a single visual stimuli.

Visual field – Area of the visual system that allows an individual to orient to specific spatial areas.

Visual inattention – Decreased awareness of the body and spatial environment on the side contralateral to the cerebral lesion despite the absence of a specific sensory deficit; visual neglect.

Visual spatial agnosia – Inability to perceive spatial relationships between objects or between objects and self, independently of visual object agnosia.

Working memory – Temporary storage and manipulation of information; short-term storage of information that is not accessible in the environment, and the process that keeps this information active for use at a later time; can deal with approximately seven pieces of information at a time.

Yoked prisms – Prism that is used to affect the client's spatial and midline awareness.

INDEX

Please visit

www.slackbooks.com
to order any of these titles!
24 Hours a Day...7 Days a Week!

Attention Industry Partners!
Whether you are interested in buying multiple copies of a book, chapter reprints, or looking for something new and different — we are able to accommodate your needs.

Multiple Copies
At attractive discounts starting for purchases as low as 25 copies for a single title, SLACK Incorporated will be able to meet all your of your needs.

Chapter Reprints
SLACK Incorporated is able to offer the chapters you want in a format that will lead to success. Bound with an attractive cover, use the chapters that are a fit specifically for your company. Available for quantities of 100 or more.

Customize
SLACK Incorporated is able to create a specialized custom version of any of our products specifically for your company.

Please contact the Marketing Manager of the Health Care Books and Journals for further details on multiple copy purchases, chapter reprints or custom printing at 1-800-257-8290 or 1-856-848-1000.

*Please note all conditions are subject to change.

CODE: 328

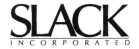

SLACK Incorporated • Health Care Books and Journals
6900 Grove Road • Thorofare, NJ 08086

1-800-257-8290 or 1-856-848-1000
Fax: 1-856-853-5991 • E-mail: orders@slackinc.com • Visit www.slackbooks.com